Minimally Invasive Orthopaedic Trauma

Minimally Invasive Orthopaedic Trauma

SERIES EDITOR

Paul Tornetta, III, MD
Professor and Vice Chairman
Department of Orthopaedic Surgery
Boston University Medical Center
Director of Orthopaedic Trauma
Boston University Medical Center
Boston, Massachusetts

EDITORS

Michael J. Gardner, MD
Associate Professor
Department of Orthopaedic Surgery
Washington University School of Medicine
St. Louis, Missouri

Jodi Siegel, MD
Assistant Professor
Department of Orthopaedics
UMass Memorial Medical Center
University of Massachusetts Medical School
Worcester, Massachusetts

Wolters Kluwer Health | Lippincott Williams & Wilkins

Philadelphia • Baltimore • New York • London
Buenos Aires • Hong Kong • Sydney • Tokyo

Acquisitions Editor: Brian Brown
Developmental Product Manager: Dave Murphy
Production Product Manager: David Orzechowski
Senior Manufacturing Coordinator: Beth Welsh
Senior Book Designer: Joan Wendt
Marketing Manager: Daniel Dressler
Production Service: Aptara, Inc.

Two Commerce Square
2001 Market Street
Philadelphia, PA 19103
LWW.com

Library of Congress Cataloging-in-Publication Data

Minimally invasive orthopaedic trauma / editors, Michael J. Gardner, Jodi Siegel.
p. ; cm.
Includes bibliographical references and index.
ISBN 978-1-4511-1474-4 (alk. paper)
I. Gardner, Michael J., editor of compilation. II. Siegel, Jodi, editor of compilation.
[DNLM: 1. Fracture Fixation–methods. 2. Fractures, Bone–surgery. 3. Musculoskeletal System–surgery. 4. Surgical Procedures, Minimally Invasive–methods. WE 185]
RD101
617.1'5–dc23

2013037718

DISCLAIMER

Care has been taken to confirm the accuracy of the information present and to describe generally accepted practices. However, the authors, editors, and publisher are not responsible for errors or omissions or for any consequences from application of the information in this book and make no warranty, expressed or implied, with respect to the currency, completeness, or accuracy of the contents of the publication. Application of this information in a particular situation remains the professional responsibility of the practitioner; the clinical treatments described and recommended may not be considered absolute and universal recommendations.

The authors, editors, and publisher have exerted every effort to ensure that drug selection and dosage set forth in this text are in accordance with the current recommendations and practice at the time of publication. However, in view of ongoing research, changes in government regulations, and the constant flow of information relating to drug therapy and drug reactions, the reader is urged to check the package insert for each drug for any change in indications and dosage and for added warnings and precautions. This is particularly important when the recommended agent is a new or infrequently employed drug.

Some drugs and medical devices presented in this publication have Food and Drug Administration (FDA) clearance for limited use in restricted research settings. It is the responsibility of the health care provider to ascertain the FDA status of each drug or device planned for use in their clinical practice.

To purchase additional copies of this book, call our customer service department at (800) 638-3030 or fax orders to (301) 223-2320.

International customers should call (301) 223-2300.

Visit Lippincott Williams & Wilkins on the Internet: http://www.lww.com. Lippincott Williams & Wilkins customer service representatives are available from 8:30 am to 6:00 pm, EST.

1 2 3 4 5 6 7 8 9 10

RRS1310

To my mother, Phyllis, who found the best in people, had compassion for all, and whose insight, guidance, and love have always made me believe that anything is possible.

Paul Tornetta, III, MD

Contributing Authors

Theerachai Apivatthakakul, MD
Professor
Department of Orthopaedics
Faculty of Medicine
Chiang Mai University
Chiang Mai, Thailand

Hrayr G. Basmajian, MD
Assistant Professor of Orthopaedic Trauma
Loma Linda University Medical Center
Loma Linda, California

Michael J. Beltran, MD
Staff Surgeon
San Antonio Military Medical Center
San Antonio, Texas

Eben A. Carroll, MD
Assistant Professor
Department of Orthopaedic Surgery
Wake Forest University Baptist Medical Center
Winston-Salem, North Carolina

Louis W. Catalano, III, MD
Assistant Clinical Professor
Department of Orthopaedic Surgery
CV Starr Hand Surgery Center
St. Luke's-Roosevelt Hospital
Columbia University
New York, New York

Cory A. Collinge, MD
Director of Orthopaedic Trauma
Harris Methodist Fort Worth Hospital
Staff Physician
John Peter Smith Orthopaedic Surgery Residency Program
Fort Worth, Texas

Peter H. DeNoble, MD
Hand and Upper Extremity Fellow
Department of Orthopaedic Surgery
CV Starr Hand Surgery Center
St. Luke's-Roosevelt Hospital
New York, New York

Jason M. Evans, MD
Assistant Professor
Division of Orthopaedic Trauma
Department of Orthopaedics and Rehabilitation
Vanderbilt University Medical Center
Nashville, Tennessee

Axel Jubel, Prof Dr med
Professor and Director
Department of Trauma and Reconstructive Surgery
Eduardus Hospital
Cologne, Germany

Christian Krettek, MD
Professor and Chairman
Trauma Department
Hannover Medical School
Hannover, Germany

G. Yves Laflamme, MD, FRCSC
Associate Professor
Department of Surgery
University of Montréal
Montreal, Quebec, Canada

Sang Ki Lee, MD, PhD
Associate Professor
Department of Orthopaedic Surgery
Eulji University College of Medicine
Seo-gu, Daejeon, South Korea

Carol A. Lin, MD, MA
Orthopaedic Trauma Fellow
Cedars-Sinai Orthopaedic Center
Los Angeles, California

Theodore Miclau III, MD
Professor and Vice Chairman
Department of Orthopaedic Surgery
University of California
Chief of Orthopaedic Surgery
San Francisco General Hospital
Director, Orthopaedic Trauma Institute
San Francisco, California

Saam Morshed, MD, PhD, MPH
Assistant Professor
Department of Orthopaedic Surgery
University of San Francisco
Director of the Clinical Research Center
UCSF/San Francisco General Hospital Orthopaedic Trauma Institute (OTI)
San Francisco, California

Rami Mosheiff, MD
Chief of the Orthopedic Trauma Unit
Orthopedic Surgery, Ein Kerem
Orthopaedic Trauma Unit
Hadassah Hebrew University Hospital
Jerusalem, Israel

Chang-Wug Oh, MD
Professor
Department of Orthopedic Surgery
Kyungpook National University Hospital
Samdok, Chung Gu, Daegu, Korea

Gil R. Ortega, MD, MPH
Site Director
Phoenix Orthopaedic Residency Program
Sonoran Orthopaedic Trauma Surgeons
Scottsdale Osborn Level I Trauma Center
Scottsdale, Arizona

Holly Tyler-Paris Pilson, MD
Resident
Department of Orthopaedic Surgery
Wake Forest University Baptist Medical Center
Winston-Salem, North Carolina

David W. Robinson, MD
Atlanta Medical Center
Orthopaedic Residency Program
Atlanta, Georgia

Dominique Rouleau, MD, FRCSC
Assistant Professor
Department of Surgery
Sacré-Coeur Hospital
University of Montreal
Montreal, Quebec, Canada

Jodi Siegel, MD
Assistant Professor
Department of Orthopaedics
UMass Memorial Medical Center
University of Massachusetts Medical School
Worcester, Massachusetts

Daniel J. Stinner, MD
Orthopaedic Trauma Surgeon
San Antonio Military Medical Center
San Antonio, Texas

Hobie Summers, MD
Assistant Professor
Department of Orthopaedic Surgery
Loyola University Medical Center
Maywood, Illinois

Yoram A. Weil, MD
Department of Orthopedic Surgery
Orthopaedic Trauma Unit
Hadassah Medical Center
Hadassah Hebrew University Hospital
Jerusalem, Israel

Patrick Yoon, MD
Assistant Professor
Department of Orthopaedic Surgery
Hennepin County Medical Center
University of Minnesota
Minneapolis, Minnesota

Bruce H. Ziran, MD, FACS
Director of Orthopaedic Trauma
The Hughston Clinic
Gwinnett Medical Center
Atlanta, Georgia

Series Preface

It is my pleasure to introduce a new series of technically based books in orthopaedic surgery. This series, *Minimally Invasive Orthopaedic Surgery,* will build on the tradition of advances that orthopaedic surgery has made and capture the exciting methods being introduced by current innovators. Just as procedures such as ACL reconstruction have undergone a near-complete transition to minimally invasive techniques from open ones, with tremendous benefit to patients, the fields of trauma surgery, spine surgery, and reconstructive surgery are seeing these changes now.

The first volume in the series, edited by Jodi Siegel and Michael Gardner, will focus on minimally invasive trauma surgery. The use of intramedullary nails was the first major stop in revolutionizing fracture care while diminishing risks. Over the past 15 years, the advent of anatomically based fixation has allowed for previously open procedures to be performed with soft tissue-sparing techniques. The idea of placing a plate up the entire femur with a 3-cm incision and poke holes was unthinkable 15 years ago and now seeing a thigh-length incision would be unimaginable! The editors have gathered experts in minimally invasive procedures and have presented them in a uniform way including the indications, setup, technical aspects of surgery, and the problem areas.

These volumes will help to introduce the novice to these important methods, and fine tune those who understand the principles and are looking for detail-oriented information, tips, and pitfalls.

I am proud to see this series take off with this volume on trauma surgery.

Paul Tornetta, III, MD

Preface

Surgical treatment of musculoskeletal traumatic injuries has evolved substantially over the last several decades. Locking plates have characterized a major change in the landscape of available implants and biomechanical principles to treat fractures. A greater understanding of soft tissue handling has also occurred. Outcome assessments have increasingly shifted from physician-centered radiographic measures to patient-centered functional outcomes. Another concurrent trend has been toward "minimally invasive" surgery, including minimally invasive fracture surgery. In order for this approach to be beneficial, several critical points require consideration. First, "minimally invasive" does not solely mean small skin incisions. Meticulously respecting the biology at the fracture site, such as minimizing periosteal stripping and muscle dissection, is paramount. Successfully performing minimally invasive trauma surgery requires a thorough understanding of the anatomy, as well as a comprehensive three-dimensional understanding of the fracture configuration. The surgeon must be able to visualize the fracture and perform the reduction without seeing them directly. This occasionally requires more reliance on fluoroscopy compared to traditional open procedures. When things begin to get difficult using these techniques, the surgeon must have a plan and a low threshold to convert to an open procedure. Second, minimally invasive techniques must never compromise the quality of the surgery, or violate the principles of fracture fixation, which still must be rigorously followed. Articular fractures require anatomic reductions and compressive rigid fixation. Metaphyseal and diaphyseal extremity fractures require restoration of length, alignment, and rotation. Minimally invasive surgery does not sacrifice fracture reduction! With experience, patience, and attention to detail, minimally invasive techniques with less soft tissue dissection can lead to patient benefits including potentially earlier mobilization and improved functional outcomes.

We would like to first thank our mentors, for their endless teaching and for helping to establish sound surgical techniques and principles which form the basis for safe and effective minimally invasive orthopaedic trauma surgery. We would also like to thank our trainees, whose constant questioning and feedback contributes to the evolution of new techniques. Finally, we'd like to thank our families for their support. We hope you enjoy this compilation.

Michael J. Gardner

Jodi Siegel

Contents

CONTENTS

SECTION 1

General

CHAPTER 1

Historical Perspective

Holly Tyler-Paris Pilson and Eben A. Carroll

THE HISTORY OF NONOPERATIVE FRACTURE TREATMENT

Before the development of antiseptic principles and surgical techniques by Joseph Lister in 1865, the mainstay of treatment for most orthopaedic fractures centered around nonoperative management, including splinting, casting, traction, and bracing. Immobilization of fractures was carried out with whatever tools and materials were available at the time. Fracture union and prevention of deformity came at the expense of prolonged immobilization with its resultant sequelae. Early fracture surgery evolved to allow and encourage bony union and prevention of malunion while avoiding the complications of long-term immobilization. The emphasis on mobilization during the healing process was espoused in the founding principles of the *Arbeitsgemeinschaft für Osteosynthesefragen*, or "the AO." Its initial philosophy focused on anatomic reduction and *soudure per primam* or primary bone healing often at a biologic cost. As fracture surgery evolved, the importance of soft tissue preservation and the primary importance of biology led to techniques which facilitated healing and function and were less invasive to bone biology.

Splinting and Casting

Early examples of nonoperative fracture management can be traced back to the ancient Egyptians. Archaeologic artifacts of fractured extremities splinted with longitudinal wooden boards were discovered by A.C. Mace during the Hearst Egyptian expedition of the University of California in 1903.[1–7]

Prior to the development of plaster-of-Paris and modern day plaster techniques, an Arab physician named Rhazes described a recipe for a casting material using clay gum mixtures, flour, and egg whites.[8,9] Variations of this recipe, including the addition of lime, honey, pork fat, vinegar, and powder of Armenian clay or plaster were concocted up through the late 18th century.[3,8–10] The benefit of this method of immobilization touted by Rhazes Athuriscus was that "... *it will be much handsomer and will not need to be removed until the healing is complete.*"[8]

In 1852, the plaster-of-Paris bandage, derivates of which are still used today, was introduced by a Russian military surgeon, Antonius Mathijsen.[11] This revolutionized the stabilization of healing fractures, providing a material which was durable and could be maintained for the duration of healing. Many subsequent methods of immobilization were invented including the copper limb curirasse described by Heister[12] and what Malgaigne called "the great machine of La Faye."[13,14] The drawback of these extensive and heavy devices, however, was that they essentially confined the healing patient to the bed for the entirety of their rehabilitation. In turn, Seutin devised the amidonné, or starched bandage,[15] allowing for earlier mobilization of the fractured extremity. Hence the debate over immobilization versus early mobilization of the fractured extremity was born. Most European surgeons favored total immobilization, with others such as Sir James Paget and Lucas-Championnière favoring Seutin's *déambulation* regimen.[16] In 1907 Championnière wrote, "*the necessity for immobilization is only relative ...... [W]hile authors attach great importance to the immobilization of a compound fracture, we find here that with small movements and an apparatus moderately immobilizing, consolidation goes on well, and no inflammatory complications result.*"[16]

Traction

Descriptions of traction applied for the treatment of fractures can be found as early as AD 130 in the writings of Galen.[2,17] He described an extension apparatus, or glossocomium (Fig. 1.1), used to temporarily treat fractured extremities until splinting could be performed by turning a handle to provide distraction. Continuous traction intended for primary fracture treatment can be found in the early writings of Guy de Chauliac (1300 to 1367);[17,18] however, it was not widely practiced until the mid-19th century. Borrowing from the traction techniques of Bardenheuer, Albert Hoffa of Wurzburg published in his book of fractures and dislocations in 1888 the use of traction for many different types of fractures including those of the femur and humerus.[19] Josiah Crosby of New Hampshire also described the use of continuous skin traction using a combination of adhesive plaster secured with a spiral bandage and weight applied to the end for the management of a femur fracture, an open tibia fracture and in two cases of clavicle fractures in children.[20] Codivilla of Bologna was the first known to apply skeletal traction via the use of an intraosseous pin, with Fritz Steinman popularizing the technique in the treatment of acute fractures.[21] Steinman, frustrated with the complications of skin traction, described using two pins driven through the femoral condyles to pull in-line traction for midshaft femur fractures in 1907.[22] Two years later, Martin Kirschner of Greifswald would describe skeletal traction using wires of a much smaller diameter.[22]

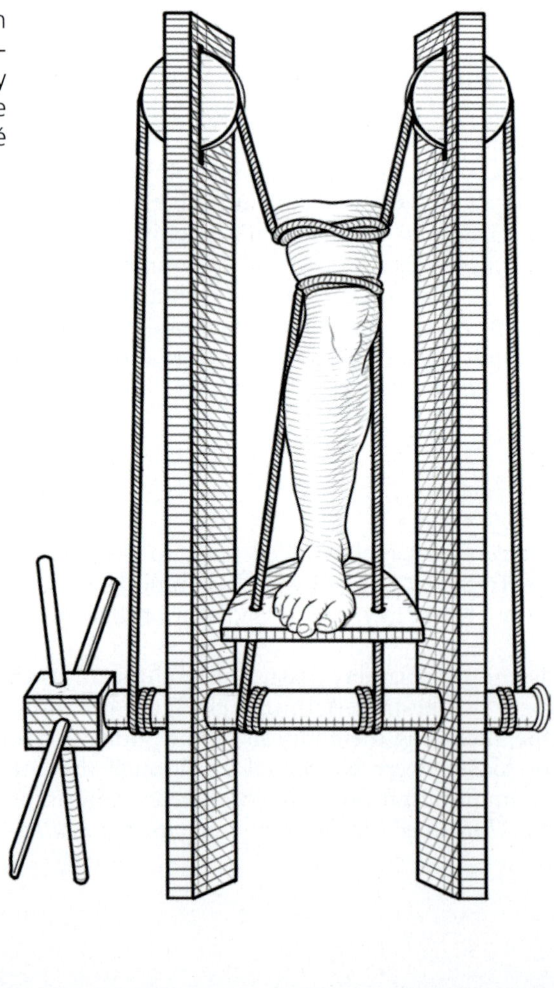

Figure 1.1 A traction apparatus called the glossocomium, described by Galen, illustrated from the writings of Ambroise Paré (1564).

Traction, though more likely to decrease the risk of malunion in healing fractures, came at the expense of prolonged periods of immobilization, as well as the risks inherent to the placement and maintenance of traction devices themselves. Aside from the obvious external drawbacks of immobilization, including bed sores, soft tissue and bone infections, and delay in return to work or war, there were other less conspicuous effects including internal signs of decompensation, such as muscle atrophy.[23]

Recognizing these limitations, Professor George Perkins of London advocated for straight simple in-line traction through a proximal tibial pin in the 1940s and 1950s, which would also allow for early mobilization of the knee using a Pyrford traction system.[15,24] Also aware of the difficulties of immobilization in healing fractures was Dowden, who in the opening sentence of his 1924 article wrote, "*The principle of early active movement in the treatment of practically all injuries and in most inflammations will assuredly be adopted before long....*"[*] Both Perkins and Dowden were among the many early advocates of mobilization of all joints of the injured limb, believing it to be even more important than precise skeletal reduction. To such pioneers it became clear that a more sophisticated means of maintaining function while the healing process occurred was needed.

EARLY OPERATIVE TECHNIQUES

Even before the introduction of aseptic surgical techniques, the internal fixation of fractures was documented as early as the 1770s. Although controversy exists regarding the first account of internal fixation of a fracture, most authors attribute it to two surgeons from Toulouse, Lapujode, and Sicre, who were said to have performed ligature, or the wire suturing of bone.[25] Screws, which undoubtedly had many applications in the mid 1800s, made their way into the repertoire of orthopaedic implants in the 1840s. Cücuel and Rigaud described the use of screw fixation in the application of traction for a depressed sternal fracture as well as for fixation of an olecranon and a patellar fracture.[15]

Early fracture surgery was mostly influenced by the development of three new technologies: Anesthesia by Morton (1846), Antisepsis by Lister (1865), and Radiography by Röntgen (1895).[26] Joseph Lister, most known for his antiseptic surgical principles, first applied these techniques using carbolic acid in the treatment of compound fractures in 1867.[27] His success in drastically reducing complications, namely death, from postoperative wound infection, and subsequent improvements in aseptic techniques, opened the door for not only fracture surgery, but also all surgical procedures in general.

The concurrent evolution in design of orthopaedic implants kept pace with the first accounts of plate fixation described by Hansmann in the late 19th century. In his 1886 article, he described his technique for applying a malleable plate in the fixation of acute fractures, pseudarthroses, and the reconstruction of a humeral enchondroma.[15] For fracture treatment, his technique involved applying the plate to span the fracture site, with screws purchasing each fracture fragment and projecting far out through the skin, for more easy removal, typically at around 4 to 8 weeks (Fig. 1.2). The end of the plate was also bent at a right angle with projection through the skin. In 1903, George Guthrie documented further use of plate fixation by Estes and Steinbach.[15] Estes used a nickel steel plate fixed to the bone with ivory pegs, whereas Steinbach utilized silver, a highly favored implant material due to its believed antibiotic properties. Ten years later Albin Lambotte (1866 to 1955) of Belgium, regarded by many as the father of internal fixation, coined the term *osteosynthesis*

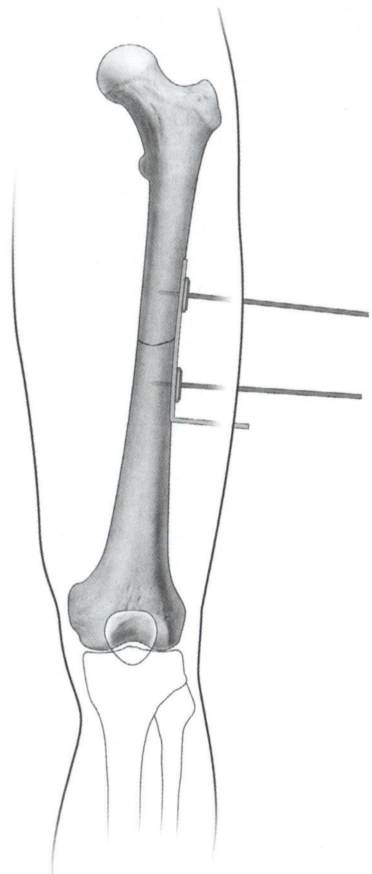

Figure 1.2 The first description of the plate fixation of fractures by Hansmann. The plate is secured to the bone by long screw shanks on either side of the fracture, which are left protruding through the skin. The end of the plate is also bent at 90 degrees and left protruding through the skin, to allow for easier removal after union. (Redrawn from: Hansmann's 1886 article, "A new method of fixation of the fragments of complicated fractures.")

[*]Dowden JW. The classic: The principle of early active movement in treating fractures of the upper extremity. *Clin Orthop Relat Res.* 2006;442:83–86.

in his classic book "*Chirurgie Opératoire des Fractures*" in 1913.[15,28] He manufactured most of his own instruments and implants, including plates and screws for internal fixation as well as an external fixation device similar in principle to the ones in use today.[28]

Another great visionary in the field of internal fixation, William Arbuthnot Lane of London, had become quite frustrated with the results of fracture management in the late 19th century. He came to understand that the firmest union did not universally lead to a good functional outcome; that a patient whose foot was in the slightest degree of malalignment could have terrible function, even if complete union was achieved.[29–31] He thus became greatly focused on the need for accuracy and maintenance of a good reduction, especially of articular injuries.

Both Lane and Lambotte were almost contemporaneously describing intramedullary screw fixation for femoral neck fractures in 1905, although various forms of intramedullary devices had been previously described by Koenig, Cheyne, Gillette, Dieffenbach, V. Langenbeck, Nicolaysen, Delbet, Schone, Muler-Meernach, Thompson, and Bircher, to whom the earliest account is attributed in 1866.[19,28,32–34] Gerhardt Küntscher, in collaboration with Professor Fischer and engineer Ernst Pohl at Kiel University in Germany, were credited with the development of the first long metallic intramedullary device, as we know it today, in the 1930s.[34,35] Further modifications by the AO group and collaboration between Klemm, Schellmann, Grosse, and Kempf resulted in the development of the current generation of interlocking nailing systems.

Many of the later implant designs of Lane and Lambotte were most likely inspired by Sherman, who introduced his own series of plates and screws in his 1926 article, drawing attention to the superior fixation obtained with parallel, threaded, self-tapping fine pitched screws.[36] This more superior fixation, he believed, would be firm enough to permit early mobilization and rehabilitation, a theme which set the foundations for the AO era.[36,37]

THE AO ERA

In 1958, the establishment of the *Arbeitsgemeinschaft für Osteosynthesefragen,* or the AO, by 13 men: Maurice Müller, Hans Willenegger, Robert Schneider, Martin Allgöwer, Walter Bandi, Ernst Baumann, August Guggenbühl, Willy Hunzicker, Walter Ott, René Patry, Walter Schär, Walter Stähli and Fritz Brussatis, revolutionized the operative management of fractures worldwide.

Although not part of the AO itself, the framework upon which its principles and concepts were formed can be attributed in part, if not entirely to the life and work of Robert Danis. Danis, regarded as the father of modern osteosynthesis, was trained as a general surgeon with interests in thoracic and vascular surgery, but later became intrigued by the internal fixation of fractures.[15] Undoubtedly of the mind-set of the "mobilizers," he stressed the following three aims of a satisfactory osteosynthesis in his 1949 publication, *Théorie et Pratique de l'Ostéosynthèse.*[38]

1. Immediate active mobilization of the adjacent muscles and joints
2. Complete restoration of the bone to its original form
3. The *soudure per primam* (primary bone healing) of the bony fragments without the formation of apparent callus

He developed a number of techniques for osteosynthesis, most of which were based on the concepts of anatomic reduction and interfragmentary compression, which allowed for primary bone healing by direct bone remodeling, termed *soudure autogène,* or self-welding.[15]

Just 8 years prior to the official establishment of the AO, a young Swiss surgeon and great admirer of Danis' work, Maurice Müller, visited him in Brussels. Danis' work had such an impact on Müller that he returned to Switzerland to share his passion for improving the internal fixation of fractures with his colleagues. Over the course of a 3-day meeting in the Kantonsspital of Chur in 1958, a group of surgeons presented various scientific papers on osteosynthesis culminating in the foundation of the AO to further the science of internal fixation.[15] This led to the establishment of an experimental surgical center, the formation of an alliance with two Swiss engineering firms to develop the AO instrumentarium, as well as the creation of a documentation center to keep a record of the combined surgical experiences of its members.[15,39]

The AO's fundamental principles focused on the restoration of anatomy and establishing absolute stability allowing for early mobilization.[40] Initially these principles favored anatomic reductions often at the expense of large soft tissue dissections and biologic insult. Examples of the complications of ignoring the soft tissue envelope are well demonstrated in the

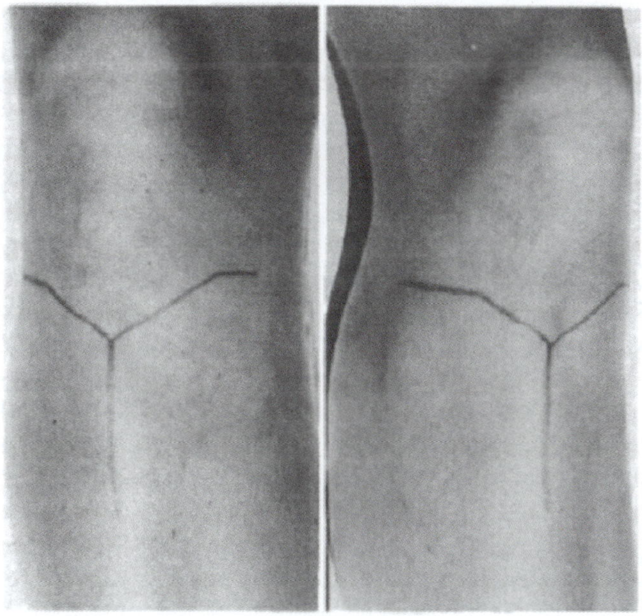

Figure 1.3 The modified anterior approach for the treatment of bicondylar tibial plateau fractures. (From: Moore TM, Patzakis MJ, Harvey JP. Tibial plateau fractures: Definition, demographics, treatment rationale, and long-term results of closed traction management or operative reduction. *J Orthop Trauma.* 1987;1: 97–119.)

initial midline anterior approach to the fixation of bicondylar tibial plateau fractures. Moore et al.[41] observed 9 wound complications (either dehiscence or infection) in their series of 11 bicondylar fractures treated with open reduction internal fixation (ORIF) through the modified anterior incision (Fig. 1.3). In a retrospective review by Young and Barrack in 1994,[42] all eight of the tibial plateau fractures in their series requiring medial and lateral buttress plating via a midline incision required a subsequent operation; seven for infection requiring multiple debridements and resulting in two amputations. The danger of focusing on anatomic reduction at the expense of the soft tissue surgical trauma was recognized.[43–46]

While the early principles of anatomic restoration, absolute stability, and immediate mobilization are still contemporary, there has been a shift toward procedures and techniques which achieve these goals but also account for the critical role of soft tissue preservation. It seems that Küntscher, who generally disfavored open fracture reductions or disturbance of the periosteum, believing that it delayed healing, was somewhat of a visionary ahead of his time in this respect.[34,35,47] It is now widely accepted that absolute stability need only be a requirement for certain fracture patterns and locations, such as intra-articular fractures.[40]

THE MINIMALLY INVASIVE ERA

The bone is like a tree, with its roots in the soft tissue.
—Unknown

Initial fracture treatment, even prior to the AO era, was aimed at precise anatomic reconstruction and fixation with primary bone healing.[48] Formation of callus was not completely understood and believed by some to be restrictive to joint motion. It was likened to a scarlet letter, an indication that the stability intended by the chosen fixation did not match that which was achieved.[47] Later studies which differentiated the types of bone healing (direct/primary vs. indirect/secondary) proved that callus was not exclusive of a good result, and was an acceptable form of healing in many fracture patterns.[48,49,50,51] The recognition that good outcomes could be achieved without the biologic cost of anatomic reduction paved the way for indirect reduction techniques and less invasive fracture treatment.

Interfragmentary compression using the early AO plates was frequently accomplished using an AO compression clamp applied externally to the steel plate under tension until all the screws were inserted.[52,53] The design limitations, including screw displacement within the hole, corrosion at the screw–plate interface and cortical osteoporosis from the stiff load-bearing steel plate, led to modifications resulting in the dynamic compression plate (DCP) (Fig. 1.4) developed by the AO in 1969.[53] The cortical osteoporosis seen at the

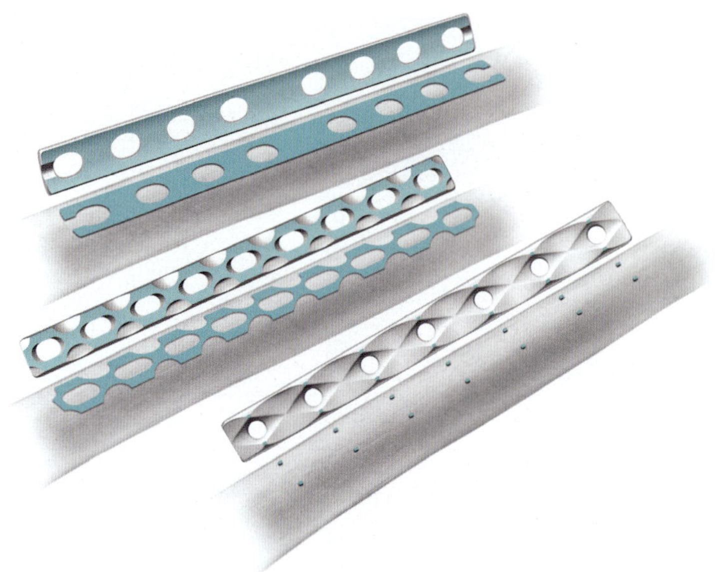

Figure 1.4 Minimally invasive implants with less direct contact with bone have evolved from the conventional dynamic compression plate (DCP), top, to the limited contact dynamic compression plate (LC-DCP), middle, and finally to the point contact fixator plate (PC-Fix), bottom.

plate–bone interface, initially attributed to stress shielding and mechanical unloading of the bone continued to be a problem, despite changing to more flexible titanium plates. Later studies,[54,55] documented the deleterious effects of the plate–bone contact area on the blood supply and contributing at least in part to this effect.

The idea that disrupting the blood supply around a healing fracture may delay, complicate, or even prevent union is a central tenet in the evolution of minimally invasive fracture surgery. These discoveries led to the development of the limited contact dynamic compression plate (LC-DCP), which in essence altered the undersurface of the plate to decrease the surface area in contact with the underlying bone and limit vascular damage (Fig. 1.4).[56] Further evolution of these concepts resulted in plates with even less surface contact with bone, the point contact fixator (PC-Fix) (Fig. 1.4).[57,58] Although intended for use as an internal plate and screw fixation system, the PC-Fix functioned more closely to that external fixator by eliminating the load transfer through the plate through a fixed-angle interface, making the screws the principal load transferring components.[59] Studies comparing the stability and sequences of healing between the DCP, LC-DCP, and PC-Fix constructs showed the superiority of the PC-Fix in terms of stability and preserving bone vitality.[57,60]

Minimally Invasive Implants and Techniques

Prior to the development of the LC-DCP, most attribute the first minimally invasive implants for fracture treatment to Brunner and Weber[61] for their wave plate in 1982 (Fig. 1.5), followed by Heitemeyer et al.[62] for their bridge plate in 1985 (Fig. 1.6). Both functioned on the same premise, that by fixing the plate to the intact bone proximal and distal to the fracture zone, bridging the fracture area with its vital soft tissue and vascular supply, successful callus formation and union would ensue. The main indications for these implants were in comminuted fractures. The wave plate was also used to stabilize pseudarthroses when applied as a tension band and was specially contoured to allow room for bone grafting at the fracture site.[61] Understanding that anatomical reduction of multi-fragmented fractures disrupts the cortical perfusion, Heitemeyer et al., designed their bridge plate to essentially disregard the comminuted fragments and focus on realignment of the proximal and distal fracture fragments. The plates were designed with five holes at each side and a continuous solid central bar overlying the fracture site. This central solid bar was also felt to make the construct more stable to torsion and bending forces. In their comparison of patients who underwent open plate osteosynthesis with anatomic realignment of all fracture fragments versus those treated with bridge plate osteosynthesis, they found much lower complication rates and faster union rates in the bridge plate group.[62]

In addition to implants, surgical techniques simultaneously evolved to preserve the blood supply to healing fractures. Indirect reduction techniques using standard implants were described by Mast et al.[63] for the internal fixation of proximal and distal femur fractures. In comminuted distal femur fractures, these authors described the use of a condylar plate used as a buttress with fixation proximal and distal to the fractures, avoiding direct exposure of the zone of injury. By leaving the comminuted fracture fragments undisturbed, they become secondarily approximated by their associated soft tissue attachments and often heal without complications. Using this specific technique and implant, however, does not provide stable fixation in the presence of coronal plane, or "Hoffa," fractures. The main goal of these techniques was to limit the exposure of the distal femoral metaphysis.[64] This concept was referred to as "biologic plating" or "biologic fixation."

Although the direct lateral exposure to the distal femur may be less damaging to the local vascular anatomy than medial dissection, the lateral exposure is not without problems of its own. Lateral dissection may still injure vital perforators and nutrient arteries.[65–67] The minimally invasive percutaneous plate osteosynthesis (MIPPO) and transarticular approach and percutaneous plate osteosynthesis (TARPO) techniques were developed to eliminate the need for elevation of the vastus lateralis muscle from the intermuscular septum through the lateral approach by employing a submuscular approach to plate insertion followed by percutaneous insertion of screws.[64,65]

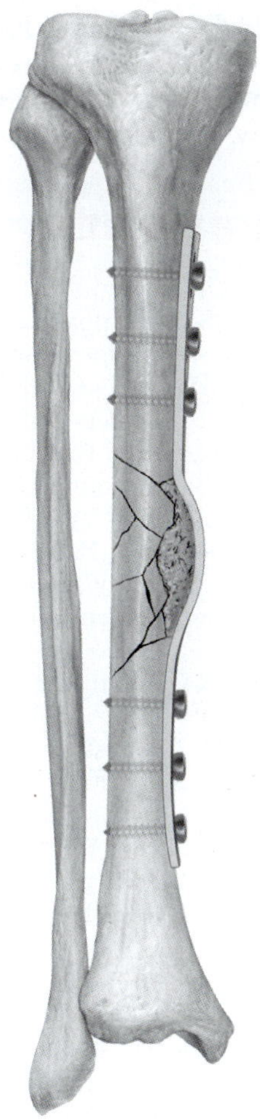

Figure 1.5 The wave plate as described by Brunner and Weber.

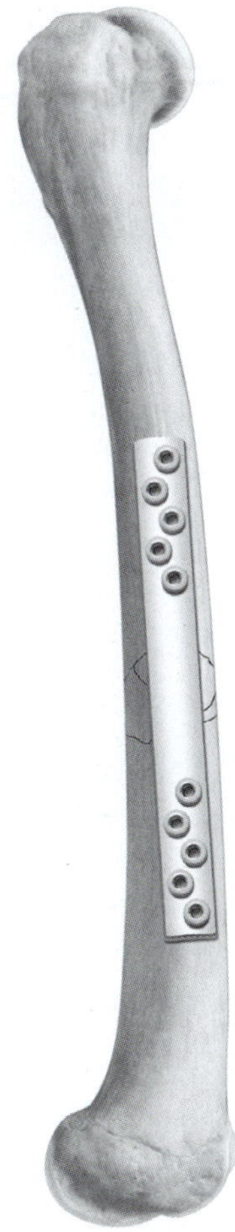

Figure 1.6 The bridge plate as described by Heitemeyer et al.

Further evolution of biologic fracture fixation culminated in the development of the less invasive stabilization system (LISS). Initially developed for treating fractures around the knee, it subsequently expanded to involve other applications.[68–70] The concept behind the LISS involved a combination of interlocked intramedullary nailing and biologic plating techniques, using the assistance of an implantation handle for submuscular plate insertion as well as percutaneous screw insertion guides.[71] Several early studies reported successful short- and mid-term results using the LISS technique in the treatment of distal femur fractures,[72–75] proximal tibia fractures,[76,77] and others.[78]

Currently, promising clinical results from minimally invasive techniques have been demonstrated in multiple locations. Minimally invasive osteosynthesis of humerus fractures has been successfully shown to be advantageous in terms of reducing iatrogenic radial nerve palsies amongst other complications,[79–81] and accelerating fracture union,[79] all while providing similar functional outcomes to traditional open osteosynthesis.[79,82] Minimally invasive reduction techniques with percutaneous screw[83] or K-wire[84] fixation for calcaneus fractures have also been described and show good to excellent results in appropriately selected patients with less severe fracture patterns. Among all, 73.9% of patients in the Rammelt study were able to return to their original occupation at an average of 6 months after their injury.[83] In general, the most significant advantage of minimally invasive techniques in calcaneus osteosynthesis is reduced wound complications, with all other outcomes being at least equivalent to standard open reduction and fixation techniques.[85,86] Satisfactory results have also been shown in the minimally invasive treatment of distal tibia, or "pilon" fractures.[87–89] Most minimally invasive techniques that have been developed for acetabular fracture fixation are centered around reducing the size of the approach rather than implant modifications.[90] With further advances in technology, image-guided techniques including robotics are being used for treatment of fractures of the pelvis and acetabulum, including the sacrum.[90–93] The main caveat when considering minimally invasive techniques for articular fractures is that emphasis should still remain on anatomic reduction of articular surfaces and rigid compressive fixation, and this should not be compromised in favor of less invasive exposures.

ACKNOWLEDGMENT

A special thanks to Simon Trach, medical student at the Ruprecht Karls Universität Heidelberg, Germany, for help with the translation of German references.

REFERENCES

1. Smith GE, Cantab MA, Syd CM. The most ancient splints. *Br Med J.* 1908;1(2465):732–734.
2. Milne JS. The apparatus used by the Greeks and the Romans in the setting of fractures and the reduction of dislocations. *Interstate Med J.* 1909;16(1):48–60.
3. Spink MS, Lewis GL. *Albucasis on Surgery and Instruments.* London: Wellcome Institute of the History of Medicine; 1973.
4. Gersdorf H von. Feldtbuch der Wundartzney. 1517. Strasbourg.
5. Shaw AB. Benjamin Gooch, eighteenth-century Norfolk surgeon. *Med Hist.* 1972;16(1):40–50.
6. Bérenger Féraud LJB. *Traité de l'Immobilisation Directe Fractures des Fragments Osseux dans les.* Paris: Delahaye; 1870:365–380.
7. Fang HC, Ku YW, Shang TY. The integration of modern and traditional Chinese medicine in the treatment of fractures. A simple method of treatment for fractures of the shafts of both forearm bones. 1963. *Clin Orthop Relat Res.* 1996;(323):4–11.
8. Austin RT. Treatment of broken legs before and after the introduction of gypsum. *Injury.* 1983; 14(5):389–394.
9. Jonas AF. The history of Plaster of Paris bandages. *Surg Gynecol Obstet.* 1956;102(2):249–252.
10. Walker CA. Treatment of fractures by the immoveable apparatus. *Lancet.* 1839;1:553.
11. Mathijsen A. The classic: New method for application of plaster-of-paris bandage. *Clin Orthop Relat Res.* 2007;458:59–62.
12. Heister L. *Chirurgie Complète.* Paris: 1739.
13. Stimson, LA. In: Henry C, ed. *A Treatise on Fractures.* Philadelphia, PA: Lea's Son & Co; 1883: 170–185.
14. Malgaigne JF. *A Treatise on Fractures.* Philadelphia, PA: JB Lippincott & Co; 1859. (Translated from the French with notes & additions by John H. Packard.)
15. Colton CL. The history of fracture treatment. In: Browner BD, Jupiter JB, Levine AM, Trafton PG, Krettek C, eds. *Skeletal Trauma: Basic Science Management and Reconstruction.* 4th ed. Philadelphia, PA: W.B. Saunders Company; 2008.
16. Lucas-Championnière J. *Antiseptic Surgery: The Principles, Modes of Application, and Results of the Lister Dressing.* University Press. 1881; 119–123. (Translated from the 2nd ed. by Frederic H. Gerrish.)
17. Guthrie D. *A History of Medicine.* London: T. Nelson; 1945:124.
18. Mellick SA. The Montpellier School and Guy De Chauliac. *Aust N Z Surg.* 1999;69:297–301.
19. Hoffa A. *Lehrbuch der Fracturen und Luxationen für Arzte und Studierende.* Würzburg: Stahel'sche universitäts-buch- & kunsthandlung; 1888.
20. Hamilton FH. *Treatise on Military Surgery and Hygiene.* New York, NY: Baillière; 1865.
21. Peltier L. The Role of Alessandro Codivilla in the development of skeletal traction. *J Bone Joint Surg Am.* 1969;51:1433.
22. Peltier L. A brief history of traction. *J Bone Joint Surg Am.* 1968;50:1603–1617.
23. Dencker H. Wire traction complications associated with treatment of femoral shaft fractures. *Acta Orthop Scandinav.* 1964;35:158–163.
24. Russell RH. Fracture of the femur. A clinical study. *Br J Surg.* 1924;11:491.
25. Evans PE. Cerclage fixation of a fractured humerus in 1775, fact or fiction? *Clin Orthop Relat Res.* 1983;(174):138–142.
26. Bartoníček J. Early history of operative treatment of fractures. *Arch Orthop Trauma Surg.* 2010;130(11):1385–1396;online publication.
27. Lister J. On the antiseptic principle in the practice of surgery. *Br Med J.* 1867;2(351):246–248.
28. Lambotte A, Schlesinger E, Murray CR. *Chirurgie Opératoire des Fractures.* Paris: Masson; 1913.
29. Layton TB. Sir William Arbuthnot Lane, Bt. C.B., M.S. *An Enquiry into the Mind and Influence of a Surgeon.* Edinburgh: Livingstone. 1956:73–82.
30. Lane WA. The classic: Operative treatment of fractures. 1914. *Clin Orthop Relat Res.* 2009;467: 1944–1947.
31. Brand R. Sir William Arbuthnot Lane, 1856–1943. *Clin Orthop Relat Res.* 2009;467:1939–1943.
32. Billroth W. *Clinical Surgery-Extracts from the reports of surgical practice between the years 1860–1876.* London: The New Sydenham Society; 1881. (Translated from the original, and edited, with annotations, by C. T. Dent.)
33. Bircher H. Eine neue Methode unmittelbarer Retention bei Frakturen der Roehrenknochen. *Arch Klin Chir.* 1887;34:91.

34. Küntscher G. *Practice of intramedullary nailing*. Springfield, IL: Charles C Thomas Publisher; 1967:32–35. (Translated from German to English by Herman H. Rinne.)
35. Böhler L. *Medullary nailing of Küntscher*. Baltimore, MD: The Williams & Wilkins Company; 1948:1–6. (Translated from German to English by Hans Tretter.)
36. Sherman WMO. Operative treatment of fractures of the shaft of the femur with maximum fixation. *J Bone Joint Surg*. 1926;8:494–503.
37. Hitzrot. Transactions of New York Surgical Society. *Ann Surg*. 1926;83:301.
38. Danis R. *Théorie et Pratique de l'Ostéosynthèse*. Paris: Masson; 1949.
39. Helfet DL, Haas NP, Schatzker J, et al. AO philosophy and principles of fracture management-its evolution and evaluation. *J Bone Joint Surg Am*. 2003;85:1156–1160.
40. Rüedi T, Murphy W. AO principles of fracture management. New York, NY: Thieme; 2001.
41. Moore TM, Patzakis MJ, Harvey JP. Tibial plateau fractures: definition, demographics, treatment rationale, and long-term results of closed traction management or operative reduction. *J Orthop Trauma*. 1987;1:97–119.
42. Young MJ, Barrack RL. Complications of internal fixation of tibial plateau fractures. *Orthop Rev*. 1994;23:149–154.
43. Mallik AR, Covall DJ, Whitelaw GP. Internal versus external fixation of bicondylar tibial plateau fractures. *Orthop Rev*. 1992;21:1433–1436.
44. Rasmussen PS. Tibial condylar fractures as a cause of degenerative arthritis. *Acta Orthop Scand*. 1972;43:566–575.
45. Covall DJ, Fowble CD, Foster TE, Whitelaw GP. Bicondylar tibial plateau fractures: Principles of treatment. *Contemp Orthop*. 1994;28:115–122.
46. Lachiewicz PF, Funcik T. Factors influencing the results of open reduction and internal fixation of tibial plateau fractures. *Clin Orthop Relat Res*. 1990;(259):210–215.
47. Böhler L, Böhler J. Küntscher's medullary nailing. *J Bone Joint Surg Am*. 1949;31:295–305.
48. Schatzker J. Changes in the AO/ASIF principles and methods. *Injury*. 1995;26(Suppl 2):B51–B56.
49. Perren SM. Biological internal fixation interface between biology and biomechanics. *Eur Cells Mater*. 2003;5(Suppl 2):22–23.
50. Perren SM. Review article: Evolution of the internal fixation of long bone fractures. *JBJS*. 2002; 84(8):1093–1110.
51. McKibbin B. The biology of fracture healing in long bones. *J Bone Joint Surg*. 1978;60-B(2): 150–162.
52. Perren SM, Huggler A, Russenberger M, et al. A method of measuring the change in compression applied to living cortical bone. *Acta Orthop Scand*. 1969;125(Suppl):5–16.
53. Perren, SM, Russenberger M, Steinemann S, et al. A dynamic compression plate. *Acta Orthop Scand*. 1969;125(Suppl):29–41.
54. Gautier E, Cordey J, Mathys R, et al. Porosity and remodeling of plated bone after internal fixation: Effect of stress shielding or vascular damage? In: Ducheyne P, VanderPerre G, Aubert AE, eds. *Biomaterials and Biomechanics 1983*. Amsterdam: Elsevier; 1984.
55. Perren SM, Cordey J, Rahn BA, et al. Early temporary porosis of bone induced by internal fixation implants: A reaction to necrosis, not to stress protection? *Clin Orthop Relat Res*. 1988;232: 139–151.
56. Perren SM, Klaue K, Pohler O, et al. The limited contact dynamic compression plate (LC-DCP). *Arch Orthop Trauma Surg*. 1990;109:304–310.
57. Borgeaud M, Cordey J, Leyvraz PF, et al. Mechanical analysis of the bone to plate interface of the LC-DCP and of the PC-FIX on human femora. *Injury*. 2000;31(Suppl 3):C29–C36.
58. Perren SM, Buchanan JS. Basic concepts relevant to the design and development of the Point Contact Fixator (PC-Fix). *Injury*. 1995;26(Suppl 2):B1–B4.
59. Tepic C, Perren SM. The biomechanics of the PC-Fix internal fixator. *Injury* 1995;26(Suppl 2): B5–B10.
60. Haasnoot E, Münch TWH, Matter P, et al. Radiological sequences of healing in internal plates and splints of different contact surface to bone. (DCP, LC-DCP and PC-Fix). *Injury*. 1995;26(Suppl 2): B28–B36.
61. Brunner CF, Weber BG. *Special Techniques in Internal Fixation*. Berlin; New York, NY: Springer-Verlag; 1982. (Translated from German to English by T. C. Telger.)
62. Heitemeyer U, Kemper F, Hierholzer G, et al. Severely comminuted femoral shaft fractures: Treatment by bridging-plate osteosynthesis. *Arch Orthop Trauma Surg*. 1987;106:327–330.
63. Mast J, Jakob R, Ganz R. *Planning and Reduction Technique in Fracture Surgery*. Berlin Heidelberg, New York: Springer; 1989;56–57.
64. Krettek C, Müller M, Miclau T. Evolution of minimally invasive plate osteosynthesis (MIPO) in the femur. *Injury*. 2001;32(Suppl 3):C14–C23.
65. Farouk O, Krettek C, Miclau T, et al. Minimally invasive plate osteosynthesis and vascularity: Preliminary results of a cadaver injection study. *Injury*. 1997;28(Suppl 1):A7–A12.

66. Farouk O, Krettek C, Miclau T, et al. Effects of percutaneous and conventional plating techniques on the blood supply to the femur. *Arch Orthop Trauma Surg.* 1998;117:438–441.
67. Farouk O, Krettek C, Miclau T, et al. Minimally invasive plate osteosynthesis: Does percutaneous plating disrupt femoral blood supply less than the traditional technique? *J Orthop Trauma.* 1999;13:401–406.
68. Schandelmaier P, Partenheimer A, Koenemann B, et al. Distal femoral fractures and LISS stabilization. *Injury.* 2001;32(Suppl 3):C55–C63.
69. Goesling T, Frenk A, Appenzeller A, et al. LISS PLT: Design, mechanical and biomechanical characteristics. *Injury.* 2003;34(Suppl 1):A11–A15.
70. Ricci W, Rudzki J, Borrelli J. Treatment of complex Proximal Tibia Fractures With the Less Invasive Skeletal Stabilization System. *J Orthop Trauma.* 2004;18(8):521–527.
71. Frigg R, Appenzeller A, Christensen R. The development of the distal femur Less Invasive Stabilization System (LISS). *Injury.* 2001;32(Suppl 3):C24–C31.
72. Weight M, Collinge C. Early results of the less invasive stabilization system for mechanically unstable fractures of the distal femur (AO/OTA Types A2, A3, C2 and C3). *J Orthop Trauma.* 2004;18(8):503–508.
73. Wong MK, Leung F, Chow SP. Treatment of distal femoral fractures in the elderly using a less-invasive plating technique. *Int Orthop.* 2005;29:117–120.
74. Fankhauser F, Gruber G, Schippinger G. Minimal-invasive treatment of distal femoral fractures with the LISS (Less Invasive Stabilization System): A prospective study of 30 fractures with a follow up of 20 months. *Acta Orthop Scand.* 2004;75(1):56–60.
75. Kolb W, Guhlmann H, Windisch C. Fixation of distal femoral fractures with the Less Invasive Stabilization System: A minimally invasive treatment with locked fixed-angle screws. *J Trauma.* 2008;65(6):1425–1434.
76. Boldin C, Fankhauser F, Hofer HP, et al. Three-year results of proximal tibia fractures treated with the LISS. *Clin Orthop Relat Res.* 2006;445:222–229.
77. Stannard J, Wilson T, Volgas D, et al. The less invasive stabilization system in the treatment of complex fractures of the tibial plateau: Short-term results. *J Orthop Trauma.* 2004;18(8):552–558.
78. Kobbe P, Klemm R, Reilmann H, et al. Less invasive stabilization system (LISS) for the treatment of periprosthetic femoral fractures: A 3-year follow-up. *Injury.* 2008;39:472–479.
79. An Z, Zeng B, He X, et al. Plating osteosynthesis of mid-distal humeral shaft fractures: Minimally invasive versus conventional open reduction technique. *Int Orthop.* 2010;34:131–135.
80. Röderer G, Erhardt J, Graf M, Kinzl L, et al. Clinical results for minimally invasive locked plating of proximal humerus fractures. *J Orthop Trauma.* 2010;24(7):400–406.
81. Jöckel JA, Brunner A, Thormann S, et al. Elastic stabilisation of proximal humeral fractures with a new percutaneous angular stable Wxation device (ButtonFix®): A preliminary report.*Arch Orthop Trauma Surg.* 2010;130:1397–1403.
82. Laflamme GY, Rouleau DM, Berry GK, et al. Percutaneous humeral plating of fractures of the proximal humerus: Results of a prospective multicenter clinical trial. *J Orthop Trauma.* 2008; 22(3):153–158.
83. Rammelt S, Amlang M, Barthel S, et al. Minimally-invasive treatment of calcaneal fractures. *Injury.* 2004;35:SB55–SB63.
84. Stulik J, Stehlik J, Rysavy M, et al. Minimally-invasive treatment of intra-articular fractures of the calcaneum. *J Bone Joint Surg.* 2006;88(12):1634–1641.
85. DeWall M, Henderson CE, McKinley TO, et al. Percutaneous reduction and fixation of displaced intra-articular calcaneus fractures. *J Orthop Trauma.* 2010;24(8):466–472.
86. Weber M, Lehmann O, Sägesser D, et al. Limited open reduction and internal fixation of displaced intra-articular fractures of the calcaneum. *J Bone Joint Surg Br.* 2008;90(12):1608–1616.
87. Borens O, Kloen P, Richmond J, et al. Minimally invasive treatment of pilon fractures with a low profile plate: preliminary results in 17 cases. *Arch Orthop Trauma Surg.* 2009;129:649–659.
88. Leonard M, Magill P, Khayvat G. Minimally-invasive treatment of high velocity intra-articular fractures of the distal tibia. *IntOrthop.* 2009;33:1149–1153.
89. Hasenboehler E, Rikli D, Babst R. Locking compression plate with minimally invasive plate osteosynthesis in diaphyseal and distal tibial fracture: A retrospective study of 32 patients. *Injury.* 2007;38(3):365–370.
90. Stöckle U, Schaser K, König B. Image guidance in pelvic and acetabular surgery—expectations, success and limitations. *Injury.* 2007;38:450–462.
91. Arand M, Kinzl L, Gebhard F. Computer-guidance in percutaneous screw stabilization of the iliosacral joint. *Clin Orthop Relat Res.* 2004;422:201–217.
92. Ebraheim NA, Coombs R, Jackson WT, Rusin JJ. Percutaneous computed tomography-guided stabilization of posterior pelvic fractures. *Clin Orthop Relat Res.* 1994;307:222-228.
93. Gay SB, Sistrom C, Wang GJ, et al. Percutaneous screw fixation of acetabular fractures with CT guidance: Preliminary results of a new technique. *Am J Roentgenol.* 1992;158(4):819–822.

CHAPTER 2

Biological Basis of Minimally Invasive Osteosynthesis

Saam Morshed, Carol A. Lin, Christian Krettek and Theodore Miclau III

INTRODUCTION

Prior to the era of aseptic technique and general anesthesia, the early treatment of fractures was almost entirely nonoperative. This avoided the risks of surgery; however, closed reduction and prolonged immobilization often led to joint stiffness, malunion, and impairment from disuse. The subsequent development of safer surgical practices led to increased operative management of fractures which initially called for anatomic reduction and rigid fixation to achieve primary cortical healing.[1] While this allowed for early motion of the limb and perhaps the avoidance of debilitating permanent stiffness or "plaster disease,"[2] the pursuit of precise anatomic reduction often resulted in significant operative trauma, increasing the risk of nonunion and infection.[3,4]

The emerging concept of "biologic fixation" aims to preserve the vascularity of the fracture and integrity of the fracture hematoma while achieving appropriate rigidity of the fracture repair construct to maximize healing potential.[5–7] This has led to the popularization of minimally invasive osteosynthesis (MIO) techniques that strive for the appropriate balance of soft tissue preservation and construct rigidity.[8–13] This chapter provides an overview of the biology of fracture healing and the evidence supporting the concept of biologic fixation.

BIOLOGY OF FRACTURE REPAIR

Fracture repair involves a coordinated sequence of events involving four distinct phases: An initial inflammatory stage, soft callus stage, hard callus stage, and remodeling. The inflammatory stage involves hematoma formation allowing inflammatory cells to infiltrate and debride the fracture site and recruit cells necessary for bone repair. A soft callus stage composed of cartilage is formed next as these progenitor cells differentiate to form osteoblasts and chondrocytes. Chondrocytes then undergo maturation and the extracellular matrix is calcified. This is followed by removal of the calcified cartilage by osteoclasts and invasion by endothelial cells. The hard callus is formed, as bone is laid down behind the infiltrating vasculature. The newly formed bone is then remodeled until morphologically and mechanically similar to its preinjury state. Each of these phases of bone repair has been well studied in murine models[14–17] and is explained in greater detail below.

At the time of fracture, torn periosteum, exposed bone marrow, and injured soft tissues bleed and create the fracture hematoma. This fracture hematoma contains inflammatory cells, including macrophages and platelets, that degranulate releasing inflammatory cytokines such as IL-1, IL-6,[18] and TNFα[19] and growth factors such as TGFβ, PDGF, and BMP.[18] These molecules act on local cells in the marrow and periosteum to proliferate and differentiate.[20] Within the first 7 to 10 days from injury, these mesenchymal cells aggregate and form condensations within the fracture hematoma and form cartilaginous tissue—the soft callus. Stem cells differentiate into chondrocytes or osteoblasts depending on the mechanical environment. Relative instability favors chondrocyte differentiation and endochondral ossification (Fig. 2.1), whereas stability favors osteoblast differentiation and intramembranous ossification (Fig. 2.2). Operative fracture fixation uses the entire spectrum from absolute rigid internal fixation to relative stability.

During this early period of fracture healing, the main extracellular components are type II collagen and proteoglycans. The proteoglycans inhibit mineralization of the mass until enough cartilage has been formed.[21] These cells undergo proliferative and hypertrophic

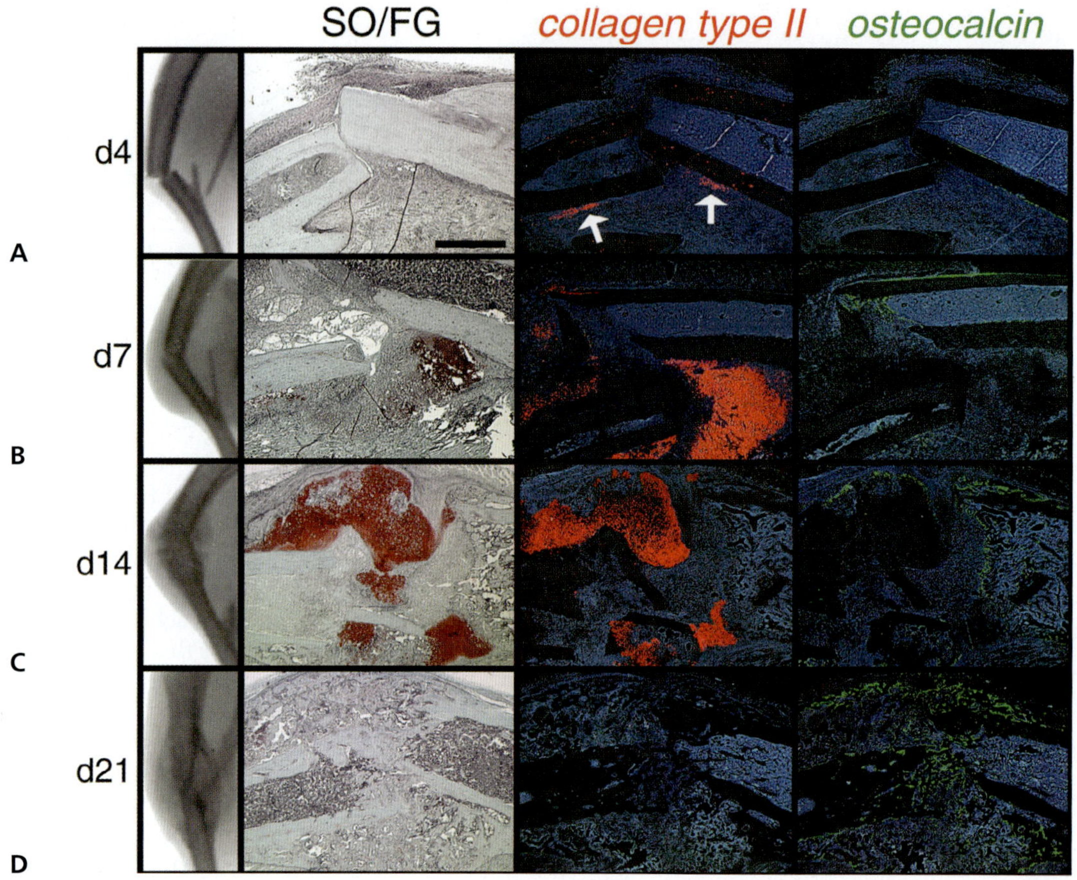

Figure 2.1 Nonstabilized fractures heal through endochondral ossification: **(A)** By day 4, radiographs show misaligned bone segments due to the lack of stabilization following fracture. SO/FG staining does not indicate the formation of cartilage or bone; however, colagen type IIa (colIIa) expression indicates that some cells are differentiating along a chondrogenic lineage (*arrows*). Osteocalcin (oc) expression reveals a small amount of new bone forming along the periosteum. **B:** By day 7, radiographs show an enlarged callus at the fracture site. SO/FG histology shows abundant cartilage at the site of the fracture, and a small amount of new bone forming along the periosteum. These histologic observations are confirmed by the widespread, strong expression of colIIa throughout the callus, and the limited expression of oc along the periosteum. **C:** By day 14, radiographs indicate the presence of a radio-opaque tissue has formed at the fracture site. SO/FG histology indicates that this radio-opaque tissue is predominantly bone replacing the cartilage callus. ColIIa transcripts continue to be detected in the fracture callus, although at much lower levels than observed at day 7. Oc is expressed throughout the callus tissues, bridging the bone segments. **D:** By day 21, radiographs indicate the bone ends are aligned to a greater extent, suggesting that the callus is undergoing remodeling. SO/FG histology indicates that most cartilage has been replaced by bone during this phase of healing. The lack of colIIa expression indicates the absence of chondrocytes. Oc is expressed throughout the callus, albeit at lower levels than observed at day 14. (From: Thompson Z, Miclau T, Hu D, et al. A model for intramembranous ossification during fracture healing. *J Orthop Res.* 2002;20:1091–1098.)

phases identical to those that take place at the growth plate. Hypertrophic chondrocytes begin releasing vesicles containing calcium and proteolytic enzymes that release phosphate ions from the surrounding matrix and degrade proteoglycans. Through the precipitation of calcium and phosphate and the decreasing concentration of neighboring proteoglycans, the callus begins to mineralize.[22] This process peaks at about 14 days and signals the beginning of vascular ingrowth into the fracture callus.[23] The parallels between growth and fracture repair continue as the calcified cartilage is identical to the primary spongiosa at the growth plate. Between 2 and 3 weeks, chondroclasts remove the calcified cartilage as well as chondrocytes that have undergone apoptosis,[24] and gradually osteoblasts convert the soft callus

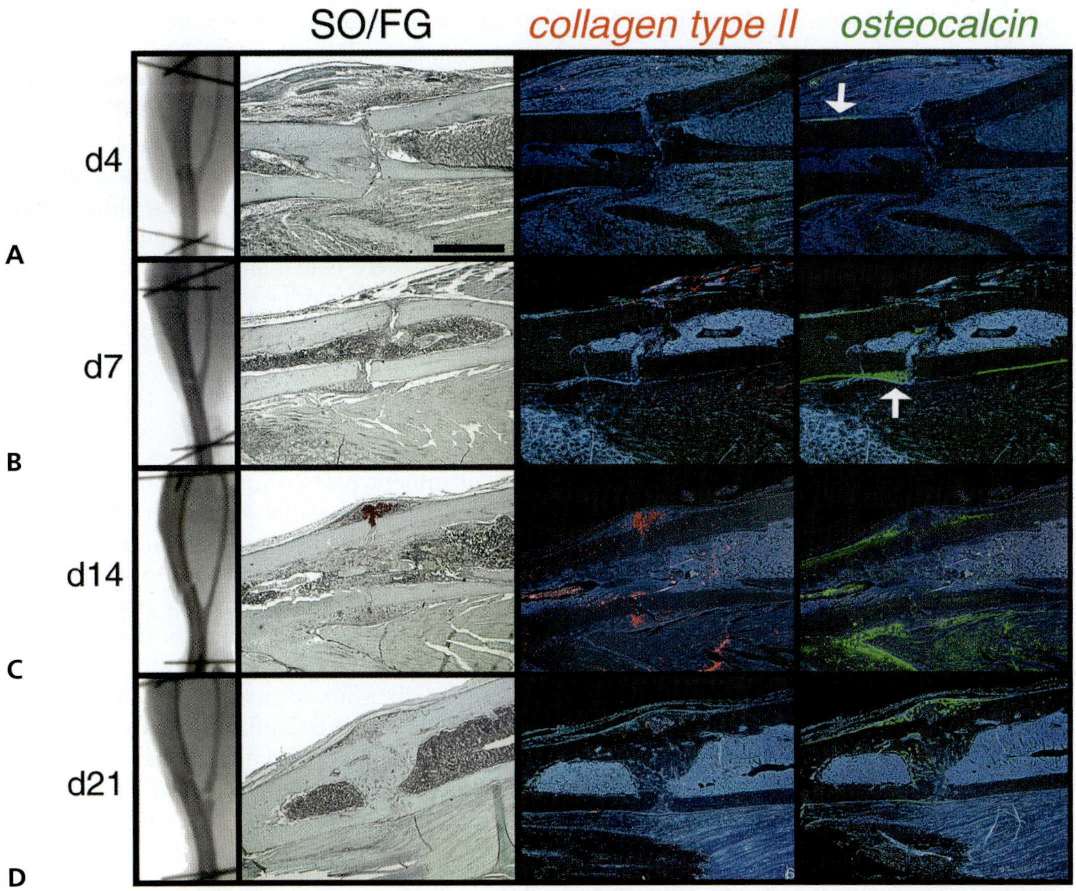

Figure 2.2 Stabilized fractures heal through intramembranous ossification: **(A)** Radiographs taken 4 days after tibial fracture reveal no evidence of callus formation. SO/FG histology confirms the lack of cartilage in the callus tissues. CollIa transcripts are undetectable in the fracture site. In an adjacent section, oc transcripts are detected in the periosteum near the fracture site (*arrow*). **B:** 7 days after fracture, radiographs fail to reveal a callus at the site of fracture. SO/FG staining of the callus tissues shows no evidence of cartilage, and some new bone at the fracture site. The lack of collIa expression confirms the absence of cartilage from the stabilized fracture callus, and oc expression substantiates that new bone has been generated in the form of a periosteal wedge (*arrow*). **C:** At day 14, radiographs indicate a small bony callus at the fracture site. SO/FG histology reveals new bone forming in the medullary canal, and a lack of cartilage. There is an extremely small region of collIa expression detectable on the anterior aspect of some fracture calluses. The lack of proteoglycan staining in an adjacent section indicates that these cells have not progressed to differentiated cartilage. Oc expression shows evidence of new bone that is bridging the fracture gap, as well as new bone in the medullary canal. **D:** By day 21, radiographs indicate that the fracture is almost healed. SO/FG staining confirms these radiographic data, as new bone bridges both anterior and posterior cortices. CollIa is not expressed at the fracture site, whereas oc transcripts indicate new bone on the anterior and posterior aspects of the fracture callus. (From: Thompson Z, Miclau T, Hu D, et al. A model for intramembranous ossification during fracture healing. *J Orthop Res.* 2002;20:1091–1098).

to the hard callus by laying down woven bone that is identical to secondary spongiosa from the growth plate. This replacement process generally is completed by 3 to 4 weeks at which point the fracture is united. Osteoclasts then begin the remodeling process and the woven bone is converted to lamellar bone.

The local soft tissues provide cellular and molecular elements that are critical to fracture repair: Skeletal progenitor cells derived from the periosteum and marrow differentiate into cartilage and bone; an extracellular matrix provides a scaffold for cells and storage space for cytokines and growth factors; and a blood supply provides the necessary cells, nutrition, and molecules essential for healing. The periosteum is of primary importance as it contributes blood supply, undifferentiated mesenchymal cells as well as the osteoprogenitor cells that eventually become bone. On its own, the periosteum is capable of bridging gaps up to one-half the diameter of bone.[25] Removal of the periosteum results in a weaker callus,[26] and removal or compression of the periosteum overlying bone can cause bone necrosis.[27–29] The external soft tissues also contribute significantly to the blood supply that supports early callus formation and development.[23,30,31] In poorly vascularized, hypoxic tissue, the differentiation and maturation of the chondrocytic tissue at the center of the callus fails and the callus cannot mature.[32,33] In addition to local vascular supply, there is evidence in animal models suggesting that the nervous system may also play a role.[34,35] The preservation of the soft tissue envelope and its vital functions is a fundamental component of biologic fracture fixation.

MECHANOBIOLOGY

In addition to fracture biology, the mechanical environment plays an important role in the cellular differentiation of the healing skeleton. Bone can successfully heal under both very rigid and relatively flexible conditions, and the exact relationship between local mechanical forces and the rate and method of fracture healing is still poorly understood. One prevailing concept as to how these factors interact is the interfragmentary strain theory proposed by Perren in 1979.[36] Interfragmentary strain is defined as the ratio of the axial fracture displacement to the fracture gap width. The theory states that the method of cell differentiation during healing is determined by the amount of interfragmentary strain at the fracture site. In support of this hypothesis are observations that absence of instability results in minimal callus formation whereas small amounts of strain induce callus formation. Strain values of 2% are tolerated by lamellar bone tissues, while hard callus or woven bone can tolerate up to 10% strain. In contrast, granulation tissue will tolerate 100% strain before rupture.[36,37] In order to obtain successful fracture union, the local environment must minimize the amount of interfragmentary strain. In the nonstabilized fracture, the increasing size and stiffness of callus reduce the amount of movement at the fracture ends, which allows for differentiation of cells to progressively stiffer tissue types. In experimental animal models, it has been shown that rigidly fixed fractures with very small gaps (i.e., areas of high strain) result in fracture ends that are resorbed prior to bony union.[38,39]

It should be noted, however, that Perren's original hypothesis only considered axial deformation, whereas in vivo fractures are subjected to multiple directional forces when loaded. This has led to research evaluating the role of hydrostatic pressure,[40] shear,[41] and tensile stresses on fracture healing, as well as the timing and nature of loading. Cyclic, compressive axial loading across a gap can increase callus size and the rate of endochondral ossification.[42–44] Studies using distraction osteogenesis models have shown that static, tensile forces favor intramembranous ossification.[45] In contrast, bending moments are known to favor cartilage formation and prevent ossification entirely.[46,47] These studies are gradually clarifying the effects of the mechanical environment on fracture healing; however, many studies rely heavily on finite element analyses and assumed material properties.[48]

It is still unclear as to exactly how much motion and force will optimize fracture healing. Some assumptions appear to be consistent between a computational model and the more complex in vivo environment. Rigid fixation will depress callus formation and differentiation in the periosteum and soft tissues,[25] whereas excessive motion and load may yield a hypertrophic nonunion.[49,50] A small amount of cyclic motion and axial load in transverse fractures will accelerate healing,[40,43,51] while shear forces in the same environment will result in nonunion.[41,47] Although these relationships are still being actively investigated, it is clear that the surgeon must find the right balance of construct rigidity and soft tissue preservation in order to maximize bone healing potential.

THE CONCEPT OF BIOLOGIC FIXATION

As the interactions between fracture biology and mechanical stability are better understood, the central paradigm of direct reduction and absolute rigidity has given way to more soft

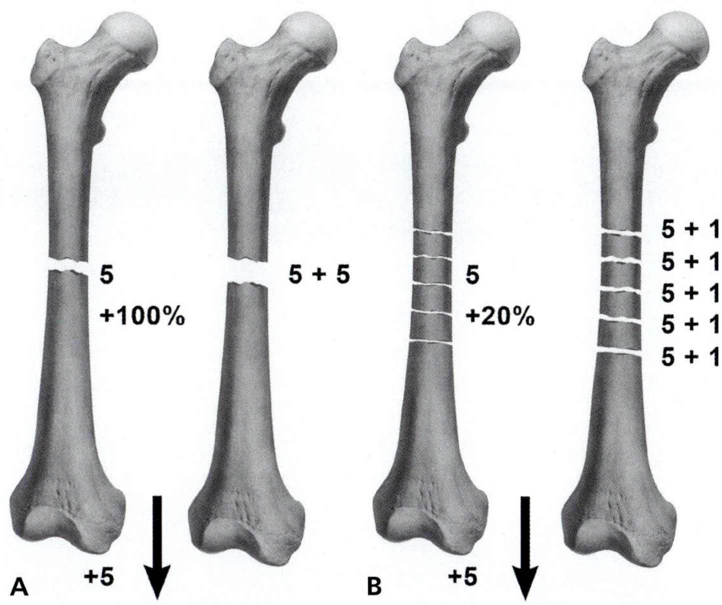

Figure 2.3 Schematic diagrams showing the distribution of a 5-unit displacement on a simple fracture **(A)** and comminuted fracture **(B)**. The displacement across the comminuted segment results in smaller interval displacements between fragments, resulting in decreased interfragmentary strain.

tissue sparing techniques. Where once the appearance of callus was thought to be a failure of fixation,[52] its presence is now better appreciated in the healing of long bone fractures via flexible "internal splints."[53] Gerber et al.[7] formalized the movement toward minimally invasive fracture fixation with the concept of "biologic fixation" in 1990, which "strives to obtain optimal rather than maximal stability with a minimum of soft tissue dissection." While articular fragments still require anatomical reduction and rigid fixation, extra-articular fractures benefit from restoration of alignment and rotation with preservation of as much of the fracture hematoma and soft tissue envelope as possible.[6,7,54]

Two key technical concepts in biologic fixation are indirect reduction and relative stability. Indirect reduction has been defined as "the blind repositioning of bone fragments through distraction accomplished with an instrument (distractor) or implant."[55] Fixation methods that impart relative stability include external fixators, intramedullary nails, and bridge plates that serve as splints. With these techniques, direct exposure of the fracture fragments can be avoided, and the periosteum and fracture hematoma are preserved.

In addition to the soft tissue preservation afforded by the lack of extensive dissection, bridge plating has the added theoretical benefit of modulating the amount of strain across the fracture site. According to the interfragmentary strain hypothesis, excessive amounts of strain will lead to the formation of fibrous tissue, and small gaps can experience large amounts of strain even with small movements. In extensively comminuted fractures that are fixed with bridge plating, the strain is effectively distributed over a much larger area and multiple fragments. As a result, the strain experienced by each fragment is proportionally reduced relative to the number of fragments[56] (Fig. 2.3).

This increases the likelihood that secondary healing will successfully occur. This theory has been supported in vivo by multiple animal studies[57–59] as well as a few clinical studies in humans. Krettek et al.[60] compared open tibia fractures which had been treated with external fixation versus those that had a supplemental lag screw used to aid with fracture reduction and found that those with lag screw fixation required bone grafting twice as often for nonunion and had significantly higher rates of refracture, often through the prior fracture site.

To assess whether these indirect reduction and biologic plating techniques improved the preservation of vascularity to bone, conventional open reduction and internal fixation were compared to the so-called "minimally invasive plate osteosynthesis (MIPO)" in cadaver femora.[61] After application of a limited contact dynamic compression plate (LC-DCP) using either MIPO or conventional plating technique, the specimens were injected with blue silicone and periosteal and medullary perfusion were evaluated (Fig. 2.4). Conventional plating disrupted up to 80% of the blood supply to the femur and the authors concluded that a minimally invasive technique using indirect reduction had far less impact on bone vascularity.

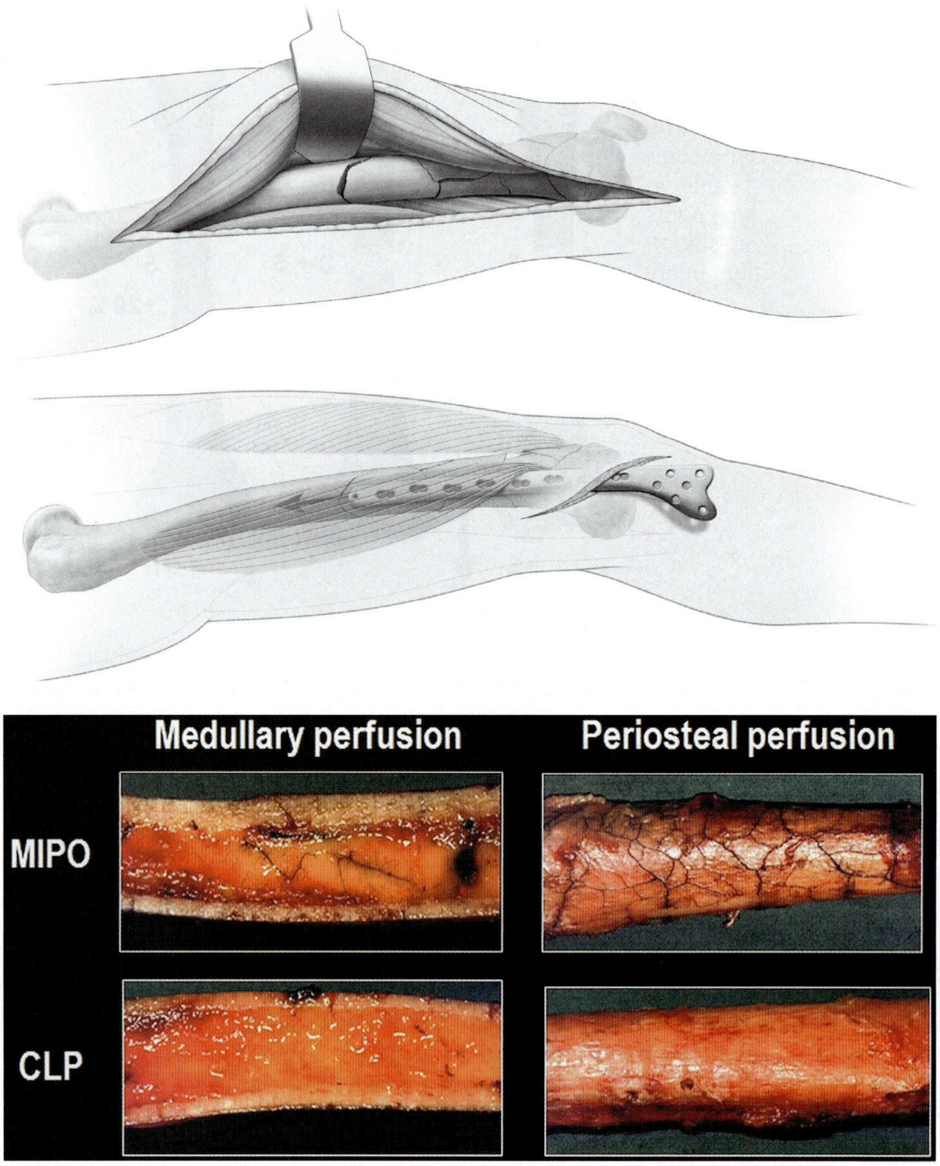

A

B

C

Figure 2.4 **A:** Extensile exposure with ligation of perforating vessels and muscle retraction. **B:** Minimally invasive application of plate. **C:** Photographs following dye injection showing medullary and periosteal perfusion. MIPO, minimally invasive plate osteosynthesis; CLP, conventional lateral plate. (From: Farouk O, Krettek C, Miclau T, et al. Minimally invasive plate osteosynthesis and vascularity: Preliminary results of a cadaver injection study. *Injury.* 1997;28(Suppl 1):A7–12).

FRACTURE REPAIR CONSTRUCTS

It is clear that adequate stability is a key factor in fracture healing, and a great deal of research has focused on how best to modulate strength and stiffness, not only in implant design but also in how the implant interfaces with bone. A fracture repair construct includes both the implant and the bone itself, and both bone and implant share the stresses experienced by the healing fracture. As the patient moves the limb and begins to bear weight, the construct must be able to withstand axial, shear, bending, and torsional loads. This is an inherently dynamic process as the amount of force each component must tolerate will change as the bone unites or is resorbed. The bone–implant interface also changes in cases of loosening or infection, or when the implant is altered, such as when a frame or nail is dynamized.

The development of contemporary biologic fixation primarily addressed complications associated with soft tissue handling during fracture fixation. The benefits of those principles had already been demonstrated with intramedullary nail fixation. For this reason, a better term for these techniques might be MIO, which would include the multitude of fixation options that share a common goal of maintaining the fundamental principles of biologic fixation.

Intramedullary nailing may represent the ideal example of MIO as the majority of fixation occurs within the bone itself without any tissue dissection. The entry site for the implant is far from the already injured soft tissues around the fracture, and there is no disruption of the fracture hematoma unless an open reduction is required. The technique has enjoyed a high degree of success particularly in the lower extremity with union rates as high as 95% to 97%.[62–68] Intramedullary nails function as internal splints creating a relatively stable environment where both the implant and the bone experience the forces of loading the extremity.[69] The construct maintains some flexibility that allows for motion at the fracture site to encourage callus formation and secondary healing, though the exact amount of motion required is still unclear. Nail geometry, and more specifically diameter, has one of the greatest influences on construct strength. Moreover, by reaming the medullary canal, a better endosteal fit may be achieved with a larger nail, thereby decreasing the working length of the construct and further increasing stability.[70] There is concern that medullary reaming jeopardizes the diaphyseal blood supply,[71] and in rare instances may cause significant pulmonary and embolic injury. However, these effects seem to have limited clinical significance and are outweighed by positive outcomes achieved with reamed intramedullary nailing.[72,73] The success of reamed intramedullary nailing despite theoretical concerns over obliteration of endosteal blood supply may be explained by the recognized importance of the periosteum, with potential increases in post-reaming tissue vascularity[74] as well as the creation of in situ bone graft[75] which can be a source of multipotent stem cells.[76] Reaming also appears to be safe in open fractures with compromised soft tissue; multiple prospective, randomized trials of reamed and unreamed tibial nails did not show significant differences in number of procedures required or rates of union.[77,78] The biologic and biomechanical advantages of intramedullary nailing make it one of the most successful and widely used forms of MIO.

In conventional plate fixation of fractures, the strength of the construct depends on the friction between the plate and the bone in the area underneath the plate that is created by screw purchase. The friction generated detrimentally impacts the periosteal and cortical blood supply beneath the plate.[29] Animal studies have demonstrated that the bone directly underneath the plate quickly becomes porous[79] regardless of the material stiffness of the implant.[80] The cause of this porosity has been attributed to necrosis of the bone under the plate[27,29,81] and has been supported by the fact that plates with smaller surface areas of bone contact produce less cortical necrosis.[82] The clinical importance of this phenomenon and design modifications meant to mitigate it are largely unknown.

The addition of locked plates to the surgeon's arsenal has added a new dimension to fracture management. With locked plating, the screw–plate interface becomes a fixed angle construct,[83] and the stability of the fracture fixation construct relies less on bone–plate friction for stability; stress is primarily transmitted through the plate itself. As such, the plate no longer must lay directly on bone for fracture fixation, allowing the plate to function more like an external fixator and leaving the periosteum intact (Fig. 2.5). The locked construct functions as a single-beam construct as there is little potential for motion between the plate and the bone, and it can be up to four times stronger than conventional plating.[84] Shearing force, which would cause conventional plates to fail, is converted to compressive forces at the screw–bone interface that is better withstood by bone tissue.[83] In locked plates, the fixation strength is the sum of all screw–bone interfaces rather than the axial pull out strength of the weakest screw.[85]

Occasionally it is preferable to use a combination of locking and nonlocking screws in fracture fixation. For example, in cases where bone–plate fixation is at risk and locked plating may be beneficial, as in the case of osteoporotic fractures, some amount of bone–plate friction may be desirable in order to obtain a reduction or achieve compression. In those cases, a nonlocking screw may be used to compress plate to bone.[86] Gardner et al.[87] compared hybrid, fully locked, and fully unlocked constructs in synthetic humeri drilled to simulate osteoporotic bone; they found that both the hybrid and fully locked constructs

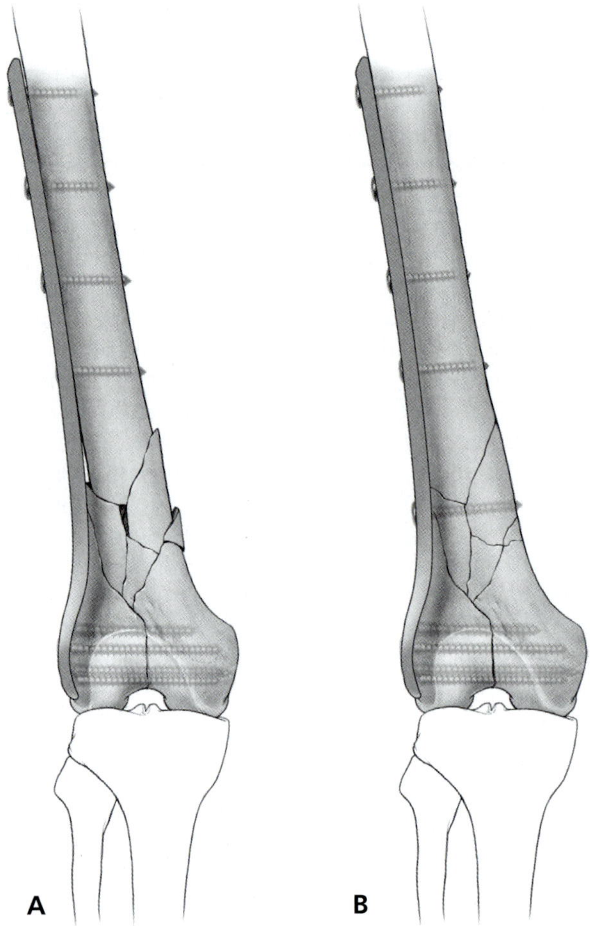

Figure 2.5 Schematic views of intra-articular distal femur fracture stabilized with direct reduction and compression of the articular surface **(A)** and indirect reduction and bridge plating of the comminuted supracondylar femur **(B)**.

maintained similar rigidity initially and after cyclic torsional loading, and that both were significantly more rigid than the unlocked model. While the principals discussed above have driven clinical practice, the evidence in support of these biologic fixation techniques is early in its development.

CLINICAL STUDIES

Over the last two decades, MIO has become more widespread with lower rates of nonunion, infection, and wound complications. Currently the MIO approach is strongly associated with locking or anatomically contoured plates, but early applications of the minimally invasive approach used conventional implants such as the dynamic condylar screw (DCS), LC-DCP,[13] or a combination of plating and external fixation.[88] Wenda et al.[89] described a submuscular plating technique using a 95-degree blade plate in 17 comminuted subtrochanteric fractures and reported that all patients had eventual consolidation, though 3 required bone grafting in a second procedure. In the distal femur, Ostrum and Geel[90] found that indirect reduction and biologic fixation techniques resulted in union in nearly all cases without the routine use of bone graft. In the tibia, Helfet et al.[91] reported a 100% union rate by 11 weeks using minimally invasive techniques and one-third tubular plates in distal tibial articular fractures, although the malunion rate was 20%. Using either a 95-degree angled condylar blade plate[92] or DCS,[93,94] angle stable fixation through a submuscular approach has led to reliable union and excellent functional results, though malunions have been reported in up to one-third of cases and are attributed to the demanding nature of these techniques and associated learning curve.

To make these techniques more accessible, multiple different implants have been designed specifically for percutaneous insertion. One of the first systems available was the Less Invasive

Stabilization System (LISS) (Synthes, Paoli, PA, USA) which uses an anatomically contoured plate, an insertion guide, and self-tapping unicortical locking screws.[95] Since the introduction of the LISS implant, multiple other systems for a variety of different fractures have been introduced. Early clinical results with this system in both the tibia and the femur have been promising. Kregor studied 103 cases of distal femur fractures treated with a LISS plate and found a union rate of 93% without bone grafting and a 3% rate of infection. There were no cases of late varus collapse or loss of distal fixation. He did report five incidences of loss of proximal fixation, two nonunions, and six malreductions primarily related to excess valgus or rotational deformities at the fracture site.[96] Weight and Collinge[97] reported 100% union and no implant failures in 22 distal femoral supra- and intercondylar fractures; they also reported 1 malunion and 2 cases of external rotation in excess of 10 degrees. Additional prospective studies have reported union rates >90% with infection rates <5%, although malalignment was also a concern.[98,99] Using the LISS for intra-articular fractures of the proximal tibia, Stannard et al.[100] found that 34 of 35 fractures healed on short-term follow-up with excellent alignment. There were two cases of infection, which occurred in patients with open fractures. Ricci et al.[101] also reported excellent union rates with maintained alignment and fixation at 2-year follow-up and no wound or infectious complications. They reported one malreduction with coronal angulation greater than 10 degrees; however, this was significantly better than the high rates reported with intramedullary nailing of proximal tibia fractures. Cole et al.[8] followed 54 complex fractures of the proximal tibia and reported that 48 had healed by 13 weeks. There were five cases of angular malreduction more than 5 degrees, and two with anterior translations of the proximal fragment of more than 1 cm. One patient had a nerve palsy that was attributed to percutaneous insertion of a distal shaft screw that injured the deep peroneal nerve. These results have spawned a wave of precontoured locked implants for nearly every anatomic location that continues to outpace the clinical evidence in support of their distribution and use.

CONCLUSIONS

While there is a lack of high quality comparative clinical data, uncontrolled case series describing successful MIO techniques for historically challenging fracture repair situations support the biologic rationale for their use. There are numerous described pitfalls that emphasize the learning curve associated with their implementation. As surgeons work to familiarize themselves with newer generations of implants designed for "percutaneous" or "minimally invasive" application, there is a danger in forgetting plate function and biologic effect of technique, which are novel factors determined by the surgeon. The utility of minimally invasive techniques with locked plates has continued to grow with successful results reported in the treatment of osteoporotic[102,103] and periprosthetic fractures,[104,105] as well as fractures in the proximal humerus.[106–108] Future clinical studies of the effects directly attributable to biologic fixation techniques are similarly challenged as implants have changed dramatically relative to historical controls. Well-designed randomized clinical trials and observational studies are needed to further research the benefits of MIO. In addition, biologic fixation techniques employing new devices as well as molecular technologies that are introduced with growing frequency need to be studied prior to widespread adoption and implementation.

REFERENCES

1. Schenk R, Willenegger H. [On the histological picture of so-called primary healing of pressure osteosynthesis in experimental osteotomies in the dog]. *Experientia.* 1963;19:593–595.
2. Schatzker J. Changes in the AO/ASIF principles and methods. *Injury.* 1995;26(Suppl 2):B51–B56.
3. Rozbruch SR, Müller U, Gautier E, et al. The evolution of femoral shaft plating technique. *Clin Orthop Relat Res.* 1998;354:195–208.
4. Rüedi TP, Lüscher JN. Results after internal fixation of comminuted fractures of the femoral shaft with DC plates. *Clin. Orthop Relat Res.* 1979;138:74–76.
5. Baumgaertel F, Gotzen L. [The "biological" plate osteosynthesis in multi-fragment fractures of the para-articular femur. A prospective study]. *Unfallchirurg.* 1994;97(2):78–84.
6. Perren SM. Biological internal fixation: Its background, methods, requirements, potential and limits. *Acta Chir Orthop Traumatol Cech.* 2000;67(1):6–12.

7. Gerber C, Mast JW, Ganz R. Biological internal fixation of fractures. *Arch Orthop Trauma Surg.* 1990;109(6):295–303.
8. Cole PA, Zlowodzki M, Kregor PJ. Less invasive stabilization system (LISS) for fractures of the proximal tibia: Indications, surgical technique and preliminary results of the UMC clinical trial. *Injury.* 2003;34:A16–A29.
9. Collinge C, Protzman R. Outcomes of minimally invasive plate osteosynthesis for metaphyseal distal tibia fractures. *J Orthop Trauma.* 2010;24(1):24–29.
10. Farouk O, Krettek C, Miclau T, et al. Minimally invasive plate osteosynthesis: Does percutaneous plating disrupt femoral blood supply less than the traditional technique? *J Orthop Trauma.* 1999;13(6):401–406.
11. Gosling T, Schandelmaier P, Marti A, et al. Less invasive stabilization of complex tibial plateau fractures: A biomechanical evaluation of a unilateral locked screw plate and double plating. *J Orthop Trauma.* 2004;18(8):546–551.
12. Guo JJ, Tang N, Yang HL, et al. A prospective, randomised trial comparing closed intramedullary nailing with percutaneous plating in the treatment of distal metaphyseal fractures of the tibia. *J Bone Joint Surg Br.* 2010;92(7):984–988.
13. Krettek C, Gerich T, Miclau T. A minimally invasive medial approach for proximal tibial fractures. *Injury.* 2001;32(Suppl 1):SA4–SA13.
14. Thompson Z, Miclau T, Hu D, et al. A model for intramembranous ossification during fracture healing. *J Orthop Res.* 2002;20(5):1091–1098.
15. Bonnarens F, Einhorn TA. Production of a standard closed fracture in laboratory animal bone. *J Orthop Res.* 1984;2(1):97–101.
16. Hiltunen A, Vuorio E, Aro HT. A standardized experimental fracture in the mouse tibia. *J Orthop Res.* 1993;11(2):305–312.
17. Ferguson C, Alpern E, Miclau T, et al. Does adult fracture repair recapitulate embryonic skeletal formation? *Mech Dev.* 1999;87(1–2):57–66.
18. Einhorn TA. Enhancement of fracture-healing. *J Bone Joint Surg Am.* 1995;77(6):940–956.
19. Kon T, Cho TJ, Aizawa T, et al. Expression of osteoprotegerin, receptor activator of NF-kappaB ligand (osteoprotegerin ligand) and related proinflammatory cytokines during fracture healing. *J Bone Miner Res.*2001;16(6):1004–1014.
20. Bolander ME. Regulation of fracture repair by growth factors. *Proc Soc Exp Biol Med.* 1992; 200(2):165–170.
21. Einhorn TA, Majeska RJ, Rush EB, et al. The expression of cytokine activity by fracture callus. *J Bone Miner Res.* 1995;10(8):1272–1281.
22. Einhorn TA, Hirschman A, Kaplan C, et al. Neutral protein-degrading enzymes in experimental fracture callus: A preliminary report. *J Orthop Res.* 1989;7(6):792–805.
23. Einhorn TA. The cell and molecular biology of fracture healing. *Clin Orthop Relat Res.* 1998;(355 Suppl):S7–S21.
24. Lee FY, Choi YW, Behrens FF, et al. Programmed removal of chondrocytes during endochondral fracture healing. *J Orthop Res.* 1998;16(1):144–150.
25. McKibbin B. The biology of fracture healing in long bones. *J Bone Joint Surg Br.* 1978; 60-B(2):150–162.
26. Grundnes O, Reikeras O. The role of hematoma and periosteal sealing for fracture healing in rats. *Acta Orthop Scand.* 1993;64(1):47–49.
27. Jacobs RR, Rahn BA, Perren SM. Effect of plates on cortical bone perfusion. *J Trauma.* 1981; 21(2):91–95.
28. Klaue K, Fengels I, Perren SM. Long-term effects of plate osteosynthesis: Comparison of four different plates. *Injury.* 2000;31(Suppl 2):B51–B62.
29. Perren SM, Cordey J, Rahn BA, et al. Early temporary porosis of bone induced by internal fixation implants. A reaction to necrosis, not to stress protection? *Clin Orthop Relat Res.* 1988;(232): 139–151.
30. Rhinelander FW. Vascular proliferation and blood supply during fracture healing. In: Brooker AF, Edwards CC, eds. *External Fixation: The Current State of the Art.* Baltimore, MD: Williams and Wilkins; 1979:9–14.
31. Rhinelander FW. The normal microcirculation of diaphyseal cortex and its response to fracture. *J Bone Joint Surg Am.* 1968;50(4):784–800.
32. Malladi P, Xu Y, Chiou M, et al. Effect of reduced oxygen tension on chondrogenesis and osteogenesis in adipose-derived mesenchymal cells. *Am J Physiol Cell Physiol.* 2006;290(4):C1139–C1146.
33. Hirao M, Tamai N, Tsumaki N, et al. Oxygen tension regulates chondrocyte differentiation and function during endochondral ossification. *J Biol Chem.* 2006;281(41):31079–31092.
34. Hukkanen M, Konttinen YT, Santavirta S, et al. Rapid proliferation of calcitonin gene-related peptide-immunoreactive nerves during healing of rat tibial fracture suggests neural involvement in bone growth and remodelling. *Neuroscience.* 1993;54(4):969–979.

35. Madsen JE, Hukkanen M, Aune AK, et al. Fracture healing and callus innervation after peripheral nerve resection in rats. *Clin Orthop Relat Res.* 1998;(351):230–240.
36. Perren SM. Physical and biological aspects of fracture healing with special reference to internal fixation. *Clin Orthop Relat. Res.* 1979;(138):175–196.
37. Hente RL, Fuechmeier B, Schlegel U. Der Einfluss einer zeitlich limitierten kontrollierten Bewegung auf die Frakturheilung. *Hefte Unfallchirurg.* 2001;282:23–24.
38. Cheal EJ, Mansmann KA, DiGioia AM 3rd, et al. Role of interfragmentary strain in fracture healing: Ovine model of a healing osteotomy. *J Orthop Res.* 1991;9(1):131–142.
39. Hutzschenreuter P, Perren SM, Steinemann S, et al. Some effects of rigidity of internal fixation on the healing pattern of osteotomies. *Injury.* 1969;1(1):77–81.
40. Carter DR, Beaupre GS, Giori NJ, et al. Mechanobiology of skeletal regeneration. *Clin Orthop Relat Res.* 1998;(355 Suppl):S41–S55.
41. Augat P, Burger J, Schorlemmer S, et al. Shear movement at the fracture site delays healing in a diaphyseal fracture model. *J Orthop Res.* 2003;21(6):1011–1017.
42. Goodship AE, Kenwright J. The influence of induced micromovement upon the healing of experimental tibial fractures. *J Bone Joint Surg Br.* 1985;67(4):650–655.
43. Kenwright J, Richardson JB, Cunningham JL, et al. Axial movement and tibial fractures. A controlled randomised trial of treatment. *J Bone Joint Surg Br.* 1991;73(4):654–659.
44. Claes LE, Wilke HJ, Augat P, et al. Effect of dynamization on gap healing of diaphyseal fractures under external fixation. *Clin Biomech.* 1995;10(5):227–234.
45. Ali MN, Ejiri S, Kobayashi T, et al. Histologic study of the cellular events during rat mandibular distraction osteogenesis. *Oral Surg Oral Med Oral Pathol Oral Radiol Endod.* 2009;107(3): 325–335.
46. Cullinane DM, Fredrick A, Eisenberg SR, et al. Induction of a neoarthrosis by precisely controlled motion in an experimental mid-femoral defect. *J Orthop Res.* 2002;20(3):579–586.
47. Cullinane DM, Salisbury KT, Alkhiary Y, et al. Effects of the local mechanical environment on vertebrate tissue differentiation during repair: Does repair recapitulate development? *J Exp Biol.* 2003;206(Pt 14):2459–2471.
48. Morgan EF, Salisbury Palomares KT, Gleason RE, et al. Correlations between local strains and tissue phenotypes in an experimental model of skeletal healing. *J Biomech.* 2010;43(12):2418–2424.
49. Bailón-Plaza A, van der Meulen MC. Beneficial effects of moderate, early loading and adverse effects of delayed or excessive loading on bone healing. *J Biomech.* 2003;36(8):1069–1077.
50. Chao EY, Inoue N, Elias JJ, et al. Enhancement of fracture healing by mechanical and surgical intervention. *Clin Orthop Relat Res.* 1998;(355 Suppl):S163–S178.
51. Claes LE, Heigele CA, Neidlinger-Wilke C, et al. Effects of mechanical factors on the fracture healing process. *Clin Orthop Relat Res.* 1998;(355 Suppl):S132–S147.
52. Allgower M, Ehrsam R, Ganz R, et al. Clinical experience with a new compression plate "DCP". *Acta Orthop Scand Suppl.* 1969;125:45–61.
53. Perren SM. Biological internal fixation: Interface between biology and biomechanics. *Eur Cell Mater.* 2003;5(Suppl 2):22–23.
54. Bone LB. Indirect fracture reduction: A technique for minimizing surgical trauma. *J Am Acad Orthop Surg.* 1994;2(5):247–254.
55. Mast J, Jakob R, Ganz R. *Planning And Reduction Technique In Fracture Surgery.* Berlin; New York: Springer-Verlag; 1989.
56. Perren SM. Evolution of the internal fixation of long bone fractures. The scientific basis of biological internal fixation: Choosing a new balance between stability and biology. *J Bone Joint Surg Br.* 2002; 84(8):1093–1110.
57. Heitemeyer U, Claes L, Hierholzer G, et al. Significance of postoperative stability for bony reparation of comminuted fractures. An experimental study. *Arch Orthop Trauma Surg.* 1990; 109(3):144–149.
58. Heitemeyer U, Hierholzer G, Terhorst J. [Value of bridging plate osteosynthesis in multiple fragment fracture damage of the femur in a clinical comparison]. *Unfallchirurg.* 1986;89(12):533–538.
59. Baumgaertel F, Perren SM, Rahn B. [Animal experiment studies of "biological" plate osteosynthesis of multi-fragment fractures of the femur]. *Unfallchirurg.* 1994;97(1):19–27.
60. Krettek C, Haas N, Tscherne H. The role of supplemental lag-screw fixation for open fractures of the tibial shaft treated with external fixation. *J Bone Joint Surg Am.* 1991;73(6):893–897.
61. Farouk O, Krettek C, Miclau T, et al. Minimally invasive plate osteosynthesis and vascularity: Preliminary results of a cadaver injection study. *Injury.* 1997;28(Suppl 1):A7–A12.
62. Allen WC, Heiple KG, Burstein AH. A fluted femoral intramedullary rod. Biomechanical analysis and preliminary clinical results. *J Bone Joint Surg Am.* 1978;60(4):506–515.
63. Callan JP. New intramedullary nail aids femur fracture healing. *JAMA.* 1979;241(11):1089.
64. Fowler SB, Riordan DC. Internal fixation of the femur with the Kuntscher intramedullary nail. *South Med J.* 1949;42(7):545–551.

65. Groh GI, Parker J, Allen WC. Fractures of the femur treated by intramedullary nailing using the fluted rod. A report of 193 consecutive cases. *Clin Orthop Relat Res.* 1992;(285):223–228.
66. Hansen ST, Winquist RA. Closed intramedullary nailing of the femur. Kuntscher technique with reaming. *Clin Orthop Relat Res.* 1979;(138):56–61.
67. Schafer D, Rosso R, Babst R, et al. [Experience with the AO universal femoral intramedullary nail for management of femur shaft fractures]. *Helv Chir Acta.* 1993;60(1–2):231–234.
68. Weber MJ. Closed intramedullary nailing of the femur with a Kuntscher nail. *J Ark Med Soc.* 1982;78(11):455–458.
69. Tarr RR, Wiss DA. The mechanics and biology of intramedullary fracture fixation. *Clin Orthop Relat Res.* 1986;(212):10–17.
70. Fairbank AC, Thomas D, Cunningham B, et al. Stability of reamed and unreamed intramedullary tibial nails: A biomechanical study. *Injury.* 1995;26(7):483–485.
71. Klein MP, Rahn BA, Frigg R, et al. Reaming versus non-reaming in medullary nailing: Interference with cortical circulation of the canine tibia. *Arch Orthop Trauma Surg.* 1990;109(6):314–316.
72. Anglen JO, Blue JM. A comparison of reamed and unreamed nailing of the tibia. *J Trauma.* 1995;39(2):351–355.
73. Nonunion following intramedullary nailing of the femur with and without reaming. Results of a multicenter randomized clinical trial. *J Bone Joint Surg Am.* 2003;85-A(11):2093–2096.
74. Schemitsch EH, Kowalski MJ, Swiontkowski MF. Soft-tissue blood flow following reamed versus unreamed locked intramedullary nailing: A fractured sheep tibia model. *Ann Plast Surg.* 1996; 36(1):70–75.
75. Frolke JP, Van de Krol H, Bakker FC, et al. Destination of debris during intramedullary reaming. An experimental study on sheep femurs. *Acta Orthop Belg.* 2000;66(4):337–340.
76. Wenisch S, Trinkaus K, Hild A, et al. Human reaming debris: A source of multipotent stem cells. *Bone.* 2005;36(1):74–83.
77. Keating JF, O'brien PJ, Blachut PA, et al. Locking intramedullary nailing with and without reaming for open fractures of the tibial shaft. A prospective, randomized study. *J Bone Joint Surg Am.* 1997;79(3):334–341.
78. Bhandari M, Guyatt G, Tornetta P 3rd, et al. Randomized trial of reamed and unreamed intramedullary nailing of tibial shaft fractures. *J Bone Joint Surg Am.* 2008;90(12):2567–2578.
79. Matter P, Brennwald J, Perren SM. [Biological reaction of bones to osteosynthesis plates]. *Helv Chir Acta.* 1974;0(Suppl 12):1–44.
80. Carter DR, Shimaoka EE, Harris WH, et al. Changes in long-bone structural properties during the first 8 weeks of plate implantation. *J Orthop Res.* 1984;2(1):80–89.
81. Uhthoff HK, Boisvert D, Finnegan M. Cortical porosis under plates. Reaction to unloading or to necrosis? *J Bone Joint Surg Am.* 1994;76(10):1507–1512.
82. Perren SM, Klaue K, Pohler O, et al. The limited contact dynamic compression plate (LC-DCP). *Arch Orthop Trauma Surg.* 1990;109(6):304–310.
83. Egol KA, Kubiak EN, Fulkerson E, et al. Biomechanics of locked plates and screws. *J Orthop Trauma.* 2004;18(8):488–493.
84. Gautier E, Perren SM, Cordey J. Effect of plate position relative to bending direction on the rigidity of a plate osteosynthesis. A theoretical analysis. *Injury.* 2000;31 (Suppl 3):C14–C20.
85. Cordey J, Borgeaud M, Perren SM. Force transfer between the plate and the bone: Relative importance of the bending stiffness of the screws and the friction between plate and bone. *Injury.* 2000;31(Suppl 3):C21–C28.
86. Gardner MJ, Helfet DL, Lorich DG. Has locked plating completely replaced conventional plating? *Am J Orthop.* 2004;33(9):439–446.
87. Gardner MJ, Griffith MH, Demetrakopoulos D, et al. Hybrid locked plating of osteoporotic fractures of the humerus. *J Bone Joint Surg Am.* 2006;88(9):1962–1967.
88. Gerber A, Ganz R. Combined internal and external osteosynthesis a biological approach to the treatment of complex fractures of the proximal tibia. *Injury.* 1998;29(Suppl 3):22–28.
89. Wenda K, Degreif J, Runkel M, et al. [Technique of plate osteosynthesis of the femur]. *Unfallchirurg.* 1994;97(1):13–18.
90. Ostrum RF, Geel C. Indirect reduction and internal fixation of supracondylar femur fractures without bone graft. *J Orthop Trauma.* 1995;9(4):278–284.
91. Helfet DL, Shonnard PY, Levine D, et al. Minimally invasive plate osteosynthesis of distal fractures of the tibia. *Injury.* 1997;28(Suppl 1):A42–A47; discussion A47–A48.
92. Bolhofner BR, Carmen B, Clifford P. The results of open reduction and internal fixation of distal femur fractures using a biologic (indirect) reduction technique. *J Orthop Trauma.* 1996;10(6): 372–377.
93. Krettek C, Schandelmaier P, Miclau T, et al. Minimally invasive percutaneous plate osteosynthesis (MIPPO) using the DCS in proximal and distal femoral fractures. *Injury.* 1997;28(Suppl 1): A20–A30.

94. Jeon IH, Oh CW, Kim SJ, et al. Minimally invasive percutaneous plating of distal femoral fractures using the dynamic condylar screw. *J Trauma.* 2004;57(5):1048–1052.
95. Miclau T, Holmes W, Martin RE, et al. Plate osteosynthesis of the distal femur: Surgical techniques and results. *J South Orthop Assoc.* 1998;7(3):161–170.
96. Kregor PJ, Stannard JA, Zlowodzki M, et al. Treatment of distal femur fractures using the less invasive stabilization system: Surgical experience and early clinical results in 103 fractures. *J Orthop Trauma.* 2004;18(8):509–520.
97. Weight M, Collinge C. Early results of the less invasive stabilization system for mechanically unstable fractures of the distal femur (AO/OTA types A2, A3, C2, and C3). *J Orthop Trauma.* 2004;18(8):503–508.
98. Schutz M, Muller M, Krettek C, et al. Minimally invasive fracture stabilization of distal femoral fractures with the LISS: A prospective multicenter study. Results of a clinical study with special emphasis on difficult cases. *Injury.* 2001;32(Suppl 3):SC48–SC54.
99. Schütz M, Müller M, Regazzoni P, et al. Use of the less invasive stabilization system (LISS) in patients with distal femoral (AO33) fractures: A prospective multicenter study. *Arch Orthop Trauma Surg.* 2005;125(2):102–108.
100. Stannard JP, Wilson TC, Volgas DA, et al. Fracture stabilization of proximal tibial fractures with the proximal tibial LISS: Early experience in Birmingham, Alabama (USA). *Injury.* 2003;34 (Suppl 1):A36–A42.
101. Ricci WM, Rudzki JR, Borrelli JJ Jr. Treatment of complex proximal tibia fractures with the less invasive skeletal stabilization system. *J Orthop Trauma.* 2004;18(8):521–527.
102. Xu LW, Ji WP, Li H, et al. [Treatment of osteoporotic distal femur fractures with less invasive stabilizing system (LISS) and high strength injectable graft]. *Zhongguo Gu Shang.* 2010;23(2): 144–146.
103. Anakwe RE, Aitken SA, Khan LA. Osteoporotic periprosthetic fractures of the femur in elderly patients: Outcome after fixation with the LISS plate. *Injury.* 2008;39(10):1191–1197.
104. Anglen J, Kyle RF, Marsh JL, et al. Locking plates for extremity fractures. *J Am Acad Orthop Surg.* 2009;17(7):465–472.
105. Tarnowski JR, Holck K. Osteosynthesis of a periprosthetic fracture of the proximal femur with the distal femur LISS system. *Acta Orthop Belg.* 2008;74(1):125–127.
106. Gardner MJ, Griffith MH, Dines JS, et al. A minimally invasive approach for plate fixation of the proximal humerus. *Bull Hosp Jt Dis.* 2004;62(1–2):18–23.
107. Roderer G, Erhardt J, Graf M, et al. Clinical results for minimally invasive locked plating of proximal humerus fractures. *J Orthop Trauma.* 2010;24(7):400–406.
108. Wei W, Zhuang Y, Zhang K, et al. [Minimally invasive percutaneous plate osteosynthesis for treatment of proximal humerus fractures with PHILOS plate.]. *Nan Fang Yi Ke Da Xue Xue Bao.* 2010;30(11):2553–2555.

SECTION 2

Specific Fractures

CHAPTER 3

Percutaneous Pinning of Distal Radius Fractures

Peter H. DeNoble and Louis W. Catalano, III

INDICATIONS

Distal radius fractures are common and various treatment options exist. Successful management must consider patient factors and fracture pattern. Percutaneous reduction and fixation are indicated for AO/ASIF extra-articular fractures A2, A3, three- and four-part fractures C1, C2. It is most effective for fractures that can be closed reduced via traction manipulation and ligamentotaxis. As a less expensive alternative to plates and screw fixation or external fixation, closed reduction and percutaneous pinning (CRPP) is currently the most cost-effective option for the treatment of distal radius fractures. In the authors' hospital system, the average cost of a 1.58-mm (0.0625-in) K-wire is $23, bringing a three- to five-wire construct to a total of $69 to $115. This compares favorably to a volar plate plus 8- to 12-screw construct, which cost an average of $1,255, and various forms of external fixators that can range from about $600 to $1,300.

Some distal radius fractures are not amenable to percutaneous treatment alone. Contraindications to CRPP include fractures with severe dorsal metaphyseal or intra-articular comminution, fractures in patients with poor bone stock, especially with fracture comminution, and AO/ASIF type B fractures (e.g., Volar Barton fracture).

PATIENT POSITIONING

The patient is positioned supine with a hand table that accommodates an outrigger for longitudinal traction (Carter Hand Surgery Table, Innovation Sport, Foothill Ranch, CA) (Fig. 3.1A). Finger traps on either the thumb and index finger or index and long fingers are attached to a wire that runs over a pulley on the traction outrigger (Fig. 3.1B). A traction of 2.27 to 4.53 kg (5 to 10 lb) is applied to the wire, and the limb is horizontal on the hand table.

REDUCTION TECHNIQUES

The mini C-arm image intensifier (Fig. 3.2) is sterilely draped and brought into the field.

Posterior–anterior (PA) and lateral images of the distal radius are obtained. The fracture is manipulated with a volarly directed pressure on the dorsal aspect of the distal fracture

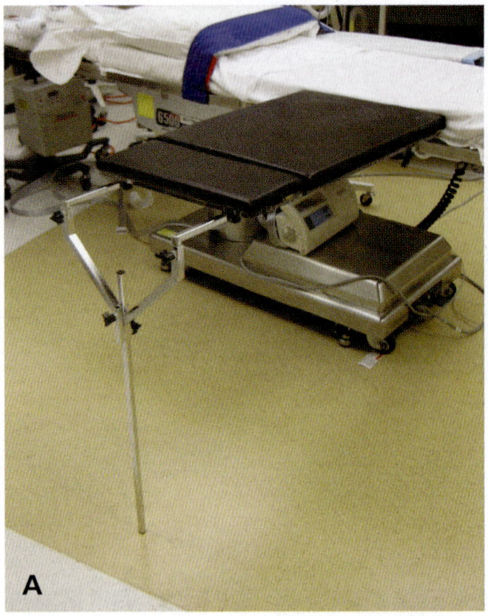

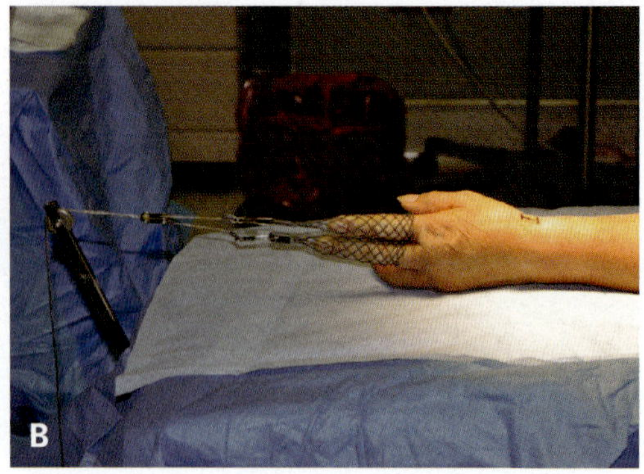

Figure 3.1 **A:** A hand table that accommodates an outrigger for longitudinal traction is helpful for maintenance of reduction throughout the procedure. **B:** Finger traps can be attached to either the thumb and index finger or index and long fingers, while a wire that runs over a pulley on the traction outrigger is attached to 2.27 to 4.54 kg (5 to 10 lb) of weight.

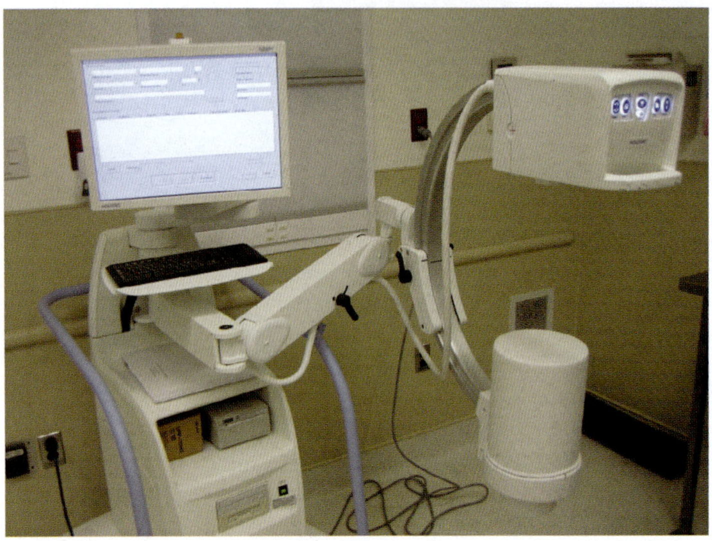

Figure 3.2 A mini-fluoroscopy unit is ideal for visualizing the distal radius and allows the surgeon and assistant to easily maneuver around it during the pin placement.

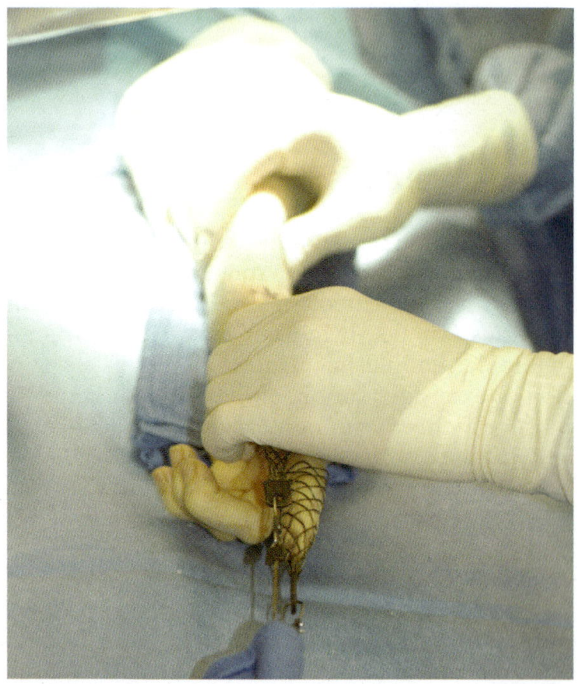

Figure 3.3 A manual reduction is performed. The surgeon provides additional distraction force with his or her left hand while the other hand stabilizes the fractured wrist proximally and applies a volarly directed force on the dorsal aspect of the distal fracture fragment.

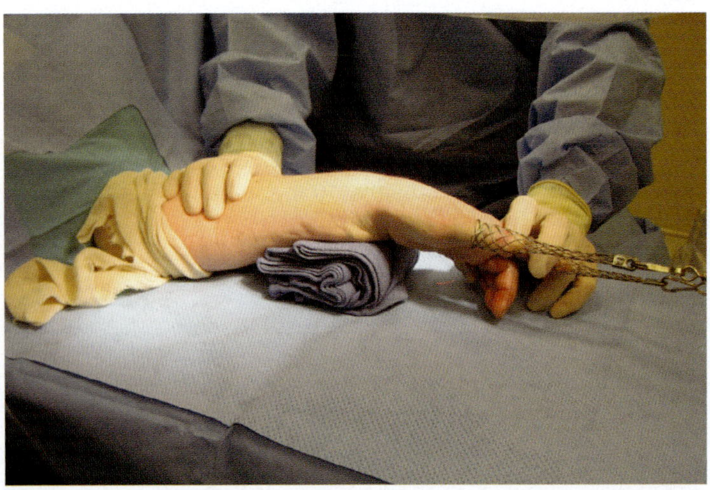

Figure 3.4 A stack of folded towels can be an effective fulcrum for reduction assistance. This can allow coronal plane correction of the distal radius via a translation force applied ulnarward through the hand and wrist.

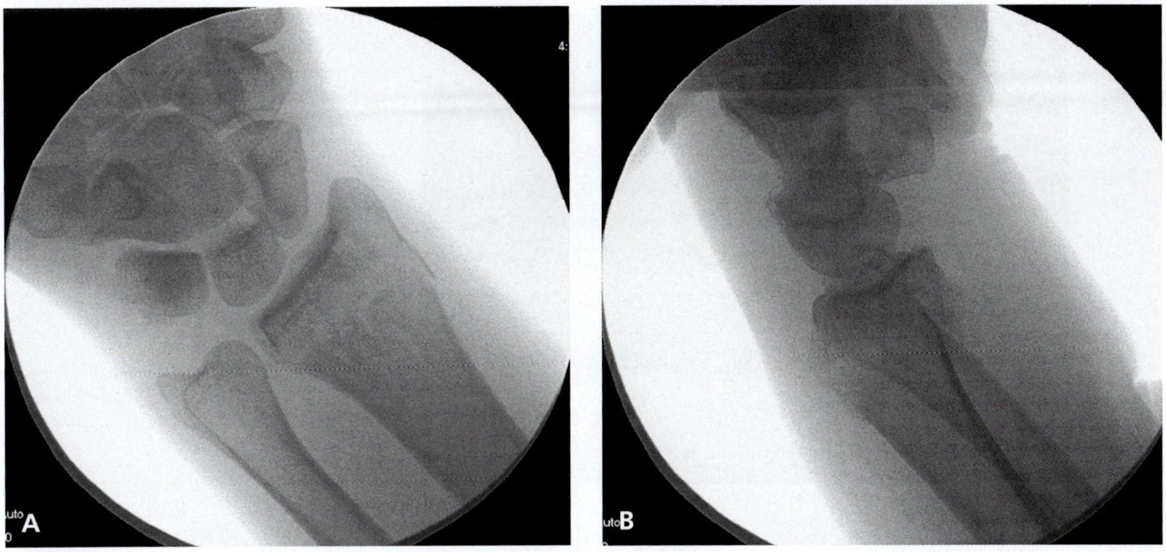

Figure 3.5 Confirm reduction in PA **(A)** and lateral views **(B)** before proceeding with pinning.

fragment in an effort to restore length and volar tilt (Fig. 3.3). In instances where there is radial translation of the distal fragment, a small bump fashioned from a folded stack of towels and is placed under the ulnar aspect of the proximal fragment to serve as an additional fulcrum for reduction. One hand stabilizes the forearm proximally while the other applies an ulnarly translating force to the wrist and hand distally (Fig. 3.4). Reduction is monitored fluoroscopically (Fig. 3.5). If good alignment is achievable via closed reduction, then the surgeon may proceed with the planned percutaneous pin fixation. If the fracture is not reducible closed, then open reduction and internal fixation may be required.

SURGICAL APPROACHES/PINNING TECHNIQUES

The authors prefer to use 1.58-mm (0.0625-in) K-wires exclusively and prefer to place pins in the radial styloid first. In order to avoid injury to the superficial sensory branch of the radial nerve, the pins are placed under direct vision using a 1.5-cm longitudinal incision extending from the tip of the radial styloid distally (Fig. 3.6). A dissecting scissor is used the spread through the subcutaneous tissue and isolate the underlying branches of the superficial radial nerve and first extensor compartment tendons (Fig. 3.7). Ragnell retractors are then used to

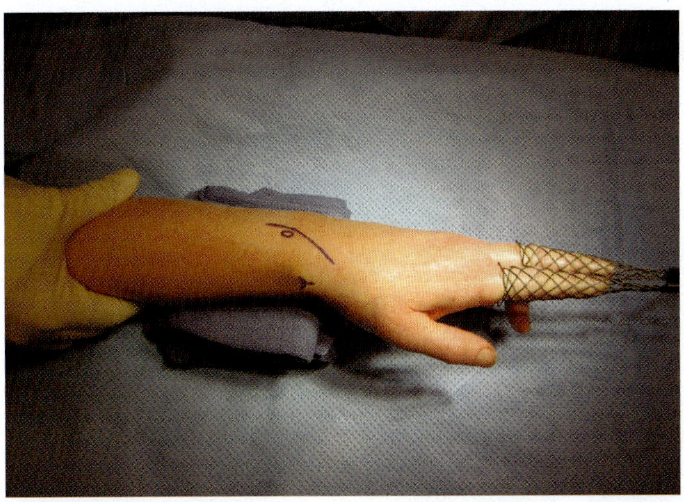

Figure 3.6 Landmarks are indicated, including the radial styloid, Lister tubercle, and the course of the extensor pollicis longus tendon. The ideal incision is 1.5 cm in length, extending from the tip of the radial styloid distally.

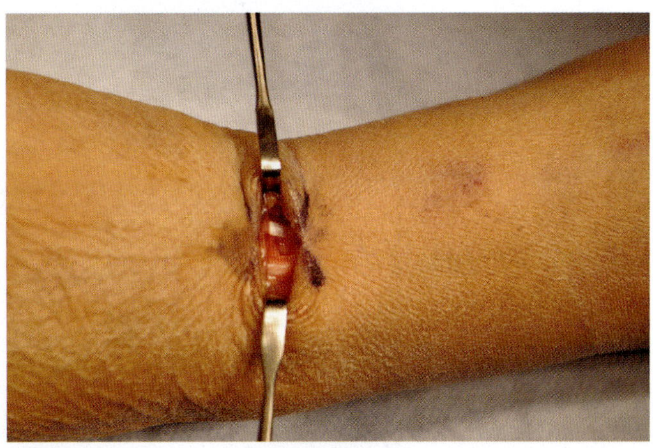

Figure 3.7 A branch of the superficial radial nerve and the extensor pollicis brevis tendon are identified in the base of the wound.

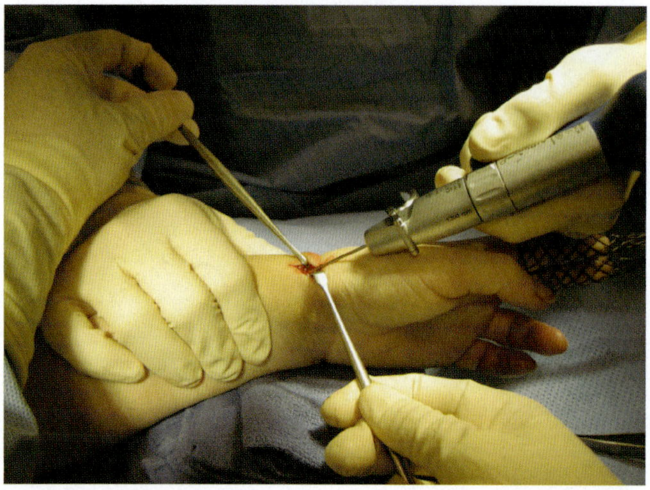

Figure 3.8 A dorsal or volar position on the styloid can be chosen for the first pin, directed in a distal-radial to proximal-ulnar direction.

bluntly retract the nerve branches and tendons. This exposure also allows the starting points to vary in the volar–dorsal direction according to the needs of the fracture pattern without risk of nerve injury.[1] The first pin is usually started at the tip of the styloid, just dorsal to the first extensor compartment (Fig. 3.8). This pin may also be placed volar to the tendons depending on the fracture pattern and the position of the sensory nerve. In addition, the trajectory of the first pin may need to accommodate for some loss of volar tilt reduction that often occurs after the initial closed reduction. Thus, the first pin should be advanced through the distal fragment in a more volarly angulated fashion in order to allow for appropriate reorientation in the sagittal plane following re-reduction. In the coronal plane, this pin is passed at a relatively shallow oblique angle to the level of the fracture site (Fig. 3.9A). Full manual reduction pressure is then reapplied, and fracture reduction is confirmed on the PA and lateral views. The K-wire is subsequently advanced into the ulnar cortex of the radius proximal to the fracture (Fig. 3.9B). Typically a second 1.58-mm (0.0625-in) K-wire is placed in a similar but slightly divergent trajectory to the first pin in both planes, maximizing construct stability. During wire placement, the first wire may substitute for a retractor, freeing an assistant's hand (Fig. 3.10). Reduction is confirmed on PA and lateral fluoroscopy (Fig. 3.11).

An alternative to this limited open approach is a percutaneous technique in which the starting points for the styloid pins are in-line with the mid-lateral coronal plane of the radial styloid, safely positioned between the two main branches of the superficial radial nerve (SRN) at this level (Fig. 3.12).[2] Without direct visualization of the nerve, however, the starting points of the wires cannot be varied dorsally or volarly as might be necessary in a smaller radius or according

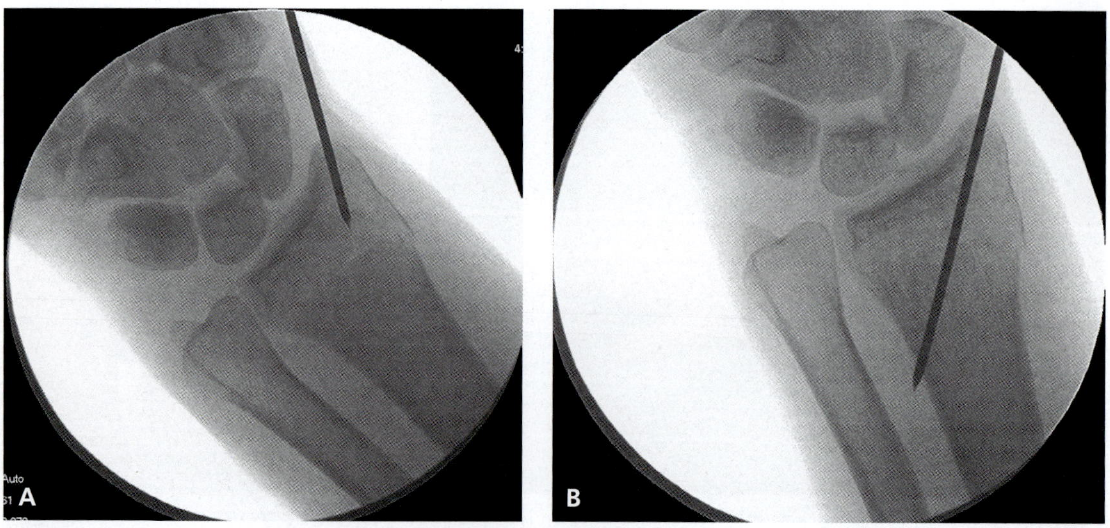

Figure 3.9 **A:** The first pin is initially advanced to the fracture site. A closed manual reduction is then performed. **B:** The wire is then advanced into the proximal ulnar cortex of the radius.

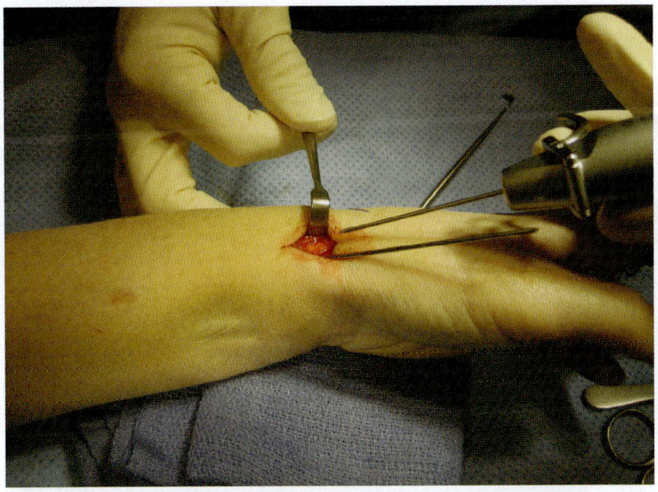

Figure 3.10 A second 1.58-mm (0.0625-in) K-wire is placed in a similar but slightly divergent trajectory to maximize construct stability.

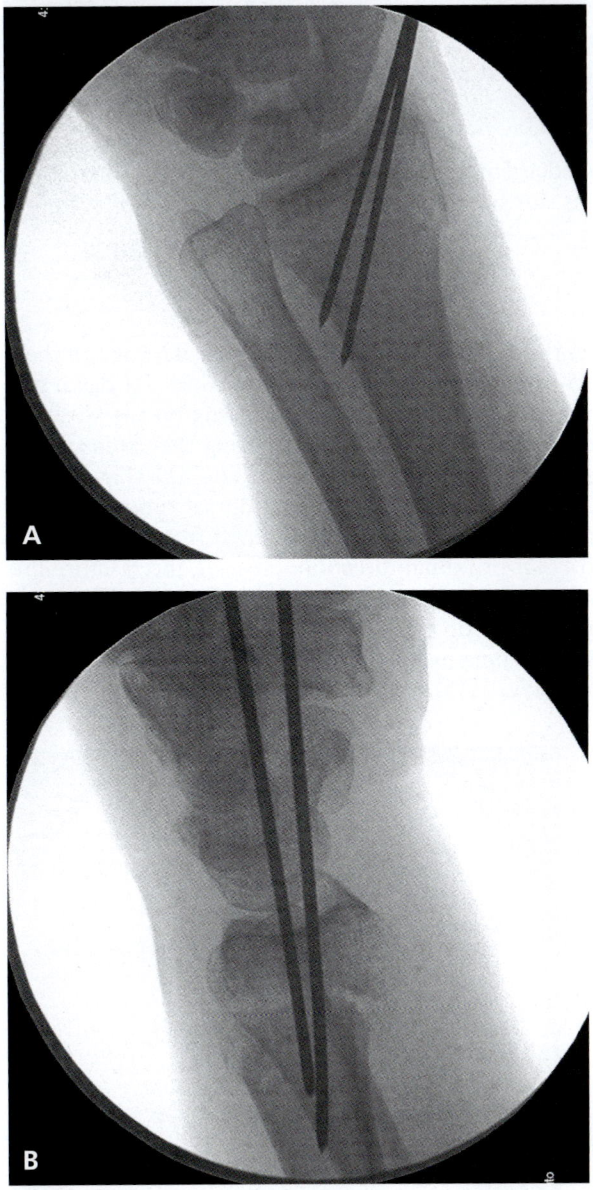

Figure 3.11 Appropriate reduction is confirmed in the PA **(A)** and lateral fluoroscopy views **(B)**.

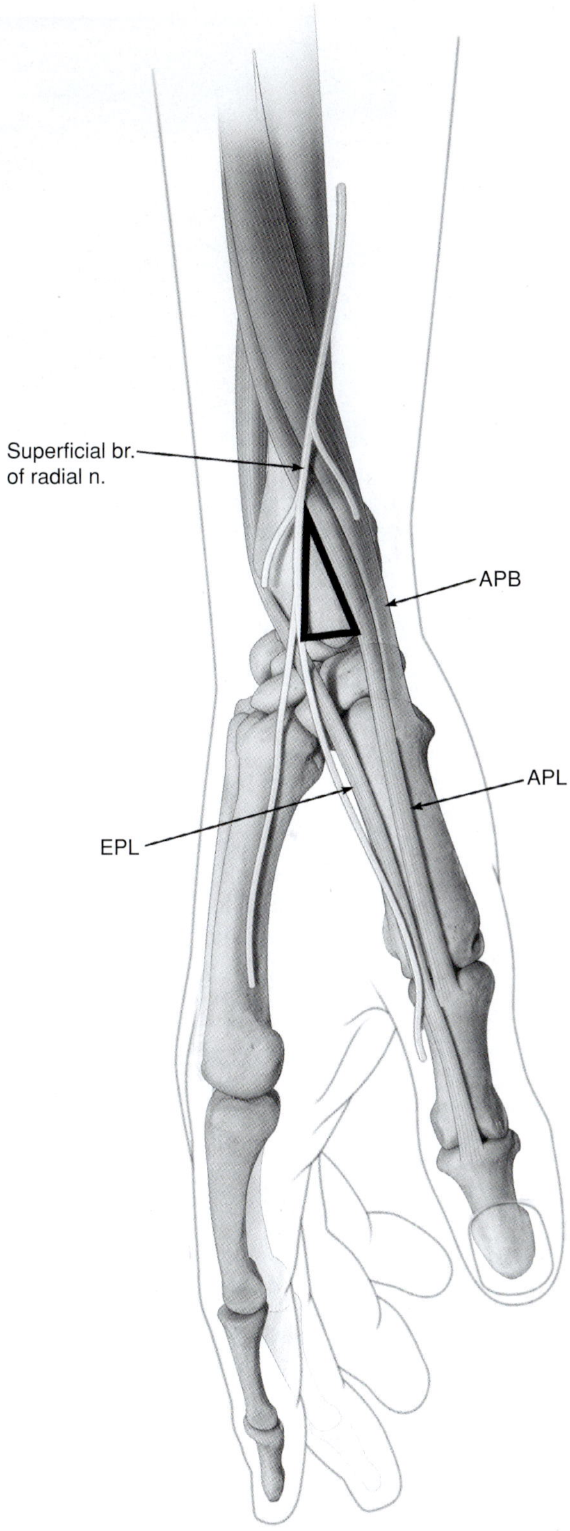

Figure 3.12 A triangular safe zone exists at the tip of the radial styloid, free of nerve branches and tendons. A longitudinal line bisecting this triangle is typically a safe corridor for percutaneous placement of K-wires.

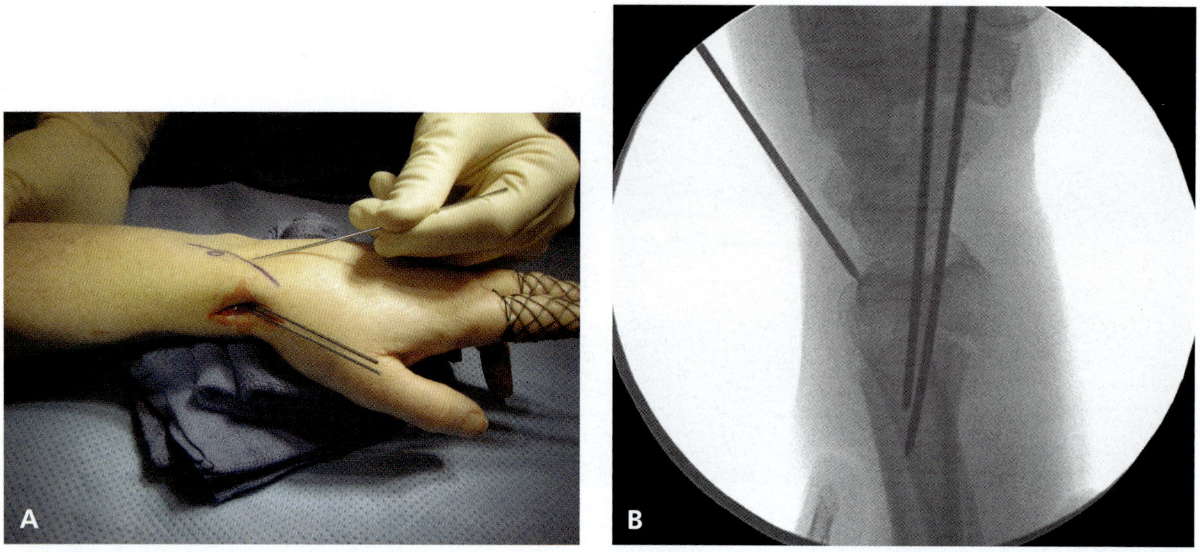

Figure 3.13 **A:** The starting point for the posterior-to-anterior pins is approximately 1 cm distal to Lister tubercle. **B:** The dorsal K-wire is started in the solid, intact subchondral bone of the dorsal rim, with care to stay extra-articular.

to specific fracture morphology. In addition, edema may obfuscate the mid-lateral coronal plane of the radius, making it harder to localize this starting point percutaneously. The authors do not routinely use this technique.

Extra-Articular Fractures

A second set of pins is placed perpendicular in the axial plane to the styloid pins. The first of these pins is started by poking a 1.58-mm (0.0625-in) K-wire through the dorsal skin just distal and radial to the distal edge of Lister tubercle (about 1 to 1.5 cm distal, depending on the swelling) (Fig. 3.13A). A starting point ulnar to Lister tubercle runs the risk of injuring the extensor pollicis longus (EPL) tendon. Good starting position is confirmed via lateral radiograph (Fig. 3.13B). It is important to begin this K-wire in the dense, solid bone of the distal dorsal rim as opposed to proximally where the cancellous bone is thinner and may be comminuted from the fracture. The wire is then driven in a dorsal-distal to volar-proximal direction, crossing the fracture line and engaging the volar cortex (Fig. 3.14). In unstable fractures, the wire can be advanced up to the fracture site first and a volarly directed reduction force can ensure good reduction before pin advancement. A second pin may also be used beginning just proximal to the first pin and directed at a slightly different angle to enhance fixation (Fig. 3.15).

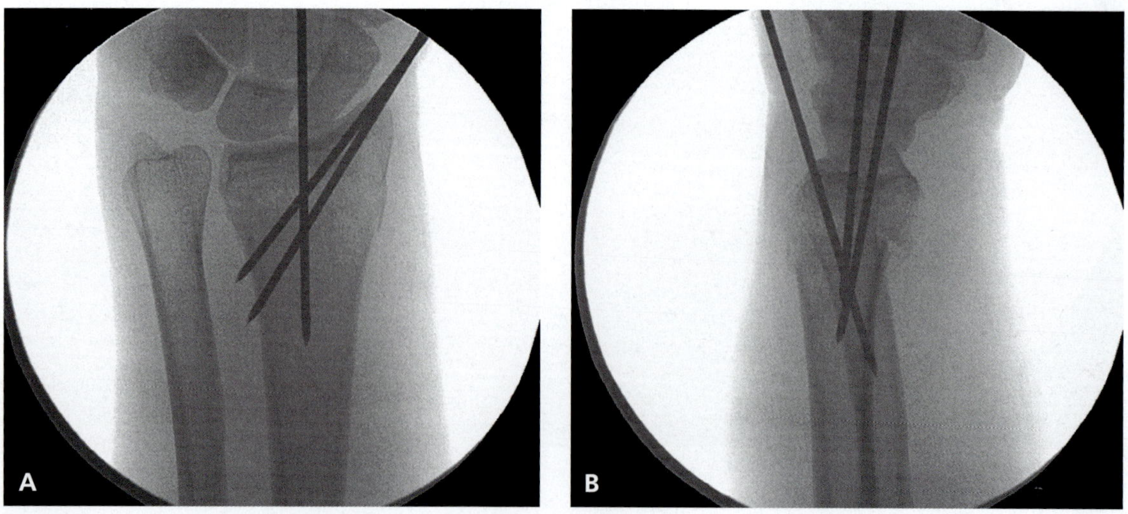

Figure 3.14 The final position of the dorsal pin, engaged in the volar cortex **(A** and **B)**.

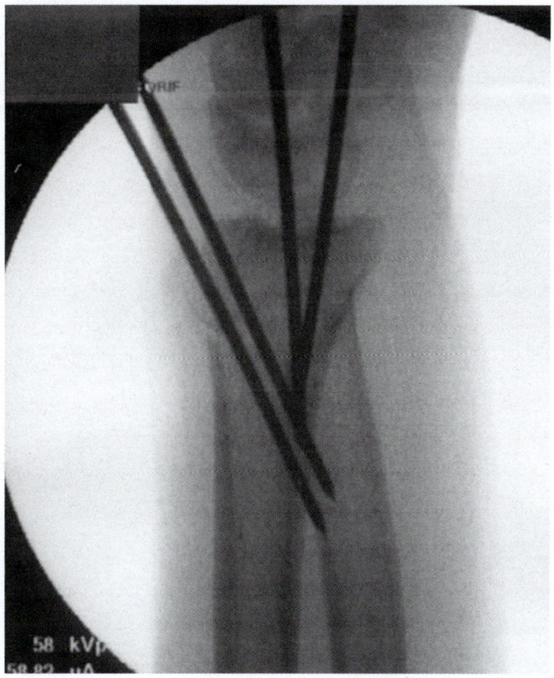

Figure 3.15 A second proximal pin may help to reinforce the volar tilt reduction.

In the case of two-part fractures with poor bone quality and minimal comminution, Kapandji-style K-wires may be used to assist in fracture reduction and augment wire fixation. These wires can be used to restore volar tilt and radial inclination. These pins are inserted percutaneously into the fracture site dorsally and/or radially. In each instance, the wires are partially engaged into the proximal far cortex. The surgeon then levers the distal fragment volarly or ulnarly until volar tilt or radial inclination is restored, respectively (Fig. 3.16). Once appropriate reduction is confirmed fluoroscopically, the wires may be advanced through the far cortex to provide a hands-free reduction force (Fig. 3.17). These wires may be retained or removed at the surgeon's discretion following placement of the standard extrafocal pins already described. While Kapandji technique with K-wires is helpful for initial reduction and supplementation of percutaneous pinning, the authors do not recommend this as an isolated technique. One recent prospective cohort study demonstrated that intrafocal pins in fractures with poor bone quality or with initially shortened fracture patterns allowed radial height subsidence at final follow-up.[3]

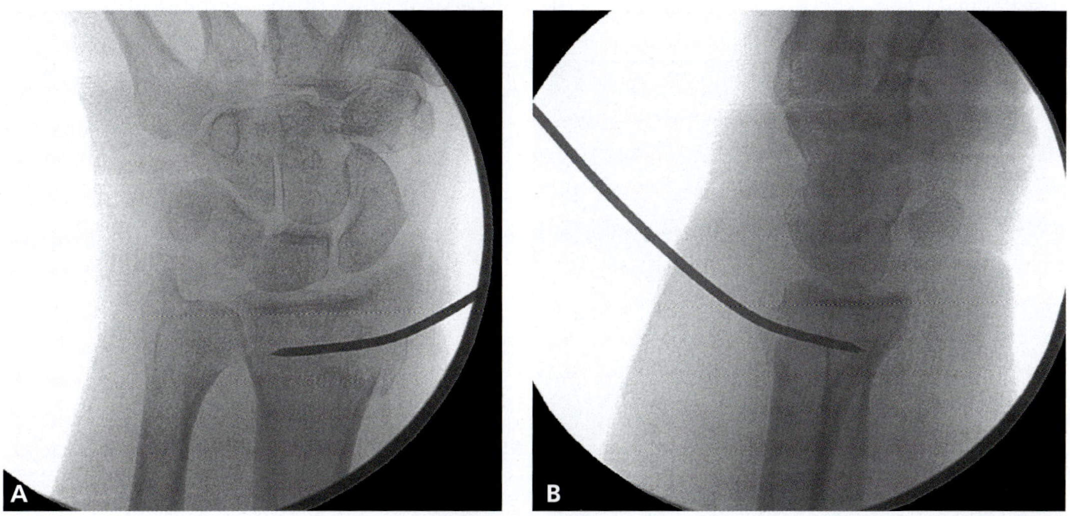

Figure 3.16 **A:** An intrafocal pin directed from the radial styloid ulnarward serves to assist the restoration of ulnar inclination. **B:** An intrafocal pin directed from the dorsal comminution proximal-volarly serves to restore volar tilt.

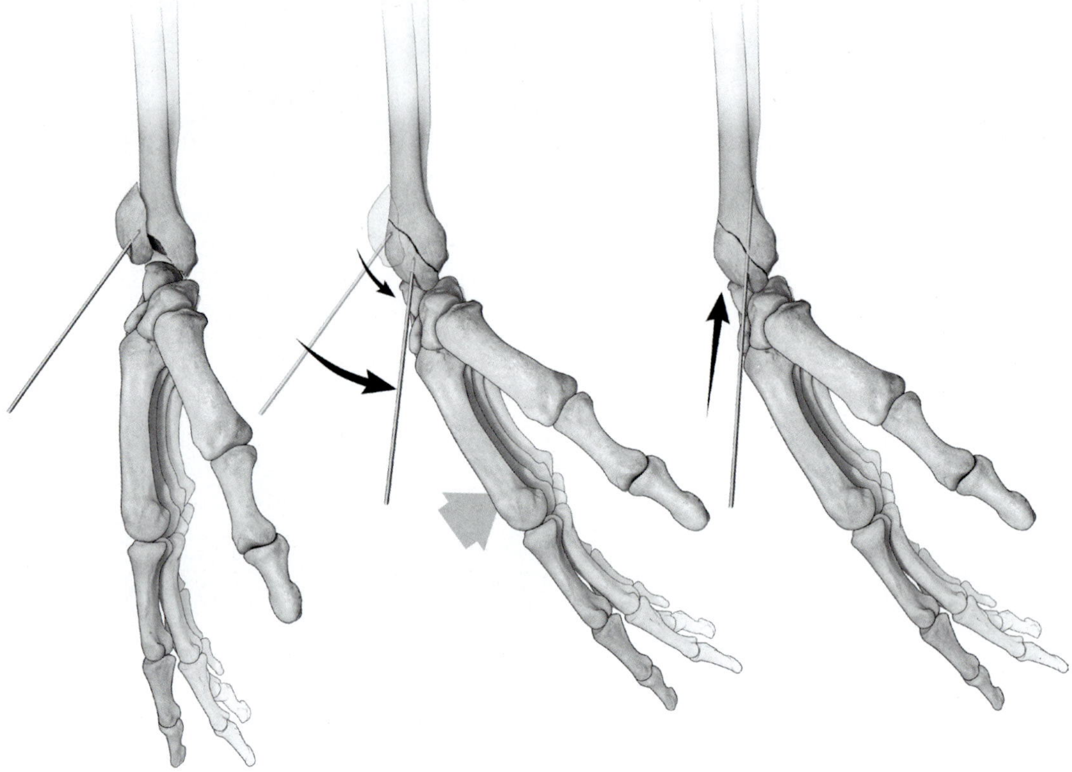

Figure 3.17 The pin is advanced through the fracture site and partially engaged in the proximal far cortex. The surgeon then uses the wire as a lever to reduce the fracture and then advances the pin securely into the far cortex.

Three-Part Fractures

Three-part fracture patterns that contain proximal subsidence of the lunate fossa with articular step-off is also amenable to percutaneous pinning. Proximal subsidence of the lunate facet is addressed by dorsal intrafocal elevation of the fragment using a 1.58-mm (0.0625-in) K-wire or a freer elevator. Once a reduction is achieved, fixation of the lunate fossa fragment can be accomplished in one of two ways. One is by placing a pin transversely across the distal radius in a radial to ulnar direction, firmly buttressing the subchondral bone of the lunate fossa (Fig. 3.18). The K-wire is lodged in the subcortical bone of the sigmoid notch of the

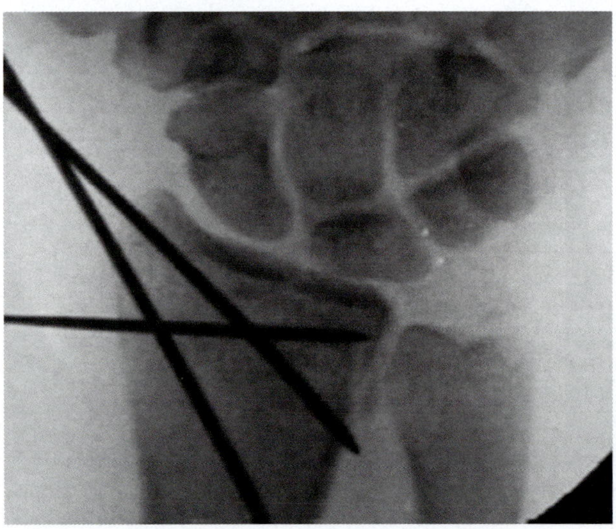

Figure 3.18 The transverse pin is located in the subchondral bone of the lunate facet, maintaining the height of this fragment. It is stopped just short of the DRUJ. DRUJ; distal radioulnar joint.

radius. Care must be taken not to penetrate into the distal radioulnar joint (DRUJ). Alternatively, a pin may be placed from the dorsoulnar corner of the distal radius, usually entering between the fourth and fifth extensor compartments, in a volar-proximal direction such that the tip of the pin engaged the volar radial cortex of the radius proximal to the fracture site.

Subacute Fractures (2 to 3 Weeks from Injury)

Fractures that are 2 to 3 weeks old may be difficult to reduce with simple manipulation and manual pressure. When the fracture is 3 weeks old or more, a 1.58-mm (0.0625-in) K-wire is not sufficiently rigid to accomplish the goal of mobilization of the fracture fragments. In these cases, a small longitudinal incision is made over the fracture line to allow entry of a 4.76-mm (3/16-in) Steinman pin with a spatula tip or a freer elevator into the fracture site. It is then swept from radial to ulnar, breaking up the healing callus. Once the fracture is sufficiently mobilized, the fracture fragment can be reduced via an intrafocal technique and stabilized with the addition of extrafocal pins as discussed previously.

Assessing DRUJ Stability

Once the fracture is stabilized, DRUJ stability is tested by shifting the ulnar head volar and dorsal relative to the distal radius with the forearm in neutral pronation/supination. If the DRUJ is grossly unstable as compared to the contralateral side in the absence of an ulnar styloid fracture, two 1.58-mm (0.0625-in) K-wires are placed transversely from the ulna to the radius, just proximal to the DRUJ. If there is instability in the presence of an ulnar styloid fracture, consideration is given to fixing the fracture, which may be done with a tension band technique. The reduction and fixation are assessed with final fluoroscopic images in at least two planes.

The pins are left superficial to the skin and are bent using pliers to prevent migration. If they tent the skin adjacent to the incision, the skin either needs to be released with a secondary incision or the pin can be cut, and, before bending it, placed through the skin adjacent to the incision obviating the need for additional incisions. The radial styloid incision is closed using interrupted 5-0 plain gut sutures.

Rehabilitation Protocol

The fracture is usually immobilized for the first 2 weeks in a sugar tong splint to allow skin around the pins to heal (Fig. 3.19). Alternatively, the wrist can be immobilized in dorsal–volar splints, which are secured with Coban (3M, St. Paul, MN), wrapped without tension. At 2 weeks, the patient is seen back in the office for repeat radiographs. A short-arm cast is applied in fractures with a stable DRUJ, or a long-arm cast for those with an unstable DRUJ that was pinned. Patients are seen biweekly to obtain new radiographs. In young adults with little comminution, the pins and cast can generally be removed at 5 weeks, while in those with poor bone stock or more extensive comminution, the pins and cast are left in place for a total of 6 weeks. Ultimately, pins are only removed once there is no longer fracture site tenderness. The cast is removed for examination of pin sites only if the patient has complaints or if there is concern for pin site infection or pin migration.

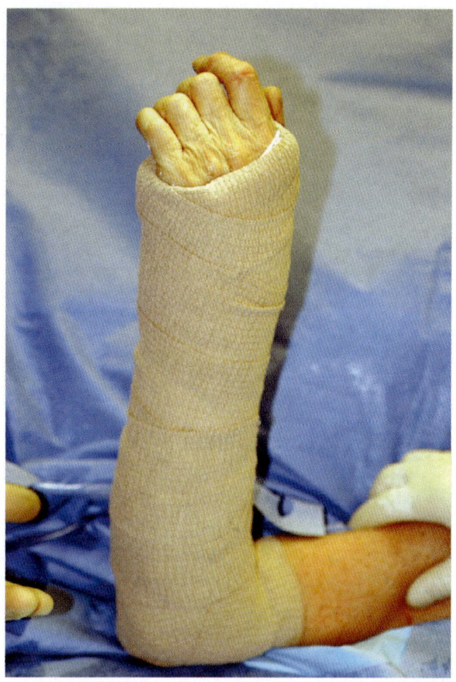

Figure 3.19 A sugar tong splint is placed, secured with Coban (3M, St. Paul, MN).

After the pins are removed, the patient is given a prefabricated removable wrist splint and is referred to a hand therapist who begins wrist range of motion exercises and scar massage. At 5 to 7 weeks, the splint is discontinued and strengthening is begun with putty and a hand gripper. At 10 weeks post-op, light resistive exercises can be started using a 0.45- to 1.36-kg (1- to 3-lb) dumbbell and progressed as tolerated. Range of motion can usually be regained by 12 weeks postoperatively. At 3 months post-op, patients can resume most activities with the exception of contact sports. Contact sports can be resumed at 4 months.

COMPLICATIONS

The authors have had few complications with this technique. The rate of pin site infection is less than 1%, in part owing to the use of a sugar tong splint for 2 weeks postoperatively. Because a 1- to 2-cm incision is used to identify the superficial radial nerve, a serious nerve injury is rare. The nerve is occasionally irritated by a pin, which typically resolves after pin removal. Fracture redisplacement is rare, occurring in 1 of 55 patients in our recent series.[4] Fracture subsidence can occur in certain situations, such as in patients with poor bone stock and comminuted fractures. Although this occurred in 13% of our patients, we have not had to reoperate any of these patients.[4]

OUTCOME

A recent randomized control trial comparing volar plate open reduction and internal fixation (ORIF) to CRPP found no significant difference between the two techniques radiographically or clinically at 12 weeks except for a lower DASH score and less ulnar deviation in the pinning group. At 12-month follow-up, DASH scores were no longer statistically different, and the only remaining difference was the CRPP group had 20% less ulnar deviation.[5] While prolonged wrist immobilization following fracture fixation was historically thought to lead to post-op stiffness, one recent randomized control trial refuted this notion. Lozano-Calderón et al.[6] compared 2 weeks versus 6 weeks of immobilization in distal radius fractures following volar plate ORIF. At 12 weeks, both groups showed no difference in ROM or reduction parameters. Likewise, Rozental et al.[5] found that at 12 weeks all range of motion parameters except for ulnar deviation was similar in the CRPP group that had been immobilized for 6 weeks when compared to volar plate ORIF that had been mobilized at 2 weeks.

In our own study, we retrospectively reviewed 54 patients with 55 AO type A2, A3, C1, or C2 distal radius fractures treated with the above described technique of CRPP. The average follow-up was 58 months. At follow-up, active wrist range-of-motion and grip strength of the injured wrist were statistically equal to the uninjured wrist with the exception of 5 degrees of wrist flexion and 4 degrees of supination. Eighty-five percent of patients were pain-free and Disabilities of the Arm, Shoulder, and Hand (DASH) scores averaged that of a healthy volunteer. There were no significant changes in radiographic reduction parameters from the initial post-op to final follow-up.

REFERENCES

1. Chia B, Catalano LW, III, Glickel SZ, et al. Percutaneous pinning of distal radius fractures: an anatomic study demonstrating the proximity of K-wires to structures at risk. *J Hand Surg Am.* 2009;34(6):1014–1020.
2. Chen Y, Zheng X, Wang J, et al. Reliable techniques to avoid damaging the superficial radial nerve due to percutaneous Kirschner wire fixation of the distal radius fracture through the radial styloid process. *Surg Radiol Anat.* 2010;32(8):711–717.
3. Oshige T, Sakai A, Zenke Y, et al. A comparative study of clinical and radiological outcomes of dorsally angulated, unstable distal radius fractures in elderly patients: Intrafocal pinning versus volar locking plating. *J Hand Surg Am.* 2007;32(9):1385–1392.
4. Glickel SZ, Catalano LW, III, Raia FJ, et al. Long term outcomes of closed reduction and percutaneous pinning for the treatment of distal radius fractures. *J Hand Surg Am.* 2008;33:1700–1705.
5. Rozental TD, Blazar PE, Franko OI, et al. Functional outcomes for unstable distal radial fractures treated with open reduction and internal fixation or closed reduction and percutaneous fixation. A prospective randomized trial. *J Bone Joint Surg Am.* 2009;91(8):1837–1846.
6. Lozano-Calderón SA, Souer S, Mudgal C, et al. Wrist mobilization following volar plate fixation of fractures of the distal part of the radius. *J Bone Joint Surg Am.* 2008;90(6):1297–1304.

CHAPTER 4

Forearm Nailing

Sang Ki Lee

Fractures of the radius and ulna should be stabilized in order to ensure axial and rotational alignment[1] and plate osteosynthesis is the treatment of choice for achieving anatomic reduction and fracture stability and preventing angular deformity or shortening.[2] An additional advantage of plating is early active motion and use of the injured extremity.[2] Functional outcomes, in addition to these benefits, have made plate osteosynthesis the procedure of choice for the treatment of both bone forearm fractures. However, although this technique usually results in adequate reduction and satisfactory healing, it has been criticized because of necessary soft tissue dissection and periosteal stripping. The fracture hematoma and blood supply are violated with surgical treatment and may result in bone necrosis and infection.[3] Experimental studies[4–7] have shown that marked osteoporosis occurs when a rigid plate is fixed to intact bone. Rhinelander,[8] Olerud and Danckwardt-Lilliestrom,[5] and Jacobs et al.[9] have shown cortical avascularity and an osteolytic process that erodes the necrotic cortical bone in dogs with compression plating. Also, a 2.3% to 4% rate of nonunion,[10,11] a 1.9% to 30.4% rate of refracture,[12–15] and a 0.8% to 2.3% rate of infection[16,17] have been reported as complications of plate fixation of forearm fractures. In an effort to avoid these problems, intramedullary nailing has been proposed as an alternative method for stabilizing forearm fractures. This technique is commonly used for other long bones, employing the principles of indirect reduction, minimal or no periosteal stripping, smaller incisions and less soft tissue dissection with decreased vascular disruption in hopes of faster fracture healing, decreased infection rate, and less need for bone grafting.[3] However, intramedullary nailing has not been widely used for fixation of forearm fractures because of its limited indications, reportedly high rates of nonunion, and need for additional immobilization. Recently, good results were reported following the treatment of forearm fractures in adults with forearm intramedullary (IM) nail.[18,19]

INDICATIONS

The indications for intramedullary nailing of both bone forearm fractures are simple diaphyseal fracture; types I, II, or IIIA open fractures; closed fracture with poor overlying skin and severe swelling; a segmental fracture; or a single bone forearm fracture. This technique should be avoided in active infection, Monteggia fractures, Galeazzi fractures, comminution and length-unstable fractures, patients who are unable to tolerate longer duration of immobilization and require early rehabilitation, open physes, and a medullary canal smaller than 3 mm. Relative contraindications include patients with osteoporosis.

PATIENT POSITIONING

Supine positioning is most useful for intramedullary nailing of forearm fractures. Both a traction device and a radiolucent table may be required to aid in reduction and evaluation. The affected arm may be placed over the patient's torso. Alternatively, lateral positioning may be used for isolated ulnar nailing.

For accessing the starting point for ulnar fractures, 90 degrees of elbow flexion, 90 degrees of shoulder external rotation, and forearm neutral position are necessary. Elbow extension also should be possible. Elevate the bed and place a padded bolster under the patient's forearm. The image intensifier should come from patient's lateral side.

For radial nailing, the forearm is pronated to allow for an entry point in distal end of the radius. The image intensifier should come from cephalad.

SURGICAL APPROACHES

The first step in forearm nailing is preoperative planning. Verify radiographically the diameter of the medullary canal of the injured bone(s). Choose a diameter nail that will be able to be inserted with minimal reaming, to minimize the risk of incarceration during insertion. Estimate screw length for reference during the procedure. It may be necessary to template the normal forearm to more accurately estimate the length.

Ulna

To expose the implant entry point, a longitudinal 1-cm long incision is made at the tip of the olecranon. Dissection is carried down sharply through the subcutaneous tissues and the triceps tendon. Care should be taken to avoid the ulnar nerve, which sits medial to the olecranon. Establish the implant insertion point by using the awl to perforate the cortex (Fig. 4.1). Multiplanar fluoroscopy is helpful when verifying proper entry point. The cannula may be used in conjunction with the awl to protect the soft tissues. Start the awl in the center of the olecranon process, directly in line with the proximal intramedullary canal of the ulna.

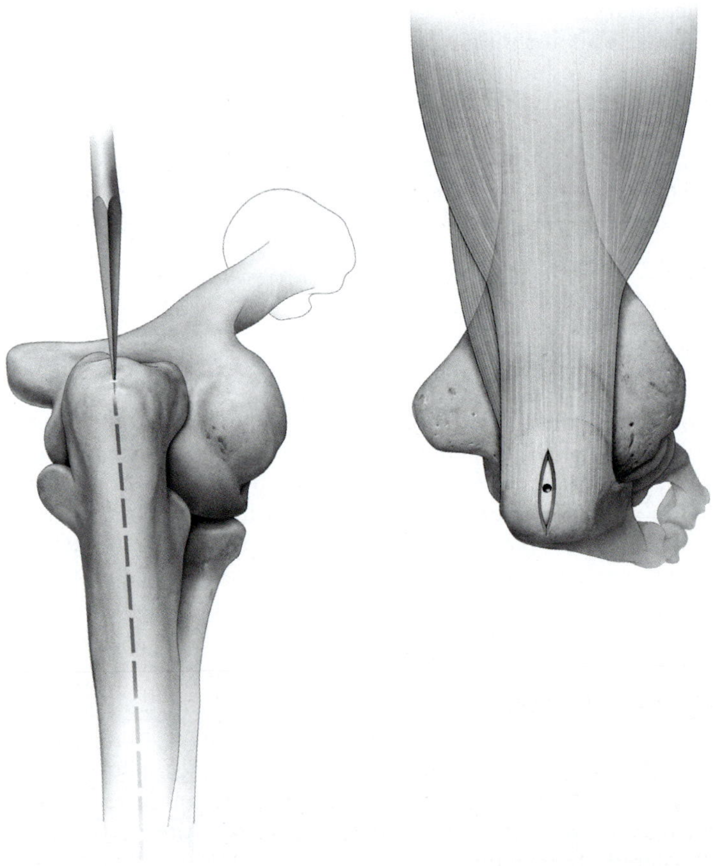

Figure 4.1 To establish the starting point for an ulnar nail, a small incision is made in the triceps insertion over the olecranon process. An awl is used to perforate the cortex and enter the medullary canal.

Radius

Make a 2.5- to 3-cm longitudinal incision along the distal radius over the fourth extensor compartment with the wrist and forearm pronated. Bluntly dissect subcutaneous tissues to avoid injury to the branches of the superficial radial nerve. The exact starting point varies depending upon the implant chosen and the specific nail design. Common nail entry points are the radial styloid between the tendons of the extensor carpi radialis longus and extensor pollicis brevis, beneath the extensor carpi radialis tendon on the radial side of Lister tubercle, or beneath the extensor pollicis longus tendon in the ulnar side of the Lister tubercle (Fig. 4.2). The author's typical entry point of choice is beneath the extensor pollicis longus tendon in the ulnar side of Lister tubercle. To utilize this starting portal, first identify and incise the extensor retinaculum, leaving the proximal third intact. Retract the extensor pollicis longus tendon to the ulnar side and extensor digitorum tendon to the radial side with a small retractor. Establish the implant insertion point by using the awl and cannula to perforate the cortex just ulnar to Lister tubercle approximately 5 mm from the articular surface. The awl should be directed proximally down the canal and inserted at an angle of 20 to 30 degrees. Care should be taken to avoid accidental penetration of the adjacent cortex and tendon injury. The cannula may be used in conjunction with the awl as a tissue protector. Fluoroscopy is helpful when verifying proper alignment.

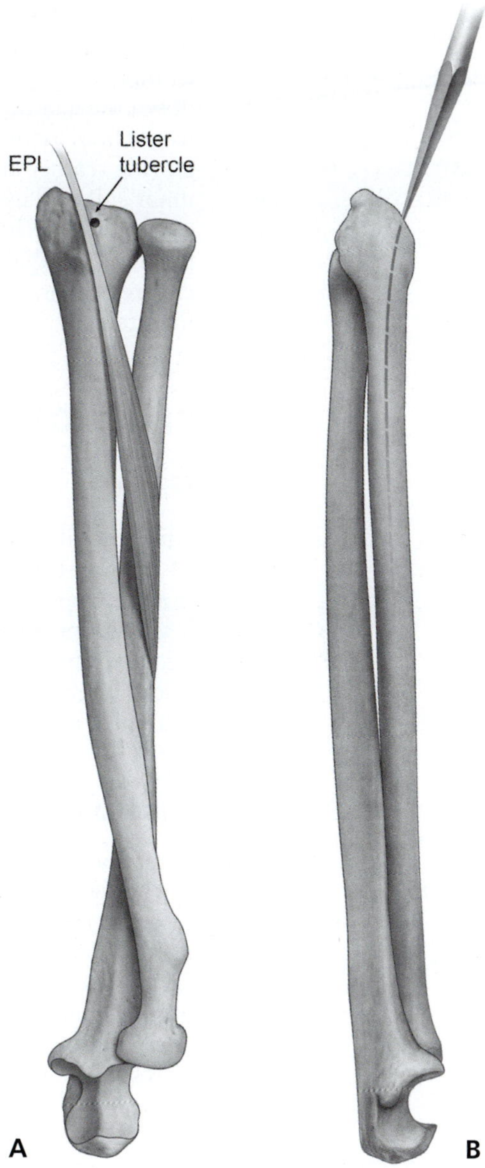

Figure 4.2 A common starting point for a radial nail is with the forearm pronated, just to the ulnar side of Lister tubercle **(A)**, 5 mm proximal to the articular surface **(B)**. EPL; extensor pollicis longus.

REDUCTION TECHNIQUE

Ulna

For ulna fractures, a handheld reamer is inserted to ream the canal and aid in the indirect reduction of the fracture without the use of a guidewire. Multiple reamer sizes are available, and typically the goal is to insert a reamer that is at least 0.5 mm larger than the planned diameter of the nail. Before advancing the reamer, manipulate the fracture under fluoroscopic control using manual traction, rotation, and translation until fracture is aligned. Rotate the angled reamer tip toward the distal fragment. If closed reduction is not possible, a small incision can be made at the fracture site to realign the medullary canals of the fracture fragments. The reamer is then inserted down the length of the ulna, and either the nail length is read directly from the reamer shaft or a mark is made on the reamer shaft and the length is measured after it is withdrawn. With the use of fluoroscopic guidance, the ulnar nail is inserted through the entry hole by hand or gently hammered into place using a mallet, and the tip of the selected nail is gently guided past the fracture site and down to the distal metaphysis. The optimal insertion depth is such that the nail tip is at the metaphyseal portion of distal ulna.

Radius

For radial fracture nailing, the nail is selected on the basis of the length and diameter of the medullary canal as measured on anteroposterior and lateral radiographs of the uninjured forearm. The nail is inserted into the medullary canal through an entry hole created with an awl in the distal end of the radius, just ulnar to the Lister tubercle and approximately 5 mm from the articular surface (Fig. 4.1). Next, a handheld reamer is inserted to ream the canal and aid in the reduction of the fracture without the use of a guidewire. It is important to protect the extensor pollicis longus and extensor digitorum tendons to avoid iatrogenic injury during reaming. Before advancement of the reamer across the fracture site, manipulate the fracture under fluoroscopic control using manual traction, rotation, and translation until fracture is aligned. A small incision at the fracture site can provide access for small reduction clamps to realign the radius if closed reduction is not possible. The chosen reamer is inserted down the length of the radius. Wrist flexion at this point facilitates reamer passage. With the use of fluoroscopic guidance, the tip of the selected nail is gently guided past the fracture site. During reamer and nail advancement, retraction of the extensor pollicis longus tendon to the ulnar side and extensor digitorum tendon to the radial side minimizes iatrogenic tendon. The nail should be inserted by hand or gently malletted into place until it is at the metaphyseal portion of radial neck. The nail position is assessed fluoroscopically in orthogonal planes to ensure that it has successfully crossed the fracture site and an accurate reduction has been maintained.

FIXATION

Ulna

After the ulnar nail is inserted, interlocking screws are inserted through the proximal end of the nail through an outrigger guide typical of most intramedullary nailing systems. The interlocking screws are inserted from lateral side of proximal ulna. Most implants provide at least two proximal interlocking screws for the ulna, and these should be utilized to impart adequate fixation stability in the proximal ulnar metaphyseal bone. Verify screw positions under fluoroscopy. These screws should not extend past the far cortex by more than 1 mm to minimize impingement on the ulnar nerve medially.

Radius

After the radial nail is fully inserted, an interlocking screw is inserted into the distal end of the nail through an attached outrigger device. This distal interlocking screw should be inserted through the existing starting portal incision, or the incision can be extended as needed depending on the patient's anatomy. Again, this screw should not extend past the far cortex by more than 1 mm to avoid iatrogenic neurovascular injury or flexor tendon impingement. Fluoroscopy should be used liberally to ensure acceptable fracture reduction and interlocking screw position (Fig. 4.3). The wound is closed, and a well-molded long arm splint is placed with the forearm in the supination or neutral position and the elbow at 90 degrees flexion.

COMPLICATIONS

When nailing the radius, the major complication is extensor pollicis longus tendon injury. Therefore, when passing hand reamers or the nail into the intramedullary canal, vigilant protection of the tendon is imperative. Other complications include infection, loss of reduction, delayed union, and nonunion. Nonunion or delayed union may occur when the tip of the nail is not securely impacted in the metaphyseal portion or when overly aggressive mobilization occurs, particularly with forearm rotation.

The interlocking screws can be prominent in the subcutaneous tissue, and can cause mechanical irritation, particularly in those systems in which distal ulnar interlocking screws are used. Early removal of these locking screws for loosening of the screw and wrist pain has been reported.[20,21] In addition, insertion of the nail and the interlocking screw through the distal part of the ulna, which has a relatively small diameter, may create a weak point around the drill hole and potentially lead to peri-implant fracture. In the radius, an additional skin incision is required when the locking screw is inserted into the proximal part of the radius, which can cause a posterior interosseous nerve injury.[20,22] Nails which have a flattened paddle-shaped distal end can avoid some of the complications associated with interlocking screws, but provide less rotational stability.

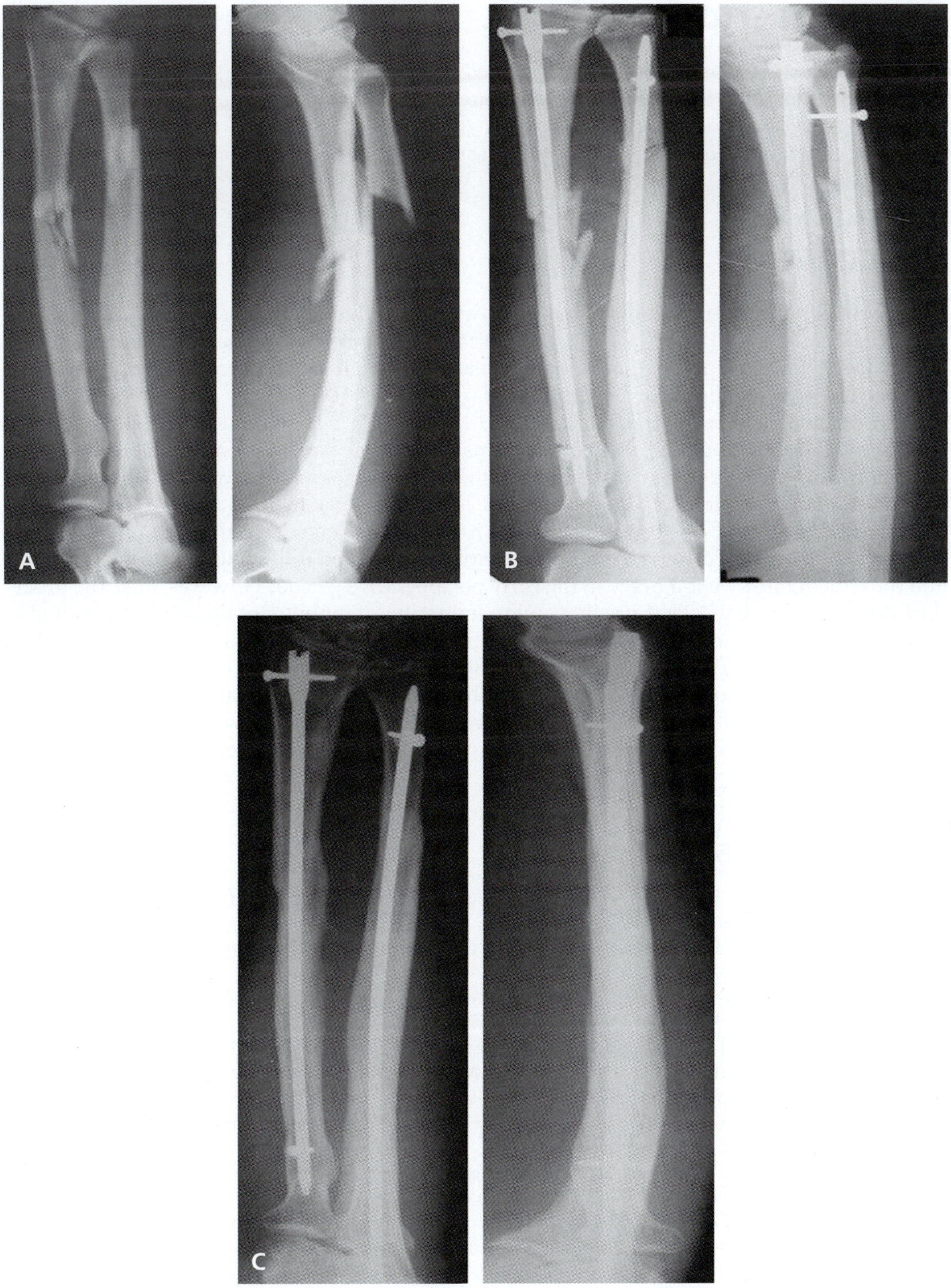

Figure 4.3 Example of interlocked nailing of an adult forearm fracture. A 51-year-old male sustained a closed displaced diaphyseal forearm fracture (AO type B3) in a traffic accident. **A:** Preoperative anteroposterior and lateral radiographs of the forearm showing a fracture of the middle one-third of the radial shaft and the distal one-third of the ulnar shaft. **B:** Fractures were reduced and fixed with interlocking intramedullary nails using a closed technique. **C:** Anteroposterior and lateral radiographs taken 12 months after the injury showing satisfactory union and alignment. Fracture union was apparent at 10 weeks after operation. (From: Gao H, Luo CF, Zhang CQ, et al. Internal fixation of diaphyseal fractures of the forearm by interlocking intramedullary nail: Short-term results in eighteen patients. *J Orthop Trauma.* 2005;19(6):384–391,with permission.)

REHABILITATION PROTOCOL

At the first postoperative office visit, a hinged elbow brace is applied with the forearm in neutral position. This limits forearm rotation for the first 6 weeks until early healing has occurred. Active range of motion exercise of the elbow is initiated. At 6 weeks postoperatively, the elbow brace is removed and active forearm supination and pronation exercises are allowed.

OUTCOMES

In general, forearm intramedullary nailing is a technically demanding procedure, and used in only selected cases. However, with appropriate patient selection, technical adequacy, and compliance with postoperative protocols, it has a very high success rate. Healing rates after primary forearm nailing have been reported at 96% to 100%.[19,20,22] The average time to fracture healing have been reported at 10 to 14 weeks.[19,20,22] In these series, mean pronation was 62 to 85 degrees, and mean supination was 80 to 87 degrees. Of note, some nail systems require intraoperative contouring of the nail to establish the radial bow, and this can impact the final forearm rotation.[20,22]

The disadvantage of this procedure is that it requires a longer duration of immobilization (until bridging callus is observed) compared with that required following plate osteosynthesis, and the patient must wear a brace in the early postoperative period. However, since the procedure does not expose the wrist or elbow joint, limitation of mobility of these joints is minimal.

The most important advantage of interlocking contoured intramedullary forearms nailing is that the nonunion rate is lower than noninterlocking systems. Several recent series have demonstrated nonunion rates equivalent to those after plate fixation, in conjunction with excellent function and patient outcomes. The restoration of radial bow is important in terms of reconstituting the normal forearm architecture and restoring of forearm rotation and grip strength.

REFERENCES

1. Markolf KL, Lamey D, Yang S, et al. Radioulnar load-sharing in the forearm. A study in cadavera. *J Bone Joint Surg Am.* 1998;80(6):879–888.
2. Hidaka S, Gustilo RB. Refracture of bones of the forearm after plate removal. *J Bone Joint Surg Am.* 1984;66(8):1241–1243.
3. Tejwani NC, Wolinsky P. The changing face of orthopaedic trauma: Locked plating and minimally invasive techniques. *Instr. Course Lect.* 2008;57:3–9.
4. Moyen BJ, Lahey PJ Jr, Weinberg EH, et al. Effects on intact femora of dogs of the application and removal of metal plates. A metabolic and structural study comparing stiffer and more flexible plates. *J Bone Joint Surg Am.* 1978;60(7):940–947.
5. Olerud S, Danckwardt-Lilliestrőm G. Fracture healing in compression osteosynthesis in the dog. *J Bone Joint Surg Br.* 1968;50(4):844–851.
6. Uhthoff HK, Dubuc FL. Bone structure changes in the dog under rigid internal fixation. *Clin Orthop Relat Res.* 1971;81:165–170.
7. Woo SL, Akeson WH, Coutts RD, et al. A comparison of cortical bone atrophy secondary to fixation with plates with large differences in bending stiffness. *J Bone Joint Surg Am.* 1976;58(2): 190–195.
8. Rhinelander FW. The blood supply of the limb bones. In: Owen R, Goodfellow J, Bullough P, eds. *Scientific Foundations of Orthopaedics and Traumatology.* Philadelphia, PA: W.B. Saunders; 1980.
9. Jacobs RR, Rahn BA, Perren SM. Effects of plates on cortical bone perfusion. *J Trauma.* 1981; 21(2):91–95.
10. Wei SY, Born CT, Abene A, et al. Diaphyseal forearm fractures treated with and without bone graft. *J Trauma.* 1999;46(6):1045–1048.
11. Wright RR, Schmeling GJ, Schwab JP. The necessity of acute bone grafting in diaphyseal forearm fractures: A retrospective review. *J Orthop Trauma.* 1997;11(4):288–294.
12. Labosky DA, Cermak MB, Waggy CA. Forearm fracture plates: To remove or not to remove. *J Hand Surg Am.* 1990;15(2):294–301.
13. Rumball K, Finnegan M. Refractures after forearm plate removal. *J Orthop Trauma.* 1990;4(2): 124–129.

14. Rosson JW, Shearer JR. Refracture after the removal of plate from the forearm. An avoidable complication. *J Bone Joint Surg Br.* 1991;73(3):415–417.
15. Bednar DA, Grandwilewski W. Complications of forearm-plate removal. *Can J Surg.* 1992;35(4): 428–431.
16. Hertel R, Pisan M, Lambert S, et al. Plate osteosynthesis of diaphyseal fractures of the radius and ulna. *Injury.* 1996;27(8):545–548.
17. Chapman MW, Gordon JE, Zissimos AG. Compression-plate fixation of acute fractures of the diaphyses of the radius and ulna. *J Bone Joint Surg Am.* 1989;71(2):159–169.
18. Crenshaw AH Jr. Fractures of the shoulder, arm, and forearm. *Campbell's Operative Orthopaedics.* Vol 3. 11th ed. St. Louis, MO: Mosby; 2008.
19. Lee YH, Lee SK, Chung MS, et al. Interlocking contoured intramedullary nail fixation for selected diaphyseal fractures of the forearm in adults. *J Bone Joint Surg Am.* 2008;90(9):1891–1898.
20. Weckbach A, Blattert TR, Weisser Ch. Interlocking nailing of forearm fractures. *Arch Orthop Trauma Surg.* 2006;126(5):309–315.
21. Hong G, Cong-Feng L, Hui-Peng S, et al. Treatment of diaphyseal forearm nonunions with interlocking intramedullary nails. *Clin Orthop Relat Res.* 2006;450:186–192.
22. Gao H, Luo CF, Zhang CQ, et al. Internal fixation of diaphyseal fractures of the forearm by interlocking intramedullary nail: Short-term results in eighteen patients. *J Orthop Trauma.* 2005; 19(6):384–391.

CHAPTER 5

Percutaneous Submuscular Plating of the Humerus

Bruce H. Ziran and David W. Robinson

INDICATIONS FOR SUBMUSCULAR PLATING

Open plating of the humerus has been the favored treatment method amongst most orthopaedic traumatologists. Humeral nailing, while still a very successful modality, is less favored amongst traumatologists, but by virtue of its strong commercial success, would imply that it is a popular modality in general orthopaedics. Why this rift in treatment exists is difficult to explain, but may be due to the minimally invasive nature of nailing and its appeal to general orthopaedic surgeons. The issues of shoulder problems may be a function of technique and implant design, and the slightly lower union rate may possibly be due to mechanobiology or fracture gaps. Open plating is ideal for fracture patterns that allow for compression and direct bone healing. However, there is also a theoretical risk that bone healing may be impaired with open reduction due to greater disruption of the fracture site vascularity and soft tissue attachments. Other associated drawbacks include greater morbidity,[1] due to a larger incision and dissection, and postoperative elbow complaints.[2,3] Plating techniques require knowledge of fracture mechanobiology, such as whether absolute stability or relative stability is the desired environment for healing. In general, the stiffer the construct created, the more anatomic the reduction required. Very stiff constructs with fracture gaps may lead to nonunion. Similarly, nonunion rates are increased with canal-filling nails and associated fracture gaps. Relative stability is achieved with long bridging plates or small, non–canal-filling nails (i.e., flexible nails). With both of these modalities, stability is sacrificed, especially with traditional plates using long spans and nonlocking screws.

Recently, submuscular (Minimally Invasive Percutaneous Plate Osteosynthesis, MIPPO) plating of humeral shaft fractures has been introduced by Livani and Belangero[4] with excellent results. Their technique utilizes a safe anterior corridor of the humerus that is relatively unpopulated with neurovascular structures. Through two small windows, proximally and distally, a plate is inserted deep to the brachialis muscle, the fracture is reduced, and stabilized to the plate. Surprisingly, even with nonlocked screws in comminuted fractures, Livani and Belangero reported excellent healing. It may be due to the preservation of fracture biology with the judicious creation of relative stability with nonrigid constructs. In order to further enhance stability, without compromising biology, Ziran et al.[5] further modified the technique to incorporate newer technology of locked screws. Other studies corroborated these findings[6,7] though it was initially reserved for fracture patterns with a low strain modulus, for example, comminuted fractures. However, other evidence has shown good outcomes using this technique even with simple fracture patterns.[5] In addition, the percutaneous technique is aesthetically more acceptable and may have the benefits of closed nailing, where the muscle envelope is less violated, but does not incur the shoulder problems associated with intramedullary nails.

The authors cannot identify any absolute contraindications to using minimally invasive technique except those applicable to traditional open reduction and internal fixation of the humerus, but caution its use with very distal humerus fractures. Proximal humerus fractures that are amenable to proximal humeral plate fixation can also be treated with the submuscular technique, but the position of the proximal plate needs to be modified to be placed anteriorly, and a long plate is required (Fig. 5.1). These plates are 3.5 mm in size, and the entire construct may not be suitable for immediate weight-bearing. Some recent studies have noted that using 3.5-mm plates for humeral shaft fractures may be acceptable in certain cases and

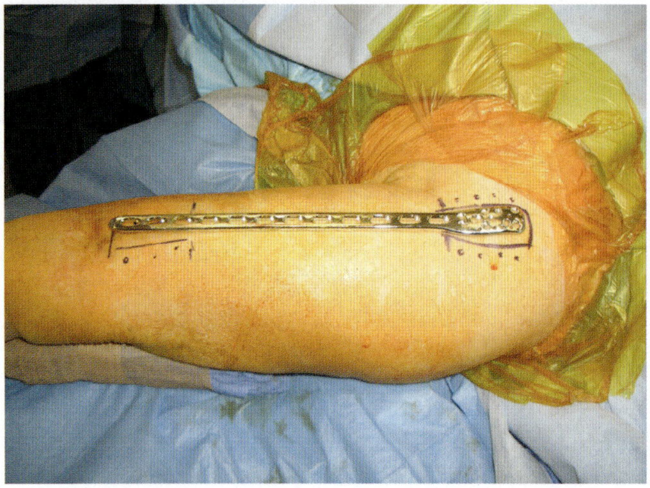

Figure 5.1 Long proximal humerus plate overlying modified anterior position.

in smaller-sized patients. While the authors prefer a 4.5-mm plate, the ability to use a single plate for such complex fractures, and in a minimally invasive method, may outweigh the disadvantage of the smaller plate. Relative contraindications include neurovascular injury requiring surgical exploration, open fractures with substantial soft tissue involvement necessitating aggressive debridement, and segmental fractures with insufficient bone proximally and distally for stable fixation.

The purpose of this present report is to describe in detail the authors' method of submuscular plating of the humerus. Since the technique may be unfamiliar to most surgeons, the authors recommend beginning with a standard open anterior approach, and then gradually decreasing the sizes of the skin portal as comfort with the technique and anatomy improve (Fig. 5.2).

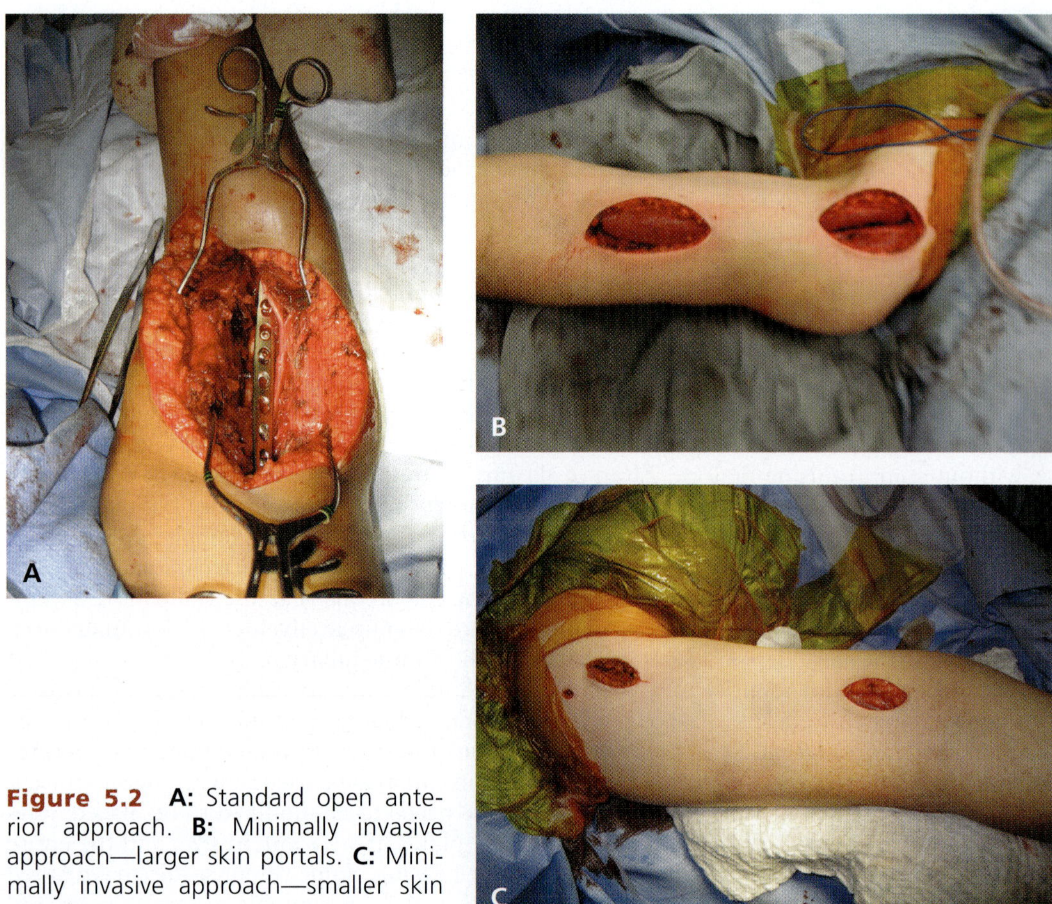

Figure 5.2 **A:** Standard open anterior approach. **B:** Minimally invasive approach—larger skin portals. **C:** Minimally invasive approach—smaller skin portals.

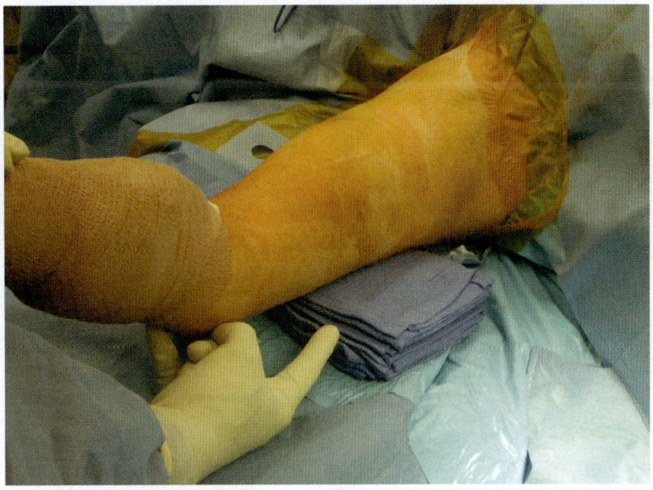

Figure 5.3 Sterile bump of towels placed under the fracture site to assist with reduction.

PATIENT POSITIONING

The room is best set up such that the scrub technician/nurse and surgical equipment are on the contralateral side of the patient or at the foot of the bed, with fluoroscopy (sterilely draped) positioned on the ipsilateral side. The patient is supine with a hand table that allows imaging from its underside (no legs). The fluoroscopy machine should be positioned to move in and out of the field from the distal aspect of the hand table. The full arm should be prepped and the patient draped from the ipsilateral nipple to the ipsilateral angle of the jaw to below the axilla. In Livani and Belangero's original technique, they positioned the arm at approximately 60 degrees of abduction, and a sterile bump (such as a stack of sterile towels wrapped with Coban) was placed under the fracture site as a fulcrum to overcome gravitational apex posterior deformity (Fig. 5.3). In our modified technique, an external fixator (mini-distractor) is used to maintain the reduction. A tourniquet is not used (or needed) since it invariably overlays the location of the proximal incision. If necessary, especially when an external fixator is not used, a third assistant may provide gentle in-line traction with the elbow flexed (this relaxes the biceps brachii, brachialis, and brachioradialis) to achieve and maintain length during the case.

SURGICAL APPROACHES

Most surgeons are hesitant to consider submuscular plating when considering the neurovascular structures of the arm. But when one looks at cross-sectional anatomy, there is a safe anterior window that can be utilized safely to apply and fix a plate to the humerus. The authors do not advocate submuscularly inserting the plate in any other anatomic corridor, such as lateral, or posterior due to the dangers of injuring a vital structure.

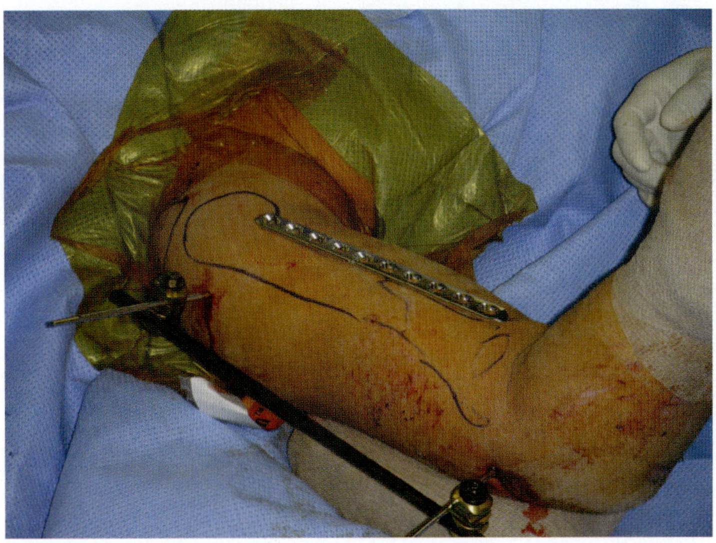

Figure 5.4 Elbow flexed to 90 degrees with plate on anterior aspect of the arm.

Identification of the skin incisions is done by placing the plate over the anterior aspect of the arm with the elbow flexed to 90 degrees (Fig. 5.4). The plate is centered over the fracture zone, utilizing fluoroscopic guidance (Fig. 5.5). The

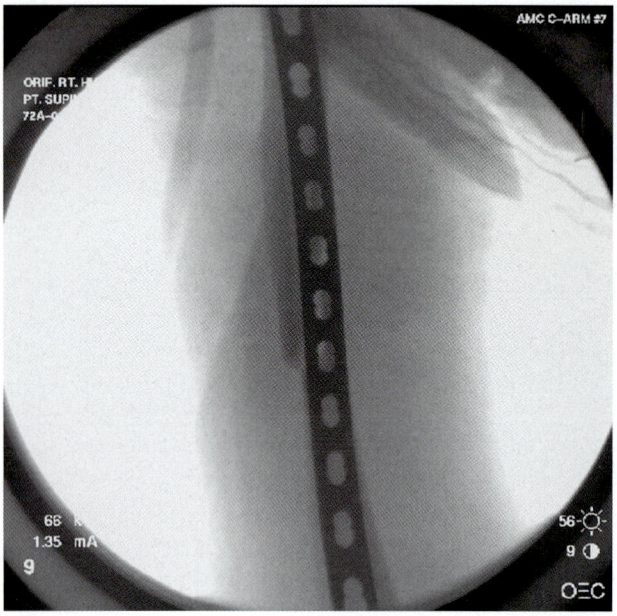

Figure 5.5 Plate centered over the fracture site utilizing fluoroscopy.

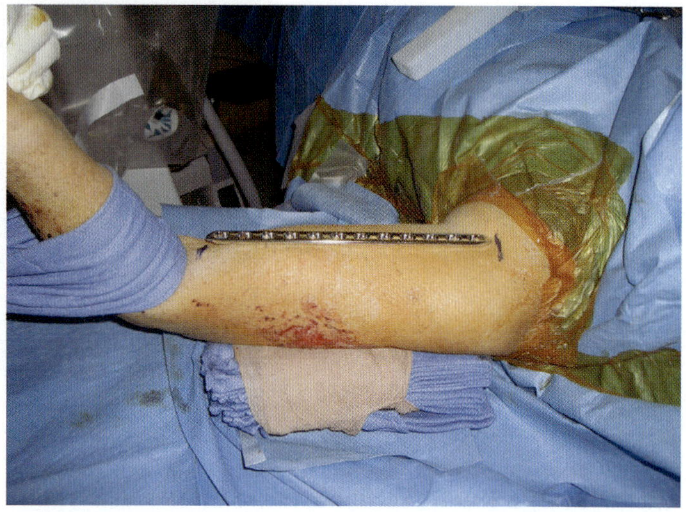

Figure 5.6 Ends of the plate marked on the skin.

appropriate length of plate is then determined depending on the caliber of plate used. For 3.5-mm systems, the plate length is usually 10 to 16 holes, while for 4.5-mm systems, the plate length is usually 9 to 14 holes (narrow plate, not wide). The ends of the plate are marked on the skin using a sterile pen (Fig. 5.6).

The order of incisions is not critical. For the proximal portal, a 2- to 4-cm incision is placed in-line with the humerus, down to the fascia. The cephalic vein may occasionally be identified and the interval is usually the distal aspect of the deltopectoral approach. The interval between the pectoralis major and the long head of the biceps brachii is identified and developed. While retracting the deltoid laterally (with care taken to protect the cephalic vein if seen), the biceps is identified as it exits from under the pectoralis major tendon (Fig. 5.7). The pectoralis may require partial release depending on the location of the fracture. The long head of the biceps serves as the anterior landmark of the proximal segment. It should be aligned with the forearm, which serves as the marker for the anterior incision in the distal segment, when the elbow is flexed. The biceps can be retracted in either direction but we

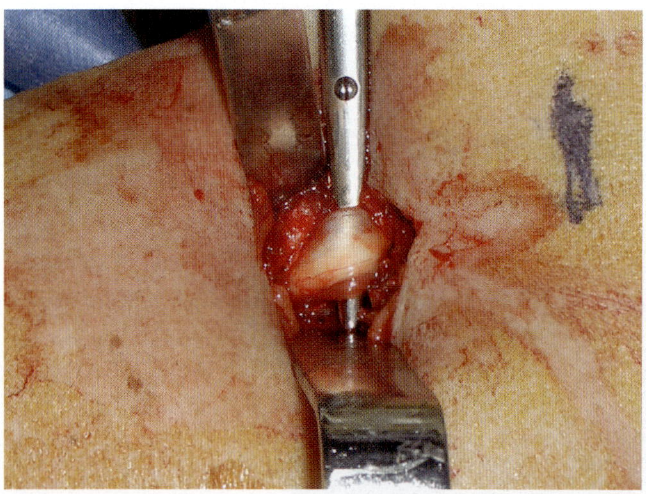

Figure 5.7 Biceps tendon in the proximal window.

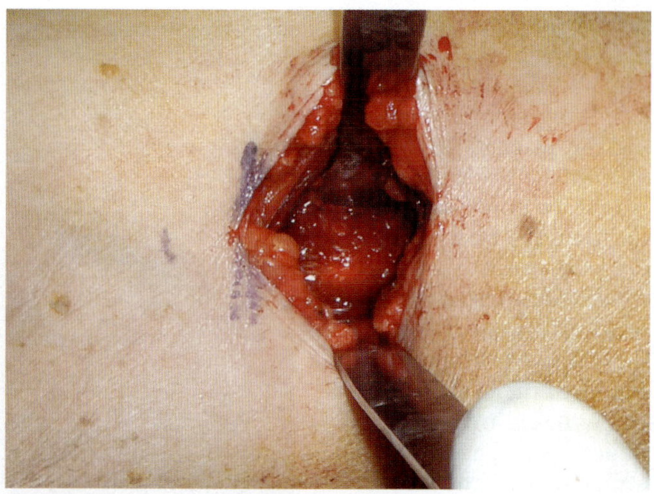

Figure 5.8 Two small Hohmann retractors centering the proximal operative window on the humerus.

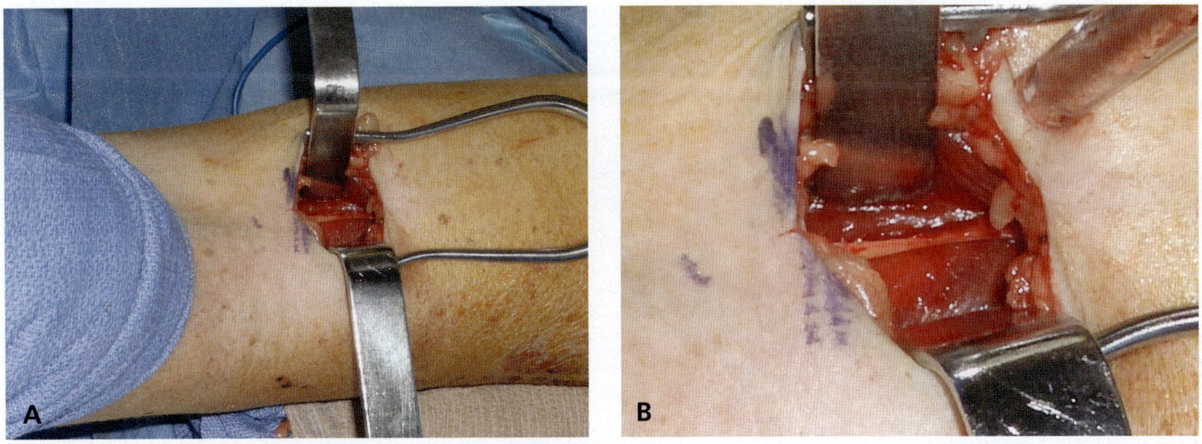

Figure 5.9 Lateral antebrachial cutaneous nerve in the distal window.

have found it easier to retract it medially. The humerus can be palpated at that point and two small wide Hohmann retractors are placed, around the humerus. The retractors protect the surrounding structures but most importantly center the operative window around the humerus (Fig. 5.8). The portal is packed with a moist laparotomy sponge and attention is directed to the distal portal.

Distally, a second 2- to 4-cm incision is made down to the fascia. This incision is utilized as a "mobile operating window." The skin is first retracted medially to identify the top of the biceps muscle and to look for the antebrachial cutaneous nerve as it exists the muscle belly (Fig. 5.9). Once identified, it is retracted medially and protected by the biceps. Then the portal is mobilized laterally to locate the interval between the brachioradialis and the brachialis. After some blunt dissection (usually with a plastic Yankauer suction tip), the radial nerve is identified here to ensure its safety (Fig. 5.10). It is unnecessary to fully mobilize the nerve or to use vessel loops since there is little work done in the nerve interval. The portal is then mobilized to its resting anterior position and the biceps is retracted medially again. A trans-muscular blunt dissection through the lateral third of the brachialis is performed until the humerus is identified and similar to the proximal exposure, two small wide Hohmann retractors are placed around the humerus to centralize the window of exposure (Fig. 5.11). Care should be taken to avoid extended or excessive retraction of these retractors due to their proximity to the nerves. Like most fracture surgery, the authors' technique calls for retraction only when needed and we discourage the use of sustained or aggressive tissue retraction. If such retraction is needed, we feel it preferable to enlarge the incision to allow more gentle soft tissue handling.

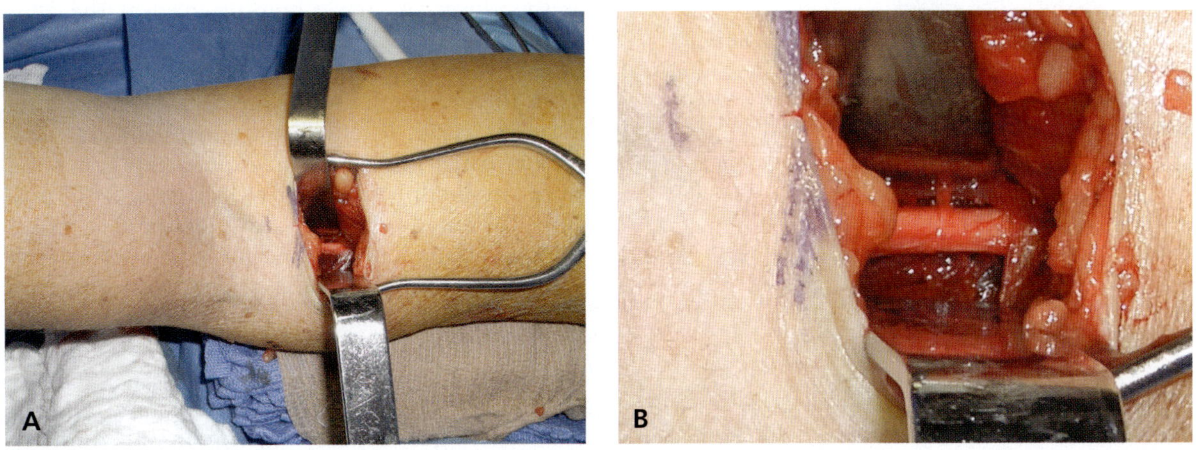

Figure 5.10 Radial nerve in the distal window.

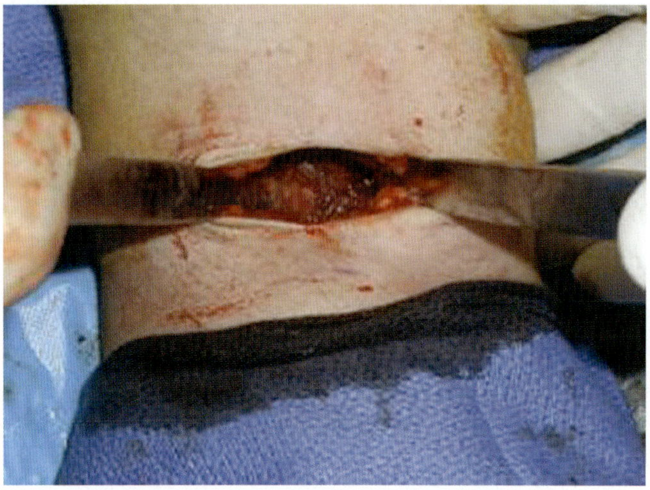

Figure 5.11 Two small wide Hohmann retractors centering the distal operative window on the humerus.

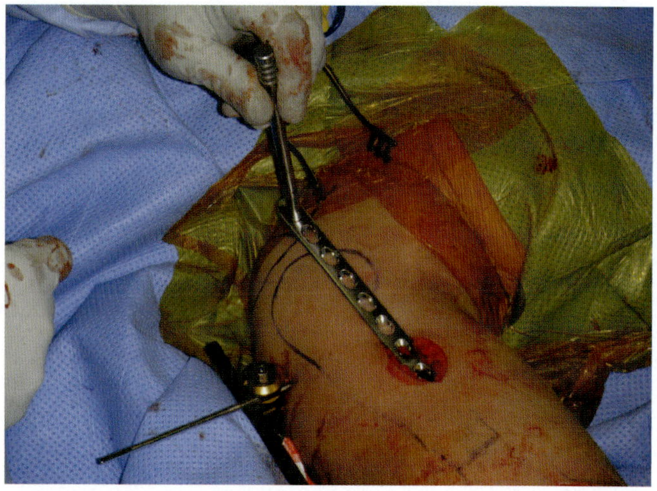

Figure 5.12 Insertion of the plate from proximal to distal.

When both portals have been developed, the plate is assembled with a long handle screwed into the most proximal locking hole. The plate is inserted from proximal to distal, using the tapered tip of the plate to dissect distally under the biceps (Fig. 5.12). The plate is advanced below the brachialis (submuscular) and on top of the humerus (extraperiosteal). The surgeon should insert a finger into the distal portal, in a proximal direction to "receive" the plate and guide it to its anterior position in the distal window (Fig. 5.13). We have found that this maneuver helps avoid inadvertent straying of the plate.

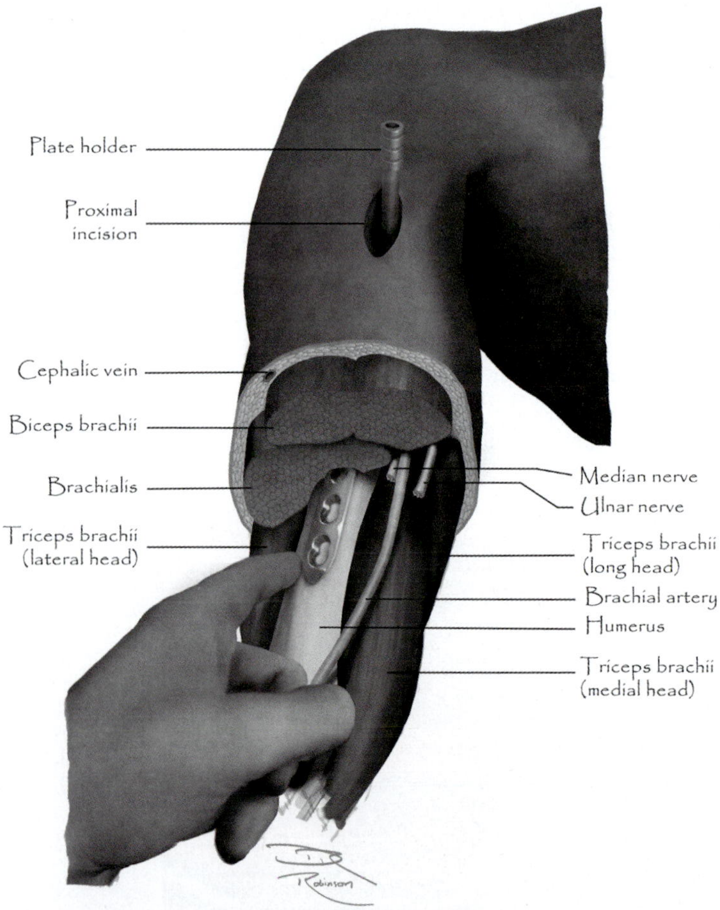

Figure 5.13 The surgeon should insert their finger into the distal portal, in a proximal direction to "receive" the plate and guide it to its anterior position in the distal window.

REDUCTION TECHNIQUES

Reduction can be achieved using a variety of methods alone or in combination. The most basic reduction technique is manual traction and a bolster as described by Livani and Belangero. The arm is held in 60 degrees of abduction with the elbow flexed and in-line traction is applied to the proximal forearm by an assistant. This also allows for rotational adjustment by internally and externally rotating the forearm. Appropriate alignment is indicated by the proximal biceps brachii tendon being in-line with the forearm when flexed at the elbow. A sterile bump placed at the apex of the fracture will help effect or maintain reduction in the sagittal plane. When this technique is used, the reduction usually has to be adjusted after plate insertion. If length and alignment are satisfactory, then provisional plate fixation can begin since small adjustments of reduction are still possible. As noted previously, absolute perfect reductions are not necessary, and invocation of relative stability will still stimulate healing with imperfect reductions. If an assistant is not available or maintaining reduction is proving difficult, a temporary two-pin single-bar external fixator can be used. The proximal pin is placed anterolateral and the distal pin placed posterolateral in the humerus (Fig. 5.14). The authors have used 4- or 5-mm

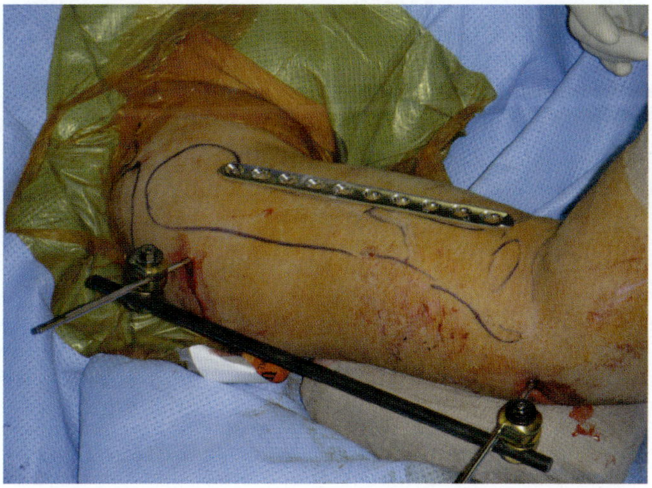

Figure 5.14 Temporary two-pin single-bar external fixator to maintain reduction.

pins proximally and 3- or 4-mm pins distally. Anterolateral pins in the proximal section minimize risk to the axillary nerve, and posterolateral pins in the distal section minimize risk to the radial nerve in the distal section. The reduction is performed and the pin clamps are tightened. Reduction should be frequently assessed fluoroscopically during the case to ensure that alignment is maintained. If it is lost, effort should be directed toward correcting the reduction prior to definitive fixation.

IMPLANT AND FIXATION

A narrow 4.5-mm plate with locking screw options (9 to 14 holes) is selected and oriented anteriorly on humerus. Length should be sufficient to provide a relatively long working length so that at least 3 to 4 empty plate holes are centered over the fracture (Fig. 5.15). Locking handles can be used in the end holes of the plate to facilitate alignment and positioning (Fig. 5.16).

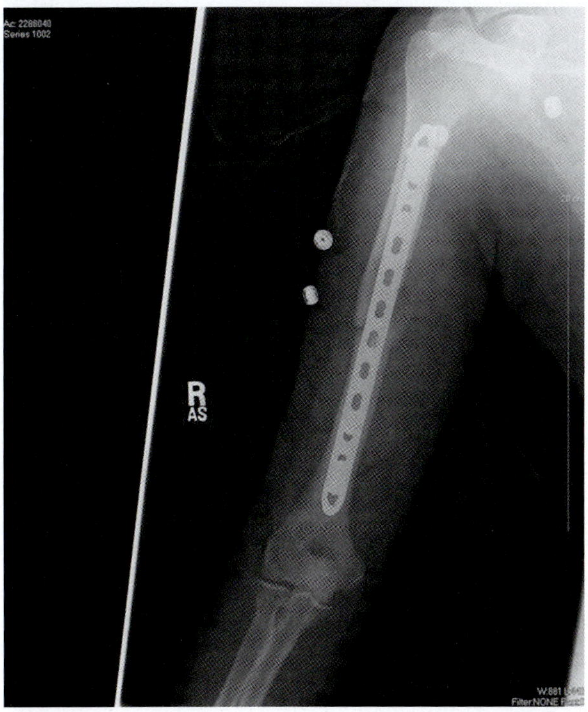

Figure 5.15 Large working length of empty screw holes centered over the fracture site.

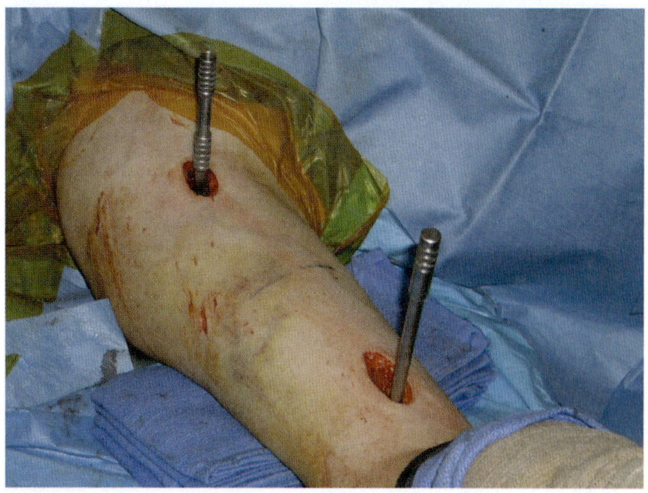

Figure 5.16 Locking handles in the end holes of the plate to facilitate alignment and positioning.

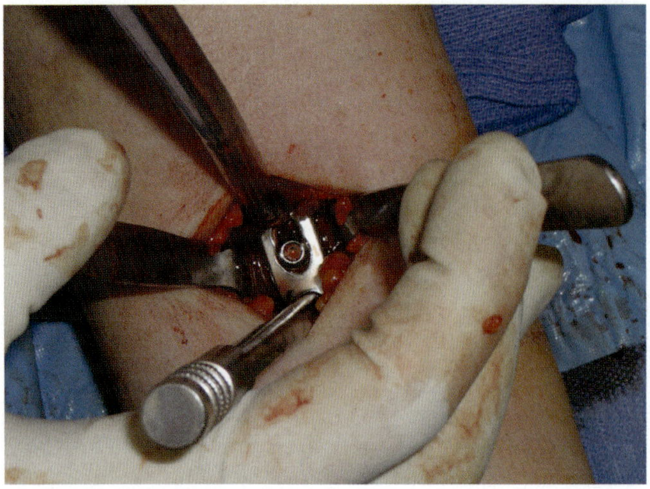

Figure 5.17 Two small Hohmann retractors placed on each side of the humerus provide access for fixation.

The two small Hohmann retractors placed on each side of the bone provide ample access to allow fixation at each end (Fig. 5.17).

The authors' technique involves achieving provisional fixation with unicortical screws before definitive fixation with bicortical locking screws. The provisional fixation is with a unicortical 4.5-mm standard cortical screw in the second hole at each end. A unicortical screw is used so that the far cortex is not compromised in the event adjustment to plate position is required. The unicortical screw is usually sufficient to approximate plate and bone, and adjustments to reduction are possible by loosening and tightening this screw. Once reduction is verified, 5-mm locking screws are placed bicortically at holes one and three at each end of the plate (Fig. 5.18). Finally, the standard screws in holes two can be converted to bicortical 5-mm locking screws if needed (Fig. 5.19).

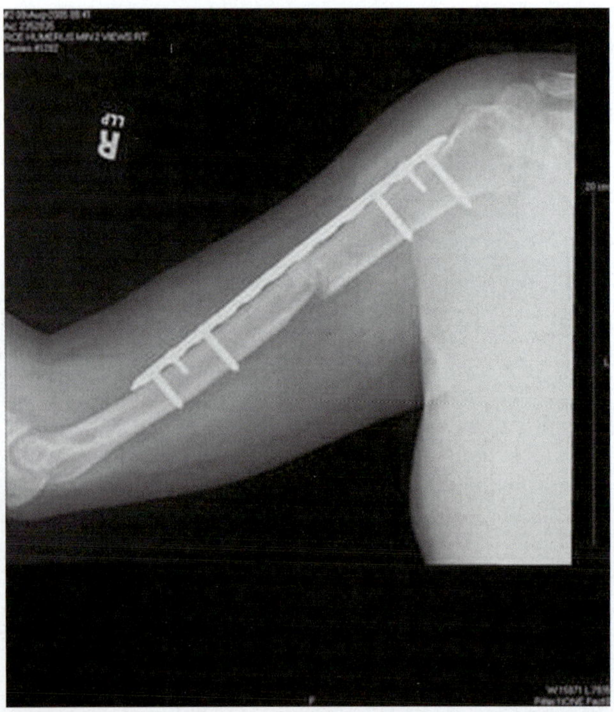

Figure 5.18 Plate fixed with a unicortical nonlocking screw and two bicortical locking screws at each end of the plate.

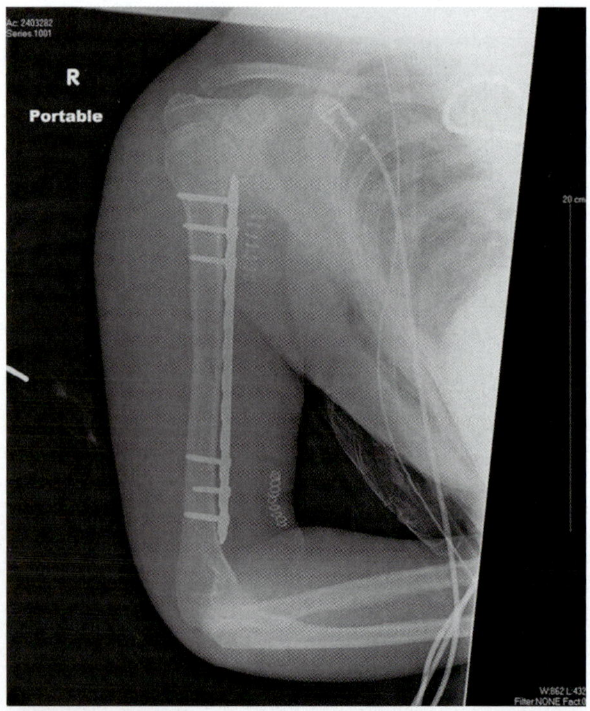

Figure 5.19 Plate fixed with three bicortical locking screws at each end of the plate.

COMPLICATIONS

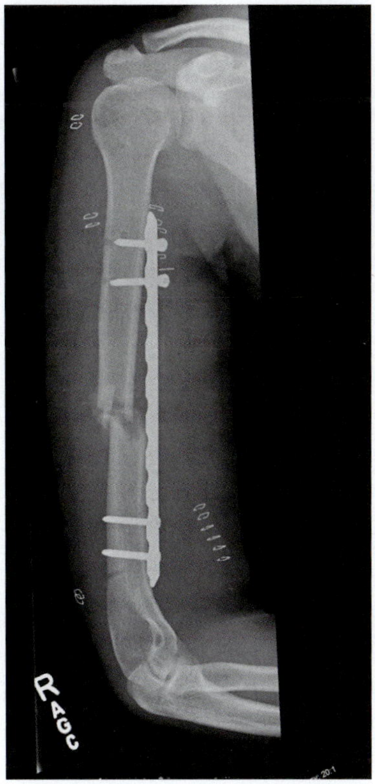

Figure 5.20 Postoperative complication showing locking screw disengagement and pull-out.

Complications from percutaneous plating of the humerus are divided into two broad categories: Intraoperative complications and postoperative complications.

Intraoperatively, there are relatively few risks outside of the general risks of surgery (bleeding, allergic reaction, anesthesia complications, etc.). Proximally, there is a risk of injury to the cephalic vein and musculocutaneous nerve. Distally, the lateral antebrachial cutaneous nerve (which exits the biceps brachii and innervates the skin over the radial aspect of the forearm) can be injured. Iatrogenic radial nerve palsies are probably due to either aggressive manipulation or retraction in the distal window. The authors have explored the iatrogenic radial nerve palsies in their series and only found what appeared to be traumatic contusions. All recovered uneventfully.

As this technique involves indirect reduction of the fracture site, consideration should be given for conversion to an open technique if appropriate reduction is unable to be achieved or maintained. Also, conversion should occur if there is greater than expected bleeding without an identifiable source or evidence indicating greater than expected soft tissue injury (such as poor muscle color/contractility).

Postoperatively, the complications include malunion (usually from poor alignment during surgery, or early implant failure), delayed union, and nonunion. The authors have also encountered hardware complications such as disengagement and breakage of locking screws (Fig. 5.20). However, these problems occurred in cases where a modified technique of using only two locking screws in only the first and second holes of the plate. Despite the advantages of locked plating systems, we feel that closely spaced screws in adjacent holes (1 and 2 from each end) do not provide the same stability as our original technique, using holes 1 and 3 as fixation points.

REHABILITATION PROTOCOL

During the initial postoperative period, patients are weight-bearing as tolerated, and are encouraged to wear a humerus fracture brace during weight-bearing activities. Radiographs are obtained at 2 weeks, 6 weeks, and 12 weeks. Fracture consolidation can be expected between 8 and 16 weeks. There is no special therapy modalities needed for this technique.

OUTCOME

The authors have found that most patients have little postoperative pain as a result of the limited dissection and lack of violation of shoulder structures. Constant and modified shoulder and elbow scores in the author's series were good to excellent and comparable to other published series, except for the notable lack of shoulder and elbow symptoms.

REFERENCES

1. Niall DM, O'Mahony J, McElwain JP. Plating of humeral shaft fractures–has the pendulum swung back? *Injury.* 2004;35:580–586.
2. Korner J, Lill H, Muller LP, et al. The LCP-concept in the operative treatment of distal humerus fractures–biological, biomechanical and surgical aspects. *Injury.* 2003;34(Suppl 2):B20–B30.

3. Sodergard J, Sandelin J, Bostman O. Postoperative complications of distal humeral fractures. 27/96 adults followed up for 6 (2–10) years. *Acta Orthop Scand.* 1992;63:85–89.
4. Livani B, Belangero WD. Bridging plate osteosynthesis of humeral shaft fractures. *Injury.* 2004; 35(6):587–595.
5. Ziran BH, Kinney RC, Smith WR, et al. Sub-muscular plating of the humerus: An emerging technique. *Injury.* 2010;41:1047–1052.
6. Apivatthakakul T, Arpornchayanon O, Bavornratanavech S. Minimally invasive plate osteosynthesis (MIPO) of the humeral shaft fracture. Is it possible? A cadaveric study and preliminary report. *Injury.* 2005;36(4):530–538.
7. Dell'Oca FAA. The principle of helical implants unusual ideas worth considering. *Injury.* 2002;33: SA1–SA27.

CHAPTER 6

Percutaneous Plating of the Proximal Humerus

G. Yves Laflamme and Dominique Rouleau

INDICATIONS

Proximal humeral fractures represent up to 5% of all fractures occurring most often in elderly patients over the age of 60 years as the result of a simple fall.[1] Even among experts, controversy exists regarding the indications for surgical management since evidence-based treatment guidelines are lacking.[2]

Percutaneous plating was developed in an attempt to address the issues of humeral head necrosis associated with open reduction through an extensive approach and insufficient primary stability associated with previous attempts at limited exposure and minimal internal fixation.[3] A locking plate provides stable fixation for early range of motion reducing soft tissue scarring and loss of the gliding surfaces.

Surgery is generally indicated when fracture instability prevents early motion or when fracture displacement is sufficiently great that functional impairment is likely. With a minimally invasive approach, indirect reduction techniques are needed to achieve an acceptable reduction. For this reason, we caution against the use of this technique for complex fracture–dislocations, head-split, four-part fractures, and nonunions of the proximal humerus. Displaced unstable two-part surgical neck fractures, isolated greater tuberosity fracture, and valgus-impacted (three- or four-part) fractures are ideal fracture types that can be easily reduced through a mini-incision especially during the learning curve period. With increased experience with this percutaneous technique, three-part fractures and some four-part fractures can be tackled but sometimes extending this approach to an extended lateral deltoid split approach is needed to obtain adequate reduction.[4] A minimally invasive incision should not be used if the best obtainable reduction is suboptimal.

PATIENT POSITIONING

The patient is positioned in a supine position on a radiolucent table with a soft bump placed behind the patient's chest. This positioning is ideal for multiply injured patients especially if cervical spine issues complicate head positioning or if associated fractures to the extremities need fixation. Simultaneous surgery is possible without the need to reposition. The entire upper extremity is draped to allow free mobility for reduction maneuvers and for optimal imaging during surgery. The setup is checked before draping with the C-arm unit brought on the opposite side to ensure complete visualization of the proximal humerus including a modified axillary view.

Alternative Positioning

The patient is placed in a beach chair position on a specialized operating room table that allows access to the shoulder. The head is immobilized in a head holder. The image intensifier is placed parallel to the table at the patient's head on the injured side. This setup allows adequate fluoroscopic visualization of the shoulder (axillary view) and conversion to a hemiarthroplasty if the fracture is unreconstructible but limits the access to the operative site.

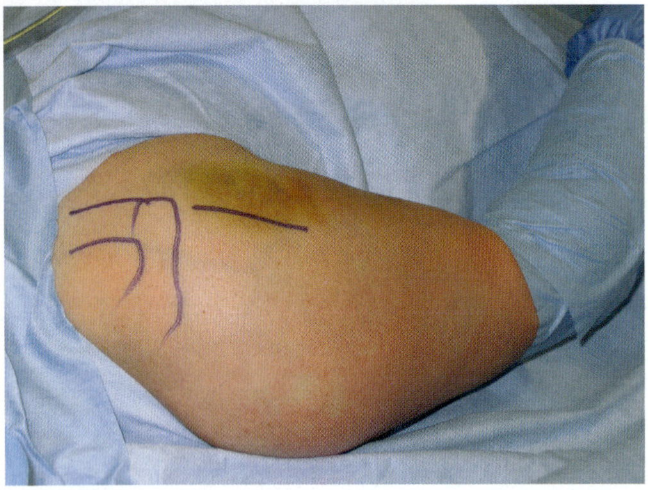

Figure 6.1 A proximal incision is first marked from the anterolateral corner of the acromion.

SURGICAL APPROACH

This minimally invasive technique allows limited disruption of soft tissue with application of the plate on the lateral side of the humeral head away from the primary vascular supply, the ascending branch of the anterior humeral circumflex artery that runs adjacent to the bicipital groove. A hypovascular bare spot of 3 cm in width was identified by Gardner et al.[5] on the greater tuberosity and a plate applied to this region may minimize iatrogenic vascular injury when treating these fractures. After proper positioning of the patient, we proceed with a direct minimally invasive lateral approach to the proximal humerus with two separate mini-incisions: The proximal window exposes the greater tuberosity and the humeral head and the distal window exposes the humeral shaft and distal part of the plate. Internal or external rotation with abduction facilitates exposure through these mobile windows.

PROXIMAL INCISION

The anterior edge of the acromion is palpated and used as a landmark (Fig. 6.1). Starting 1 cm distal from this point, a direct lateral longitudinal incision is made distally for 4 cm in-line with the middle of the humeral head. The subcutaneous tissue is incised, and the deltoid fascia is visualized and transected parallel to the underlying deltoid muscle fibers. The deltoid muscle fibers are bluntly split until the underlying subdeltoid bursa is exposed. Finger dissection is then needed to elevate the deltoid muscle from the proximal humerus. The fracture lines are able to be palpated at this point, but it is critical to identify the axillary nerve (Fig. 6.2).

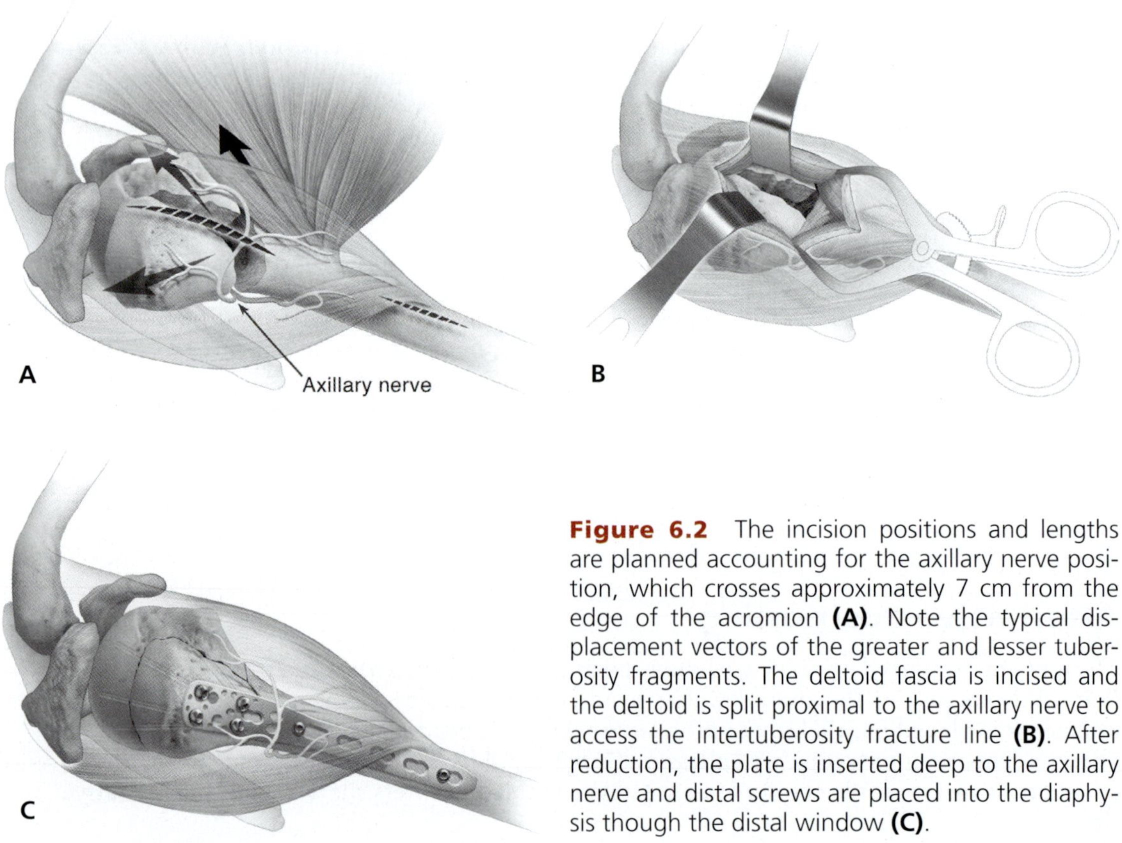

Figure 6.2 The incision positions and lengths are planned accounting for the axillary nerve position, which crosses approximately 7 cm from the edge of the acromion **(A)**. Note the typical displacement vectors of the greater and lesser tuberosity fragments. The deltoid fascia is incised and the deltoid is split proximal to the axillary nerve to access the intertuberosity fracture line **(B)**. After reduction, the plate is inserted deep to the axillary nerve and distal screws are placed into the diaphysis though the distal window **(C)**.

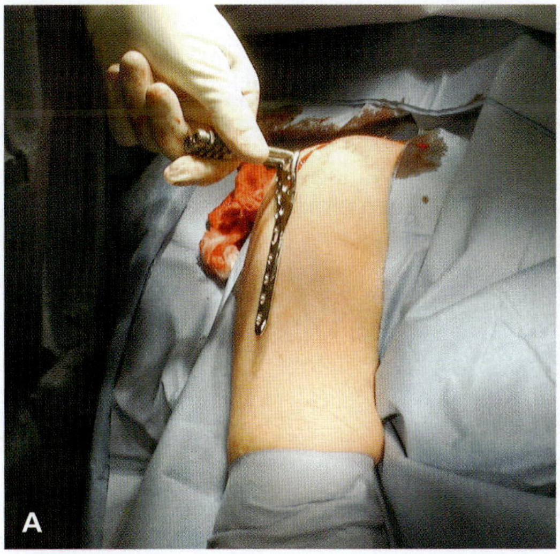

A

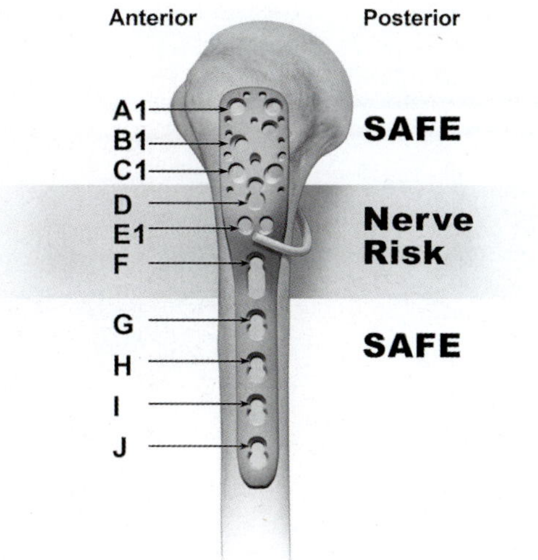

B

Figure 6.3 A plate can be used as a template to estimate the axillary nerve position and the safe zones for the incisions **(A)**. After assessing the appropriate plate position relative to the humerus, the axillary nerve risk zone can be determined **(B)**.

The average distance from the lateral edge of the acromion to the axillary nerve is 7 cm (range, 62 to 85 mm).[6] This cord-like band is located in the posterior aspect of the wound as it exits the quadrangular space and then runs on the undersurface of the deltoid around the humerus as it innervates the deltoid muscle. If scarring or hematoma prevents palpation of the nerve, the surgeon should consider extending the incision and directly identifying the nerve using the extended lateral or anterolateral (AL) deltoid splitting approach.[4,5]

DISTAL INCISION

Mapping the second window is facilitated by the plate used as a template over the skin (Fig. 6.3). A 2-cm incision is made in-line and distal to the previous incision and is centered over the distal three screw holes (Fig. 6.4). The correct location is confirmed using fluoroscopy. The subcutaneous tissue and deltoid musculature are bluntly dissected. This incision is well below the course of the axillary nerve.

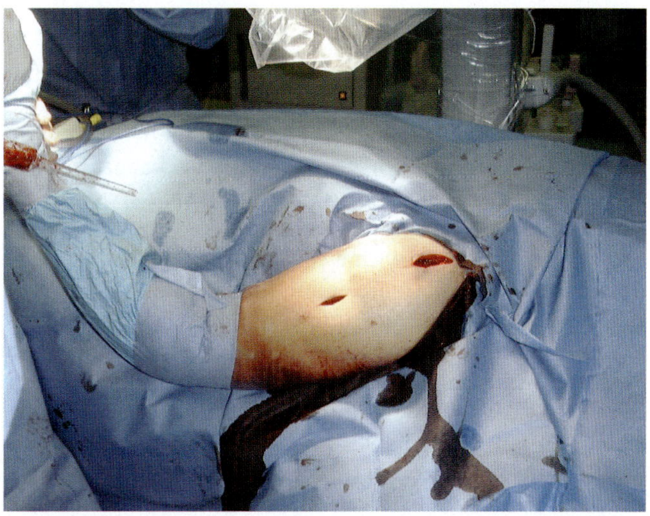

Figure 6.4 The proximal and distal incisions are made, one proximal and one distal to the crossing axillary nerve.

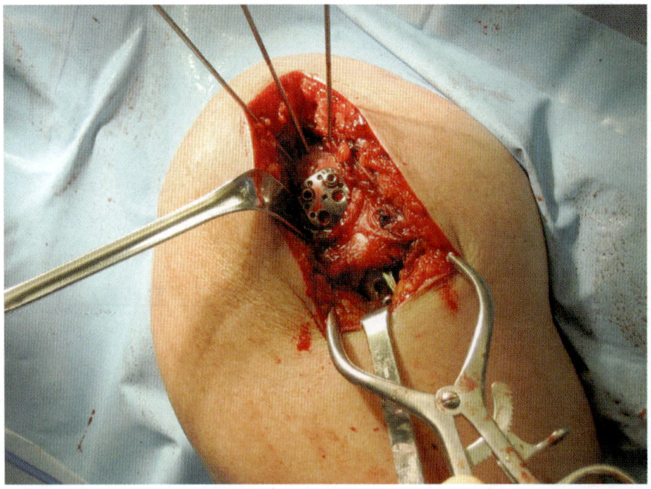

Figure 6.5 As an alternative to the percutaneous approach, the anterolateral acromial approach can be used, which connects the skin bridge between the proximal and distal incisions but utilizes the same deep proximal and distal windows in relation to the axillary nerve.

ALTERNATIVE APPROACH

The extended AL acromial approach allows minimally invasive access to the proximal humerus. The AL acromial approach uses the anterior deltoid raphe between the anterior and middle deltoid heads as a surgical plane, which allows direct visualization of the axillary nerve.[5] With the shoulder in neutral rotation, an approximately 10-cm incision is made beginning at the AL corner of the acromion and carried distally. After splitting the raphe approximately 6 cm distally in the wound, the axillary nerve is identified and protected (Fig. 6.5). This is our preferred approach for complex fractures or nonunions of the proximal humerus. The axillary nerve is visualized and can be mobilized to insert the inferomedial oblique "calcar" screws.

REDUCTION TECHNIQUES

The key to minimally invasive surgery is the ability to obtain acceptable reduction using indirect reduction techniques. As many surgeons have emphasized, normal anatomy is not crucial to normal function in the shoulder. However, optimizing stability by achieving adequate medial support is essential to prevent loss of reduction.[7] Varus reduction also correlated with fixation failure and poor outcomes and should be avoided.[8] Knowledge of the deforming forces on the fracture fragments must be understood in order to use appropriate reduction maneuvers.

VARUS TYPE

The proximal window allows access and is used to assist reduction of the tuberosities and humeral head. The humeral head and shaft reduction is the first step whether the greater tuberosity is involved or not. The humeral shaft nearly always assumes a position of anteromedial displacement due to the deforming force of the pectoralis major, which causes the humeral head to assume a relative retroverted position. As described for closed reduction, longitudinal traction with a posteriorly directed force is applied to the arm to reduce the apex anterior deformity. To aid reduction, a small Cobb elevator (or a Hohmann retractor) is introduced in the fracture site anterolaterally between the overlapping fragments and tilted downward correcting the translational displacement like a "shoehorn maneuver" to lift up the head over the shaft (Fig. 6.6). Placement of a Hohmann retractor anteromedial to the shaft may also help offset the deforming adduction force created by pectoralis major. Adequacy of the reduction is verified using the C-arm fluoroscopy. Once the reduction is achieved with good medial calcar contact or realignment, a K-wire can be inserted anteriorly from the shaft into the head (or from head to shaft) to temporarily stabilize the head–shaft fracture.

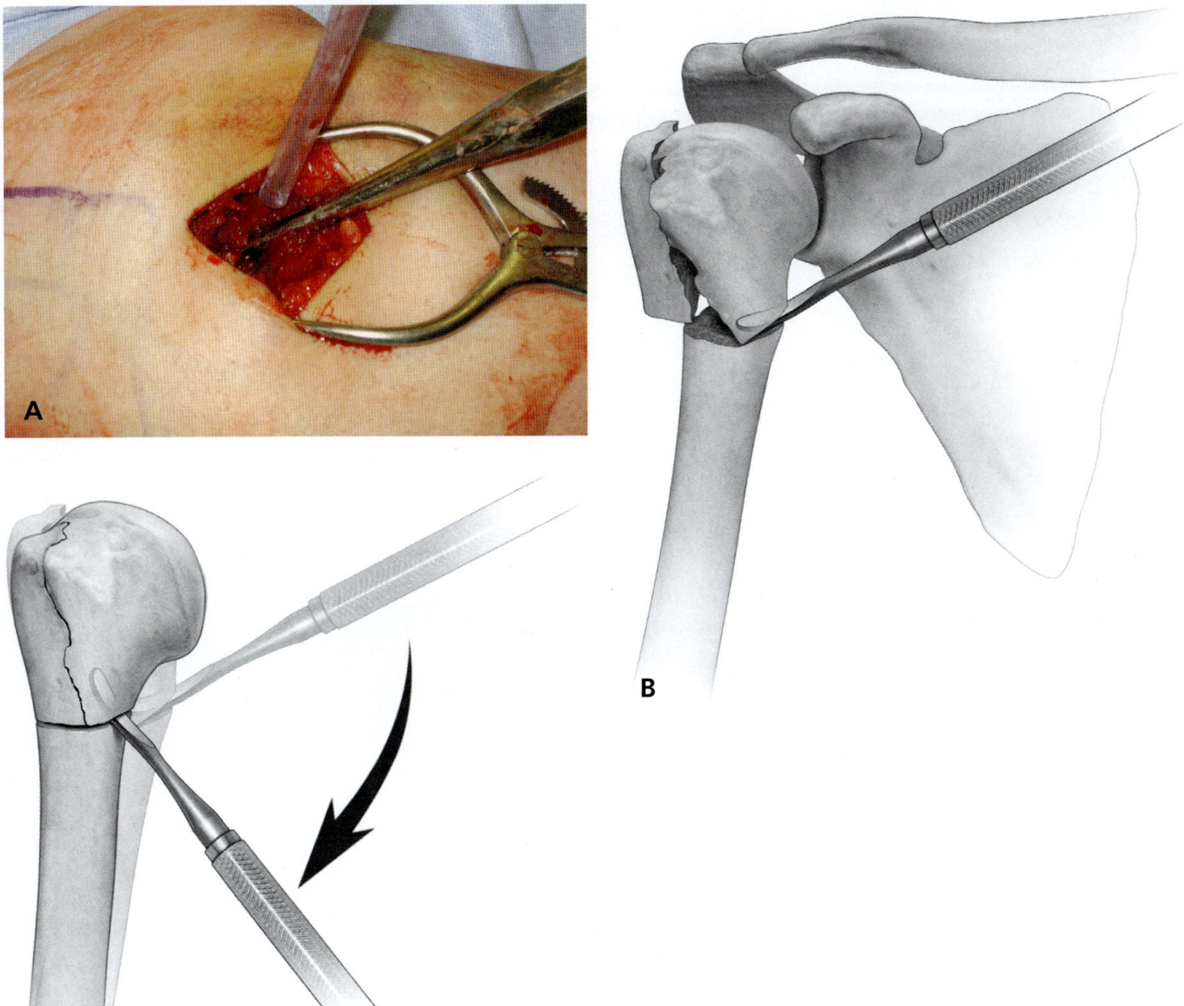

Figure 6.6 Clinical photograph **(A)** and schematic demonstrating the "shoe-horn" maneuver **(B** and **C)** to reduce the common antero-medial deformity in fractures of the surgical neck.

With the head–shaft segment reduced, the greater tuberosity fragment, if present, can be manually reduced. The displaced fragment is found posterosuperiorly to the humeral head due to the external rotation and abduction imposed by supraspinatus, infraspinatus, and teres minor. External rotation and abduction is needed during this reduction technique. The greater tuberosity is grasped with a Kocher forceps and reduced anteriorly and distally into its anatomic position and held with provisional K-wires inserted away from future plate placement. Provisional sutures are useful in the cuff to help control and manipulate the fragment. We always secure the rotator cuff attached to the greater and lesser tuberosity fragment with nonabsorbable stay sutures.

VALGUS TYPE

A valgus-impacted fracture is reduced by applying a medial force to the superolateral aspect of the humeral head and using the medial soft tissues as a hinge. In the absence of lateral displacement of the humeral head fragment, the humeral head is likely to remain viable. Caution is needed in order to maintain the intact medial soft tissue attachment often found between the humeral head and shaft. Several instruments can be used such as a blunt dissector, but after disimpaction we usually prefer using our thumb to gently elevate the humeral

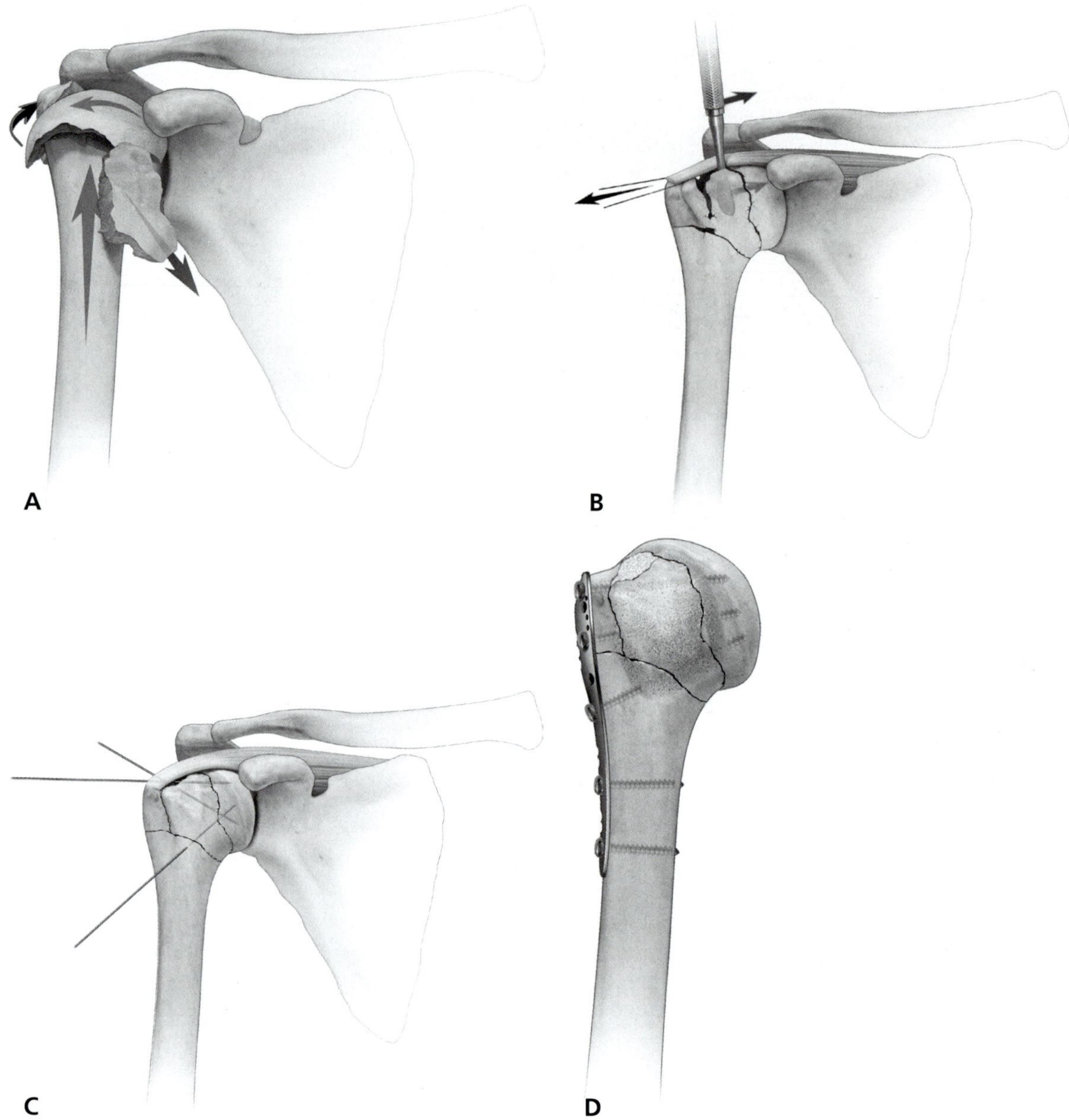

Figure 6.7 In valgus fracture patterns **(A)**, the humeral head is elevated toward the glenoid with an elevator **(B)** and maintained with K-wires **(C)**. The rotator cuff sutures are used to mobilize the tuberosity fragments into position. The plate is then inserted and screws are placed into the humeral head. Bone graft substitute may be used to fill large metaphyseal voids to augment support of the humeral head fragment **(D)**.

head articular fragment onto the glenoid surface, using the glenoid as a template (Fig. 6.7). Lateral displacement must be avoided since the medial periosteal vessels that perfuse the articular segment may be ruptured, and avascular necrosis (AVN) is more likely to result. Once the humeral head is reduced to approximately 130 degrees of head–neck angle, the greater tuberosity is pulled out from the posterior aspect of the shoulder and brought back into its bed, after which it serves to maintain reduction of the humeral head. Temporary stabilization is achieved with 1.6- or 2-mm K-wires that are inserted from the GT fragment across the fracture into the calcar. Nonabsorbable sutures are then passed through the posterior and superior rotator cuff tendons and secured to the plate to add additional mechanical support.

The most common pitfall is over-reducing the greater tuberosity into the void created by the severe impaction of the cancellous osteopenic bone. This leads to altered rotator cuff

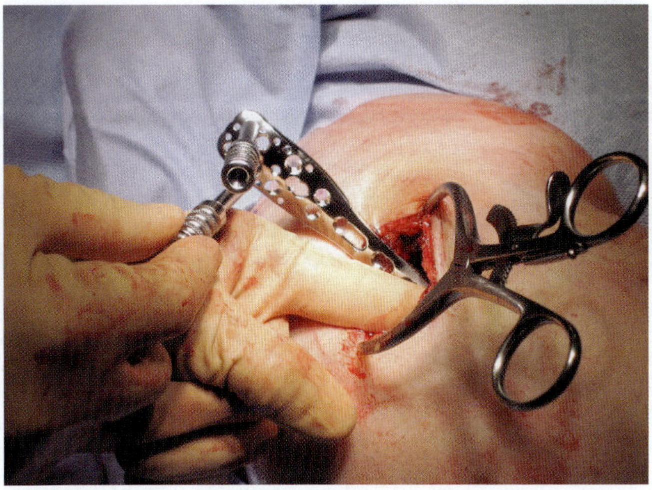

Figure 6.8 Once the position of the axillary nerve is clearly identified, the plate is inserted along the humeral shaft, deep to the axillary nerve.

biomechanics with reduced offset. Calcium phosphate cement may be a solution to fill in the void, as it provides good resistance to axial loading and head collapse. The superior locking screws engaging in the best bone are the most important to prevent collapse and loss of reduction in valgus.

PLATE INSERTION

During plate insertion, the most important consideration is to keep the plate directly along the bone to prevent entrapment of the axillary nerve under the plate. The *first step* is to identify the axillary nerve and to protect it from entrapment by positioning the index finger on the nerve during insertion of the plate on the proximal humerus (Fig. 6.8). If the nerve is not palpated, a separate deltopectoral approach or an extended AL acromial should be used. Furthermore, the attachable insertion guide block that is present on several plating systems cannot be safely used because the distal edge impinges directly on the axillary nerve when insertion is percutaneous. Locking screw sleeves can be anchored into the proximal holes to perform as a handle to aid with insertion. Similar low-profile, precontoured locking plates with multiple screw options can also be used. Plates with targeting devices are available to facilitate distal screw insertion but can be bulky and limit the access to tactile palpation and reduction maneuvers.

The plate is positioned on the proximal lateral humerus with the angulation of the plate positioned at the inferior portion of the greater tuberosity. To prevent acromial impingement, the superior edge of the plate should sit 5 mm lower than the greater tuberosity. To control the articular fragment, we typically use two joysticks (2-mm K-wires) starting medial to the greater tuberosity getting purchase in the articular fragment (Fig. 6.8). Once satisfactory plate placement is attained, the proximal fracture fragments are provisionally fixed by placing a K-wire, drill bit, or a fully threaded cancellous screw through any one of the proximal humeral head screw holes and into the humeral head.

PLATE REDUCTION

Anatomically contoured proximal humerus plates may be used as a reduction tool to buttress the humeral head. Through the distal window, a conventional 3.5-mm screw or a push–pull device is tightened slowly to bring the diaphysis in close contact with the plate (Fig. 6.9). The length of this screw needs to be long enough to engage the far cortex and may be exchanged for a shorter screw after additional screws are in place. The plate may translate on the diaphysis in the sagittal plane during this indirect reduction technique. An axillary view should be checked at this point to ensure the sagittal plane reduction and plate position remains acceptable. Adding a K-wire (or a second cortical screw) in a distal hole prevents

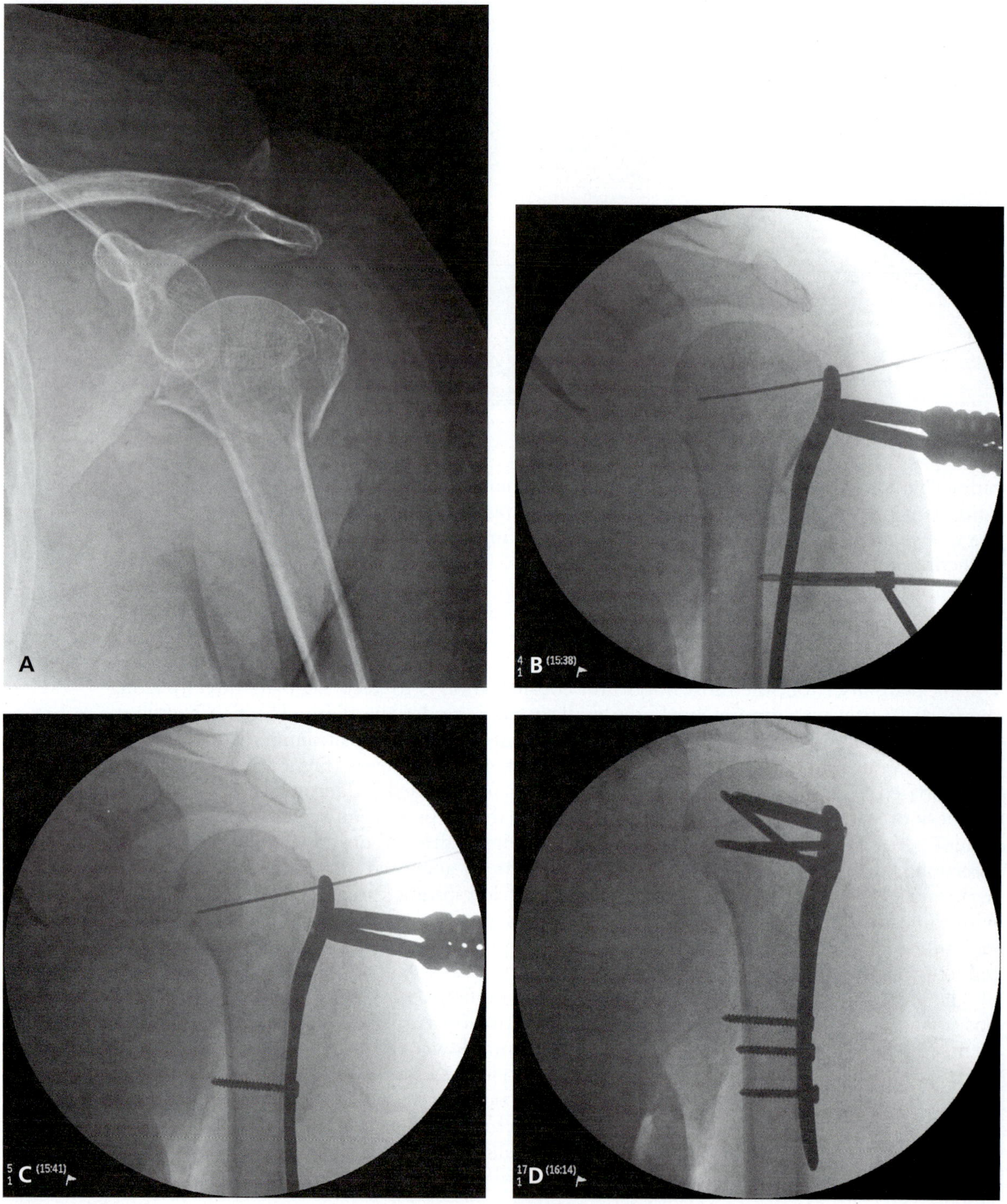

Figure 6.9 A very effective reduction technique is using the plate as a reduction tool. This is a case example of an elderly patient with a valgus fracture **(A)**. The humeral head is elevated and the tuberosities are reduced. The plate is then inserted **(B)**. A cortical reduction screw is then placed through the plate into the humeral shaft to reduce the bone to the plate **(C)**. Final fluoroscopic views show anatomic reduction **(D)**.

rotation. Readjustment and fine tuning the humeral head position is possible with the K-wires (joysticks) fixed in the articular fragment before fixation with screws. If varus still persists, a pointed reduction forceps is engaged between the superior aspect of the tuberosity and the plate to derotate the head by creating compression. Tactile verification through both incisions and fluoroscopy must confirm the plate position on the shaft and lateral surface of the head before proceeding to definitive fixation. Incorrect placement of the plate to far anteriorly on the humeral head and residual apex anterior angulation are common pitfalls to remember. With a deltoid splitting approach, the plate should sit on the lateral surface and not the usual AL surface close to the bicipital groove recommended for the deltopectoral approach.

DEFINITIVE PLATE FIXATION

The *second step* to prevent axillary nerve injury is to fix the plate with screws positioned in the safe zone. The most proximal six holes and two most distal screws (those distal to the slot hole) pose little danger to the axillary nerve. In the proximal window, a minimum of four locking screws are inserted and tightened sequentially. Additional screws should be added in osteopenic bone or with comminution of the calcar. Abduction of the arm offers better visualization through this mobile window especially for the screw in row D. A total of six proximal locking screws can be safely secured if desired (Fig. 6.10).

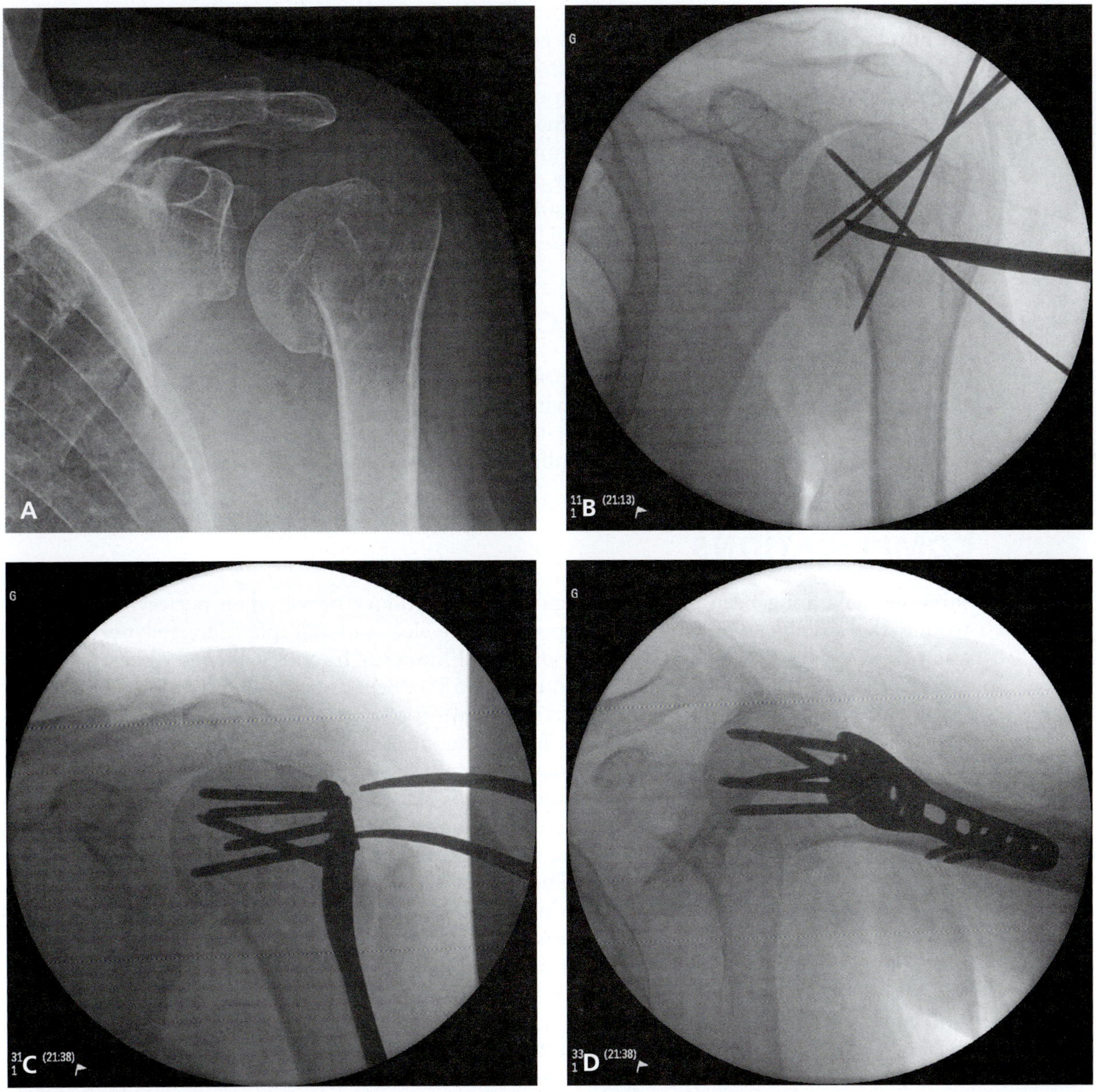

Figure 6.10 Case example of a patient with a varus injury pattern **(A)**. The humeral head is reduced with an elevator, and maintained with K-wires **(B)**. Screws are placed into the head through the proximal window **(C)**, and subsequently placed into the diaphysis through the distal window. An overall excellent reduction was obtained **(D)**.

The most common pitfall with the use of locking plates in the proximal humerus is iatrogenic screw penetration into the articular surface. To prevent the severe morbidity of such a complication, we recommend the following.

1. Exceptional vigilance while placing subchondral humeral head screws using live fluoroscopic imaging throughout a full range of motion. Every screw needs to be verified to be extra-articular individually, especially with divergent screws.
2. Tap drilling to enhance proprioceptive feedback and to avoid penetrating the subchondral bone. In osteopenic bone, we drill the near cortex and then use the depth gage with a twisting motion to advance up to the subchondral bone eliminating the risk of joint perforation.
3. Shorten screws by subtracting 3 to 5 mm from the measured screw length allowing some fracture settling. Additional screws can be used to compensate for reduced stability.
4. After surgery, fracture collapse can also lead to screw penetration. Optimizing stability by achieving adequate medial support and avoiding varus is essential.

In the distal window, three 3.5-mm conventional screws that usually measure 26 to 28 mm are used to secure the plate distally. In osteopenic bone with thin cortices, one 3.5 mm locking screw may be added to protect the cortical screws from shear forces.

Once fixation is stable, live fluoroscopy with full rotation confirms the correct placement and length of each screw. All temporary fixation devices are carefully removed and/or replaced. Tension band sutures (the same sutures used to initially mobilize the tuberosities) around both tuberosity fragments are anchored to the plate holes. The deltoid fascia and subcutaneous tissues are repaired with a nonabsorbable suture, and the skin edges reapproximated with staples or a running subcuticular stitch. A sterile dressing is applied, and the arm placed in a sling.

REHABILITATION PROTOCOL

Patients are started on immediate postoperative active range of motion of the shoulder and elbow. A standardized protocol begins with pendulum exercises and then active-assisted exercises until clinical and radiographic evidence of healing. At this point, the addition of strengthening and proprioception exercises are allowed which typically takes about 8 to 12 weeks.

COMPLICATIONS

Surgeons have long been cautioned regarding the axillary nerve when performing surgery around the shoulder. Visser et al.[10] reported that electromyography-detected nerve injury was present in up to 82% of displaced proximal humerus fractures treated operatively and nonoperatively; the axillary nerve was injured in 58%. Because the deltoid muscle is the main flexor and abductor of the arm, loss of innervation to this muscle can significantly affect patient function. Before employing this percutaneous technique clinically, we conducted an anatomic study on 12 cadaveric specimens to evaluate its feasibility and safety. To prevent injury to the axillary nerve with this technique, it is important that the axillary nerve be identified and protected by positioning the index finger on the nerve during insertion of the plate on the proximal humerus. Furthermore, screws should be positioned in the safe zone away from the course of the axillary nerve. The extended AL acromial approach of the proximal humerus was recently described by Gardner et al.[5] as a minimally invasive approach for plate fixation. This anatomic study has demonstrated the predictability of the position of the axillary nerve as it crosses the anterior deltoid raphe. Subsequently, their approach was used in 16 patients with no axillary nerve injury.

In our series of 34 patients, the axillary nerve was identified in all cases under the deltoid 1 to 3 cm distal to the end of the proximal wound margin. There was no case of axillary nerve palsy or paresthesia. Two reoperations were performed: One to remove an intra-articular screw and one for plate removal for acromial impingement. No cases of AVN were identified at follow-up of 19 months. However, fracture configuration is the most important determining factor for developing AVN and the selection of two- and three-part fractures with a high proportion of impacted valgus-type fracture may explain the absence of AVN. This selection of only fractures with good prognosis may also explain the overall low complication rate like loss of reduction and screw penetration.

Recent studies have reported that one of the most frequent complications with locking plates in the proximal humerus is screw penetration missed at the time of surgery or postoperatively with fracture collapse. Techniques to minimize this complication are discussed earlier in the text. With the unpredictable functional results of shoulder hemiarthroplasty, many surgeons are expanding indications for ORIF, including four-part fractures, head-split patterns, and fracture–dislocations. Higher complication rate should be expected with these fractures.

OUTCOME

Patients can expect to return to a function close to normal after percutaneous plate fixation of the selected proximal humerus fractures (surgical neck and valgus-impacted). Functional outcome results corresponded to a normal age-adjusted score. The average Constant-Murley score increased from 50 to 77 during the first year and plateaued at 82 (SD16). The DASH score improved from 41 to 26 between 2 weeks and the final follow-up (mean follow-up: 19 months). With analysis of subcategories of the Constant score, it was observed that relative scores were better in pain (85%) and in power (87%) categories compared with activity (76%) and mobility (75%) subscales. The patients had an average range of motion of 143 degrees of shoulder abduction (range, 110 to 180 degrees) and 155 degrees of anterior flexion (range, 110 to 180 degrees). All 34 fractures healed within the first 6 months. There was no loss of reduction or hardware failure. Similar results were published in two recent studies using percutaneous plating.[9,11]

REFERENCES

1. Kannus P, Palvanen M, Niemi S, et al. Osteoporotic fractures of the proximal humerus in elderly Finnish persons: Sharp increase in 1970–1998 and alarming projections for the new millennium. *Acta Orthop Scand.* 2000;71:465–470.
2. Gibson JN, Handoll HH, Madhok R. Interventions for treating proximal humeral fractures in adults. *Cochrane Database Syst Rev.* 2001;(1):CD000434.
3. Laflamme GY, Rouleau DM, Berry GK, et al. Percutaneous humeral plating of fractures of the proximal humerus: Results of a prospective multicenter clinical trial. *J Orthop Trauma.* 2008;22(3): 153–158.
4. Robinson CM, Khan L, Akhtar A, et al. The extended deltoid-splitting approach to the proximal humerus. *J Orthop Trauma.* 2007;21(9):657–662.
5. Gardner MJ, Griffith MH, Dines JS, et al. The extended anterolateral acromial approach allows minimally invasive access to the proximal humerus. *Clin Orthop Relat Res.* 2005;434:123–129.
6. Smith J, Berry G, Laflamme Y, et al. Percutaneous insertion of a proximal humeral locking plate: An anatomic study. *Injury.* 2007;38(2):206–211.
7. Gardner MJ, Weil Y, Barker JU, et al. The importance of medial support in locked plating of proximal humerus fractures. *J Orthop Trauma.* 2007;21(3):185–191.
8. Agudelo J, Schürmann M, Stahel P, et al. Analysis of efficacy and failure in proximal humerus fractures treated with locking plates. *J Orthop Trauma.* 2007;21(10):676–681.
9. Röderer G, Erhardt J, Graf M, et al. Clinical results for minimally invasive locked plating of proximal humerus fractures. *J Ortho Trauma.* 2010;24(7):400–406.
10. Visser CP, Coene LN, Brand R, et al. Nerve lesions in proximal humeral fractures. *J Shoulder Elbow Surg.* 2001;10(5):421–427.
11. Gallo RA, Hughes T, Altman G. Percutaneous plate fixation of two- and three-part proximal humerus fractures. *Orthopedics.* 2008;31(3):237–242.

CHAPTER 7

Minimally Invasive Operative Treatment of Displaced Midclavicular Fractures with a Titanium Elastic Nail

Axel Jubel

INDICATIONS (Table 7.1)

Elastic Stable Intramedullary Nailing (ESIN) is indicated in displaced fractures of the central third of the clavicle (Allman type I)[1] in skeletally mature patients. Displacement is defined as the absence of cortical contact between the main proximal and distal fragments. Conservative treatment of displaced fractures in adults is associated with an increased risk of malunion and nonunion.[2–5]

In polytraumatized patients, operative stabilization of mid-third clavicle fractures may be necessary to facilitate nursing and to maximize the recovery and rehabilitation potential. In open clavicle fractures, fracture stabilization should be done after soft tissue and osseous debridement to reduce the incidence of infection. In fractures with associated vascular injury, ESIN is indicated after vascular repair, to prevent repair damage by fracture motion. Patients with additional lower extremity fractures that do not allow full weight-bearing can be mobilized on crutches after operative stabilization with an elastic titanium nail.

Regarding the fracture pattern, strong indications for ESIN are all types of simple fractures (two fragments) and simple wedge comminuted fractures.[6–8] According to the OTA/AO classification system[9,10] the indications for ESIN comprise type B1 and type B2 fractures which correspond to type 2B1 fractures of the Robinson[11] classification system.

Indications for ESIN in complex or comminuted fractures (type B3 of the OTA/AO classification or type 2B2 of the Robinson classification system) or fractures of the proximal or distal third of the clavicle (Allman type II and III)[12] are less clear. In these patterns, there is a high risk of secondary shortening due to the fact that this implant is not interlocked and is length unstable, relying on intact cortices to prevent shortening. These fracture patterns are typically treated with plate fixation.[8] In proximal and distal third clavicle fractures, generally there is not sufficient length of the short fragment to provide stable fixation of an intramedullary implant.

Accurate radiographic assessment of the clavicle is essential for correct analysis of displacement and the fracture type. The clavicle should ideally be radiographed in two projections: Upright anteroposterior with the arm hanging to allow gravity to demonstrate true displacement of the fragments, and 30 to 45 degrees craniocaudal tilt projection. The fracture can then be correctly classified according to the OTA/AO or Robinson classification system and the treatment indications determined.

The ESIN procedure is also indicated in symptomatic hypertrophic nonunions after midclavicular fractures as an alternative to plate fixation,[13] whereas pathologic fractures and fractures in osteoporotic bone are best treated with plate fixation.

TABLE 7.1. Indications

	Good Indications	No Indications
Localization	Central 4/5th	Lateral and medial fractures
Fracture Type	Simple and wedge comminuted	Complex comminuted
Nonunion	Hypertrophic nonunion	Atrophic nonunion

PATIENT POSITIONING

The patient is positioned on a radiolucent operating table in the supine position. Clear intraoperative imaging in two orthogonal projections must be possible, which can be particularly difficult with the patient in the beach chair position. An image intensification device or C-arm is mandatory for correct placement of the titanium nail. A folded, soft radiolucent bump placed under the scapula allows for shoulder retraction, facilitating both closed and open reduction.

To have sufficient room to rotate the image intensifier, the table must be positioned such that the C-arm can be brought in ipsilateral to the fracture. This may require rotating the OR table so that the patient's head is directed toward the middle of the operating room and the table pushed on its stand also toward the middle of the room (Fig. 7.1). Thus, the clavicle can be imaged in two planes perpendicular to each other (craniocaudal and caudocranial). These are similar to pelvic inlet and outlet views. Long ventilation tubing may be necessary for this position. The anesthesiologist and anesthesia machine are placed at the foot of the patient. Alternatively, the table may remain straight with the patient's head at the anesthesia machine, the patient's healthy arm tucked by the side, and the C-arm brought in from the contralateral side. The downside of this positioning is the surgeon needs to work under the C-arm.

The arm and the entire shoulder girdle on the injured side is sterilely prepared and draped, including the sternal notch medially (Fig. 7.2). This allows the arm to be manipulated to facilitate indirect reduction maneuvers. The arm is initially placed beside the body. The surgeon stands on the uninjured side to introduce the nail from medial to lateral. The assistant and the base of the C-arm are positioned on the injured side.

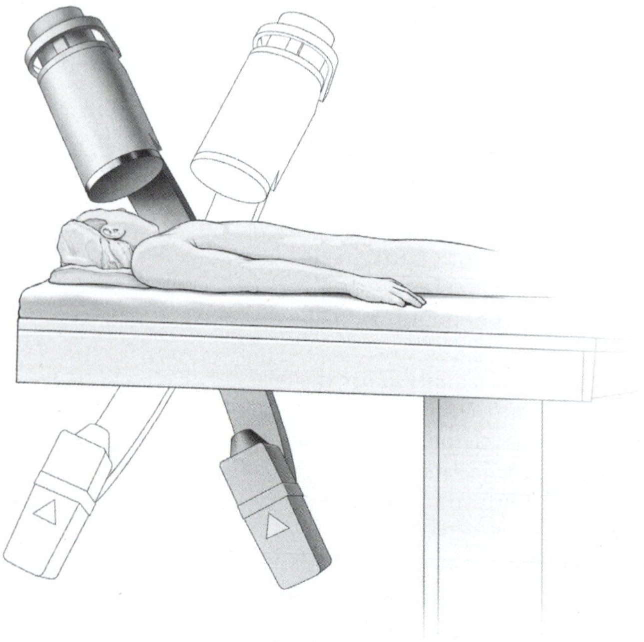

Figure 7.1 The patient is positioned supine on a radiolucent table. The C-arm is brought in from the ipsilateral side and tilted cranial and caudal to obtain near orthogonal views of the clavicle.

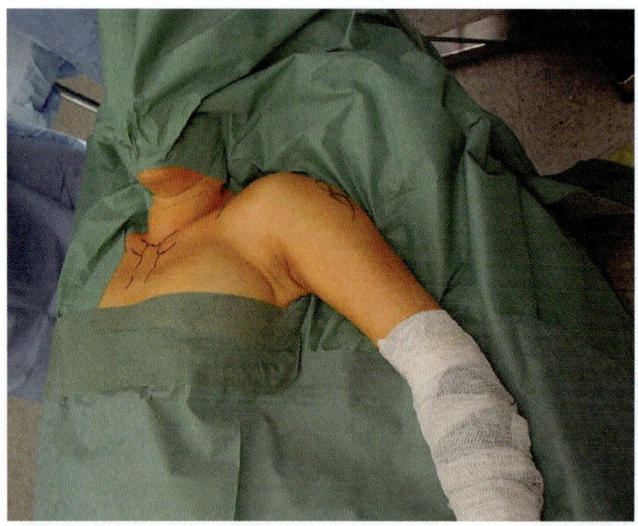

Figure 7.2 The patient's entire upper extremity, including the contralateral sternoclavicular joint, is prepared and draped.

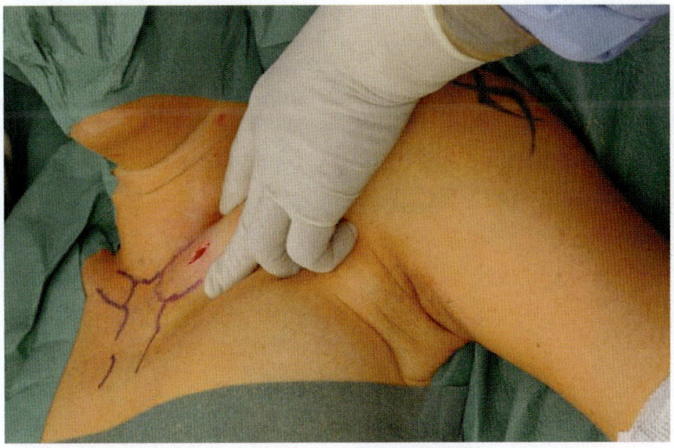

Figure 7.3 A 1- to 2-cm skin incision is made just lateral to the sternoclavicular joint on the injured side.

SURGICAL APPROACH

A skin incision of 1 to 2 cm is made just lateral to the sternoclavicular joint (Fig. 7.3). By applying manual pressure on the supraclavicular fossa, the skin is displaced cranially preventing the incision from being directly over the end of the nail. The subcutaneous fat is dissected down to the clavicle with scissors and the ventral cortex of the clavicle is exposed without disrupting the periosteum. Two small Langenbeck retractors are inserted and the superior and inferior margins of the sternal clavicle are identified. Approximately 2 cm lateral to the sternoclavicular joint, a 2.5-mm drill guide is placed over the center of the clavicle, and a unicortical hole is drilled into the ventral cortex (Fig. 7.4). At this position, the ventral clavicle cortex is enveloped by skin and subcutaneous tissue only. There are no muscle fibers or tendinous origins or insertions. The apex of the dome-shaped cortex is identified to ensure the drill is positioned in the center of the radius. This minimizes the risk of perforation of the posterior cortex. The 2.5-mm drill hole is then enlarged using a 30-degree angulated awl.

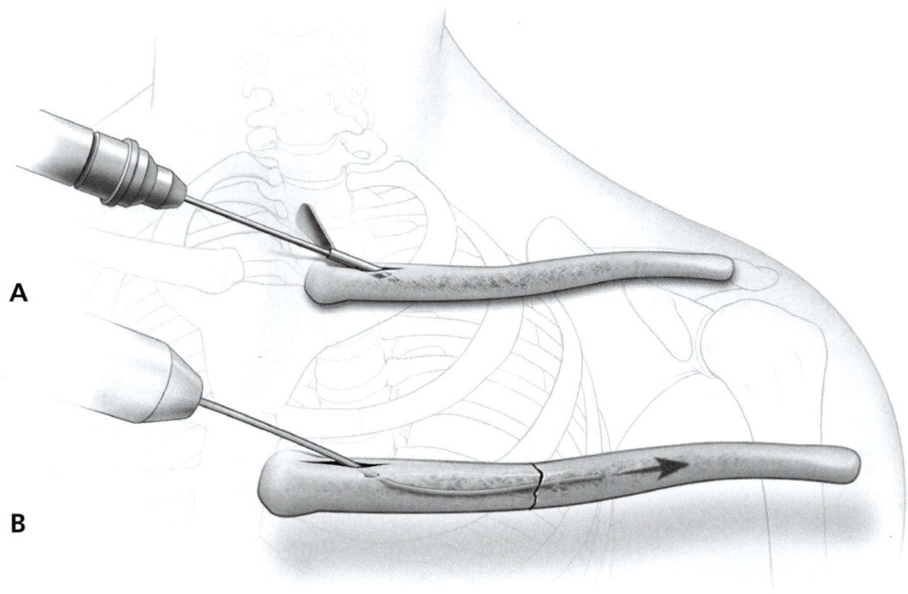

Figure 7.4 A 2.5- or 3.5-mm drill is inserted unicortically at a laterally directed 45-degree angle **(A)**. This serves as the eventual nail insertion portal **(B)**.

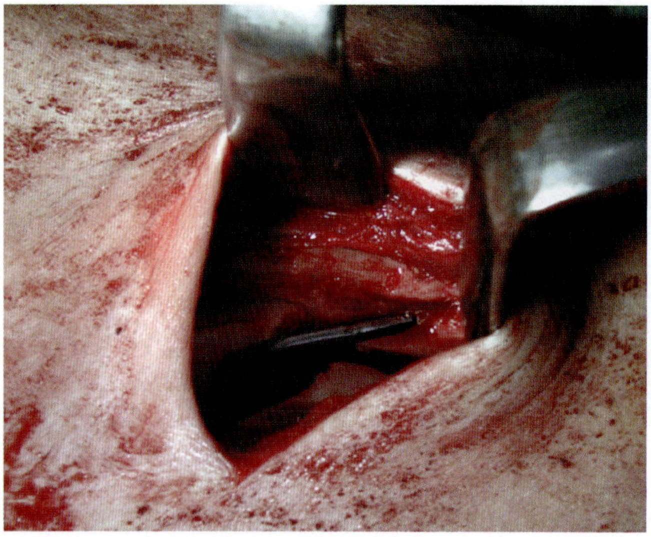

Figure 7.5 Open reduction through a small incision is required in many acute fractures. The nail tip can be seen here at the fracture site prior to reduction.

OPEN REDUCTION

Closed reduction maneuvers are attempted initially. Shoulder retraction can provide a distraction force at the fracture site, restoring length. Typically the medial fragment is displaced proximally due to the pull of the strap muscles, and manual force can help restore this deformity. Fractures that are over 1-week old can be difficult to reduce with closed methods.

If closed reduction is unsuccessful, a 2- to 3-cm long additional incision is made in the Langer line at the lateral end of the medial main fragment. The subcutaneous fat is incised together with the underlying platysma muscle leaving thick soft tissue flaps. With acute fractures, the platysma muscle, the fascia, and the periosteum over the fracture site are often disrupted and do not require any further division (Fig. 7.5). The middle branches of the supraclavicular nerve run under the platysma muscle. There is no need for dissection of these nerves. Together with the platysma muscle the branches can be secured under a small Langenbeck retractor or a lid hook. In some cases they need to be incised to obtain optimal access to the fracture site. In many cases, trapezius muscle fibers are interposed between the main fragments. These muscle fibers are carefully removed using an elevator. Muscle and soft tissue attachments are elevated only as needed to visualize the fracture site. Small butterfly fragments usually found anteriorly should be left intact to their soft tissue attachments.

REDUCTION TECHNIQUES AND FIXATION

Acute Fractures

Under image intensification the smallest diameter of the medullary canal is estimated to assure correct nail size. As a general rule, the nail diameter should be two-thirds of the narrowest diameter of the medullary canal. If the fit is too loose, fixation may be compromised and migration or secondary loss of reduction is possible. If the fit is too tight, iatrogenic comminution or difficulty inserting the nail may occur. Generally a 2.5-mm diameter nail (in women) and a 3-mm diameter (in men) provide sufficient stability.

For insertion, the titanium is mounted on a Jacobs chuck with a T-handle or a specialized insertion chuck (Fig. 7.4B). With oscillating movements by the surgeon's hand, the nail is advanced up to the fracture site without perforating the cortex. The bent tip of the nail acts as runner and prevents penetration of the dorsal cortex (Fig. 7.6). To ensure correct placement of the nail, fluoroscopic control is used. During nail passage through the medial fragment, the angled nail tip typically needs to be angled anteriorly to "bounce" of the posterior cortex, due to the anterior starting portal.

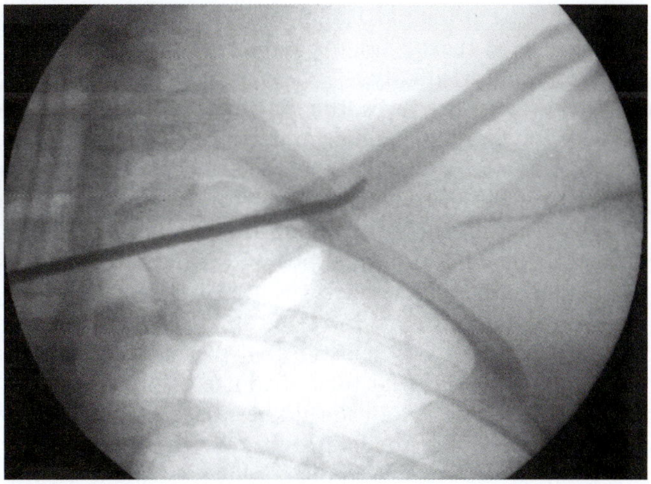

Figure 7.6 Fluoroscopy taken immediately after insertion of the nail into the medullary canal. The tip serves as a runner and prevents perforation of the opposite cortex.

The reduction is effected indirectly by manipulation of the medial fragment with the nail mounted on the chuck. The chuck acts as a joystick and the lateral end of the medial fragment can easily be moved in all directions. The manipulation of lateral fragment is effected by moving the free draped arm. External rotation of the arm leads to an anterior movement of the medial end of the lateral fragment, whereas internal rotation results in posterior translation. External rotation and elevation of the arm leads to a dorsal rotation and caudal movement of the lateral fragment. Forearm traction in a caudal direction and adduction leads to cranial displacement of the medial end of the lateral clavicle. Depending on the required displacement, the arm is manipulated by the assistant, while the surgeon manipulates the medial fragment with the chuck. In addition, the bent tip of the nail can be used as a reduction finger. The accuracy of the reduction can be directly visualized or palpated and secured under the skin between the thumb and the index finger. Serrated reduction forceps that crush the periosteum should be avoided.

The insertion and advancement of the nail into the lateral fragment is checked under image intensification in the craniocaudal and caudocranial planes; the planes should be orthogonal to each other. In transverse fractures, closed reduction is generally successful. In the presence of long oblique fractures or wedge comminuted fractures especially with a displaced vertical butterfly fragment closed reduction can be difficult to achieve.

If the closed reduction fails in oblique fractures, an attempt can be made to align the fragments with a percutaneously placed sharp reduction forceps (Fig. 7.7). If this maneuver is unsuccessful, a 3- to 4-cm long additional incision is made over the fracture site to enable a direct manipulation of the main fragments and the nail tip. The soft tissues are dissected

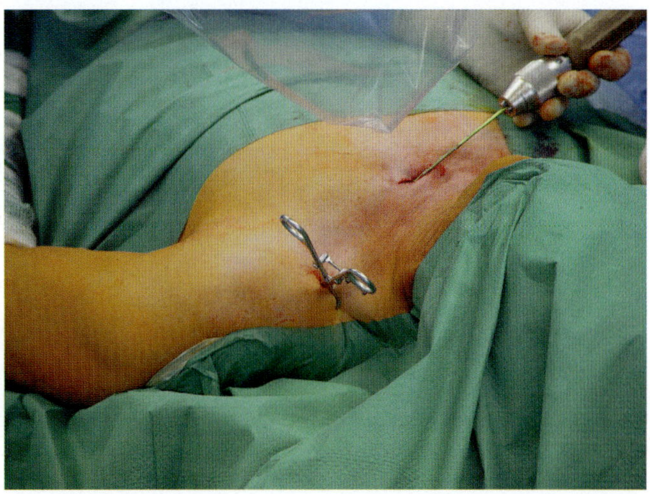

Figure 7.7 Percutaneous reduction can be performed with a sharp reduction forceps in oblique or spiral fracture patterns.

to expose the principal fragments. At this point the "personality" of the fracture is reassessed and the reason for the failure of closed reduction is analyzed. Each case needs to be approached individually.

In transverse fractures, the tip of the nail is introduced into the entrance of the medullary canal of the lateral fragment under direct view and palpation. If the medullary canal is obliterated, an opening should be made either with a 2.5-mm drill bit or a small awl without perforating the cortex. The ability to work with the proximal and distal fragments is facilitated by elevating the ends of the main fragments through the incision with an elevator or a small bone forceps. In addition, exposing the lateral fragment is facilitated by external rotation of the arm. Long oblique fractures are often best reduced using one or two sharp small bone forceps to secure reduction.

After reduction, the elastic nail is advanced into the lateral fragment using a torsional motion while advancing for a distance of 4 to 5 cm past the fracture site, just lateral to the conoid tubercle. The nail should be seated a minimum of 3 cm distal to the fracture to ensure adequate fixation of the lateral fragment.

Although the clavicle appears almost straight on the caudocranial, or "outlet," view, on the craniocaudal, or "inlet," view, the bone appears as an S-shaped double curve when viewed from above. Approximately 2 cm proximal to the lateral end, at the conoid process, the clavicle turns anteriorly (Fig. 7.8A, B). In addition, the pyramidal- or prismatic-shaped cross section of the medial part of the clavicle becomes flatter at the lateral end, as the cylindrical medullary canal becomes obliterated. Care must be taken to prevent dorsolateral cortex perforation at the dorsal convexity of the lateral fragment. Using fluoroscopic visualization in a craniocaudal view so that the clavicle can be seen from above, the tip of the nail may be placed precisely. To prevent cortex perforation the sharp tip of the nail is rotated away from the dorsal cortex so that it can glide like a runner on the inner surface.

In cases of wedge comminuted fractures, intercalary fragments are not detached from their soft tissue connections and are loosely reapproximated without internal fixation. Large vertically displaced butterfly fragments are carefully mobilized and reduced preserving the soft tissue attachments. Single and large butterfly fragments can be apposed to the main fracture fragments with sutures. For this fixation, a small elevator or a curved Overholt clamp is passed underneath the clavicle in an anterior to posterior direction. A no. 1 PDS (Ethicon) resorbable suture mounted on a CTX needle is passed through the soft tissue attachments of the butterfly fragment and passed around the medial main fragment. In these cases extreme care has to be used to avoid injury to the neurovascular structures and the pleural dome when passing the suture underneath the clavicle. The needle is directed toward the elevator that protects the underlying structures, or the suture may be grasped with a clamp and passed underneath the clavicle. To cerclage the butterfly fragment securely, one suture around each main fragment should be used. If more complex fracture comminution is discovered intraoperatively, the author recommends conversion to plate osteosynthesis.

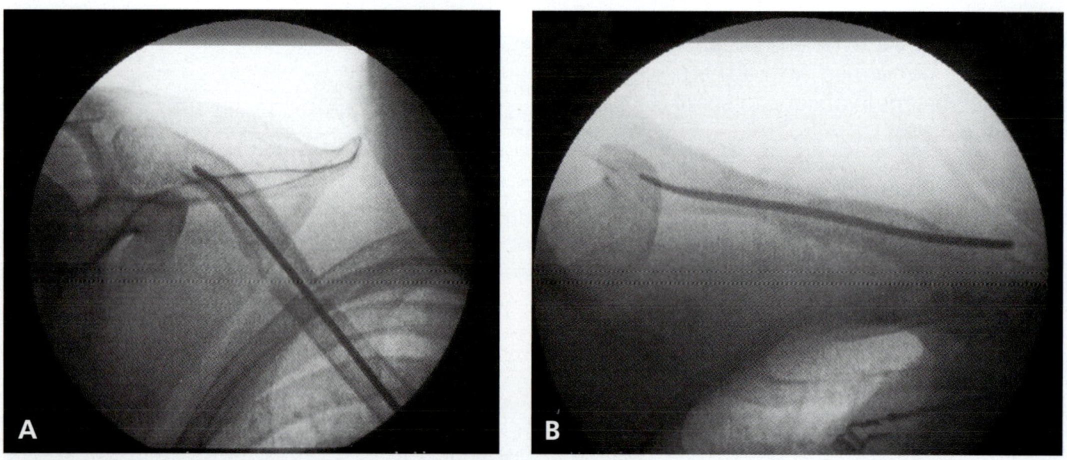

Figure 7.8 Craniocaudal **(A)** an anteroposterior view **(B)** showing final correct placement of the nail. Note the apex posterior curve of the distal clavicle.

After sufficient engagement of the lateral fragment, the nail can be shortened so that its end lies under the skin. The medial end of the nail is cut 2 to 3 mm proud of the cortex with a wire cutter. To prevent painful skin irritation it is essential that the protruding end is not bent. The intramedullary position of the nail is checked under image intensification and radiographs are taken.

The medial wound is irrigated and closed with one or two interrupted subcuticular stitches using 4-0 or 3-0 Monocryl sutures (resorbable) and Steri-Strips. If open reduction has been performed, it is important to close the periosteum and fascia overlying the fracture with simple or figure-of-eight no. 1 absorbable sutures. The platysma muscle is reapproximated using 2-0 absorbable sutures. Wound closure is performed with a subcutaneous 3-0 resorbable Monocryl suture and subcuticular interrupted stitches using 4-0 or 3-0 Monocryl sutures (resorbable) and Steri-Strips.

Nonunion

Symptomatic nonunion is treated with a similar technique as for acute fractures; however, several minor modifications are required. Positioning and draping is performed as described above. The iliac crest or alternative site should be prepared and draped for harvesting of autograft. The author uses the same surgical approach as used for open reduction as described above. The skin incision required is usually more extensive than for acute fractures. It is necessary to incise the periosteum overlying the nonunion site longitudinally. The nonunion is exposed circumferentially with a small elevator. Using a rongeur the fibrous tissue is removed to identify native healthy bone of the lateral and medial fracture ends. With a small osteotome, the hypertrophic callus is resected, morselized, and saved for use as a bone graft. The ends of the lateral and the medial fragments are decorticated at 1 to 2 cm. Under image intensification the main fragments are then reduced. ESIN is possible in cases only without a bony defect. If there is a bony defect that renders the nonunion site unstable, the author recommends a structural bone graft and plate fixation.

In nonunions, it is nearly always necessary to reconstitute the medullary canal. This can be achieved with a 2.5-mm drill bit. The nail is inserted from medial to lateral in the technique described for acute fractures. After stabilization, the morselized callus is packed about the fracture site. The periosteum and the platysma muscle are carefully reapproximated to assure a sufficient blood supply to the fracture site. Wound closure is performed as described above.

COMPLICATIONS (Table 7.2)

Severe intraoperative complications, like iatrogenic damage to the underlying vascular structures or injury to the pleural dome, are extremely rare and have never been observed by the author.[6,14] To the author's knowledge none of these complications have been described in the literature with elastic clavicle nailing thus far. Transient paresthesias can be observed in 1% to 2% of cases and may be caused by lengthening of the clavicle during the reduction maneuver or by reduction of vertically displaced butterfly fragments.[7,15]

The main intraoperative difficulty during this procedure is the inability to achieve a closed reduction, which occurs in 40% to 50% of patients.[7,15] In this situation, open reduction should be performed as described above. Functionally and subjectively there is no difference between closed and open reduction.[16]

Perforation of the cortex of the lateral fragment increases the risk of implant migration. In most instances of dorsolateral cortical perforation, a beach chair position has been used. In this patient position, a true craniocaudal fluoroscopic view is not possible. For this reason, the author highly recommends supine positioning as described above. If dorsolateral perforation occurs and is noticed intraoperatively, repositioning of the nail under fluoroscopic control is still possible. If dorsolateral perforation occurs and is not noticed, the nail is at risk of migrating laterally and tenting the skin within the first few postoperative weeks.

Determination of the correct entry point of the nail is essential. If the entry point of the nail is placed too medially there is a risk of irritation of the sternoclavicular joint. If the entry point is placed too laterally the anchorage of the nail in the proximal fragment may be compromised. Irritation of the sternocleidomastoid muscle may result from placing the nail too cranially.

TABLE 7.2. Problems and Complications

Problem/Complication	Frequency (%)	How to Prevent—What to Do?
Closed Reduction Impossible	40–50	Open reduction is necessary
Dorsolateral Cortex Perforation	2	Use image intensification to view the nail and the clavicle from above (Fig. 7.9A) Reposition the nail under fluoroscopic control
Clavicle Split	<1	Use correct nail size Never use a diameter >3.5 mm
Painful Skin Irritation Medial	4–8	Do not leave the end >2–3 mm Do not bend the end
Implant Migration	1	Use correct nail size Never use a diameter <2.5 mm
Implant Breakage	1	Never use a diameter <2.5 mm Do not use an end cap
Transient Nerve Palsy	1–2	Carefully mobilize vertical butterfly fragments
Loss of Reduction	2–3	Respect indications: No comminuted fractures
Operative Revision	2–4	Shortening of the protruding end Change to fixed angle plate
Nonunion	1	Do not leave gaps >5 mm Leave the nail in situ as long as the patient has no complaints
Refracture	<1	Leave the nail until definitive radiologic fracture healing is observed; 6–12 (24) mo

In adults, the diameter of the nail should not be <2.5 mm; otherwise adequate stability may not be achieved and, in addition, the implant may break or migrate. If the nail does not obtain sufficient cortical contact in the main fragments, there is a high risk of secondary shortening (telescoping effect) or medial migration.

The main postoperative problem is a painful skin irritation caused by the protruding end of the nail, typically medially if lateral perforation has not occurred. The medial end of the nail should be cut short such that it is just proud of the bone. It should not be bent or be longer than 5 mm to minimize the risk of skin irritation. In most cases, a bursa will develop within the first 6 weeks after surgery over the nail insertion site. When the bursa covers the nail end, the pain will be minimal. Painful soft tissue irritation of more than 6 weeks may be an indication for nail shortening under local anesthesia. Some authors advocate the use of small end caps to prevent skin irritation and nail migration.[17,18] According to the author's experience, these end caps are unnecessary. Inserting the cap increases the risk of either fracture to the anterior clavicle cortex at the insertion point of the nail or nail breakage. The large diameter of the cap itself can cause soft tissue irritations. An end cap may be advantageous in comminuted fracture types to minimize shortening, but this has yet to be demonstrated.

Nonunion (1% to 2%) is a rare complication after ESIN. If the patient has no pain or other complaints, the nail should be left in situ. According to the author's experience, radiologic fracture healing even after 2 years is possible. If the patient has pain at least 6 months postoperatively and radiographic union has not occurred, nonunion revision surgery is recommended. The nail should be removed and plate fixation is applied after excision of the nonunion and bone grafting.

Refracture is a known complication after plate fixation. After ESIN, this complication is extremely rare. To prevent refracture, it is essential to leave the implant in situ until complete radiologic bridging is observed in two planes. According to the author's experience this may often take 6 to 12 months.

REHABILITATION PROTOCOL

Postoperative immobilization or a sling after ESIN of midclavicular fractures is not necessary. Movements of the arm and return to activities of daily living should be based on the patients' comfort level. Strenuous activities such as pulling, lifting, or pushing should be

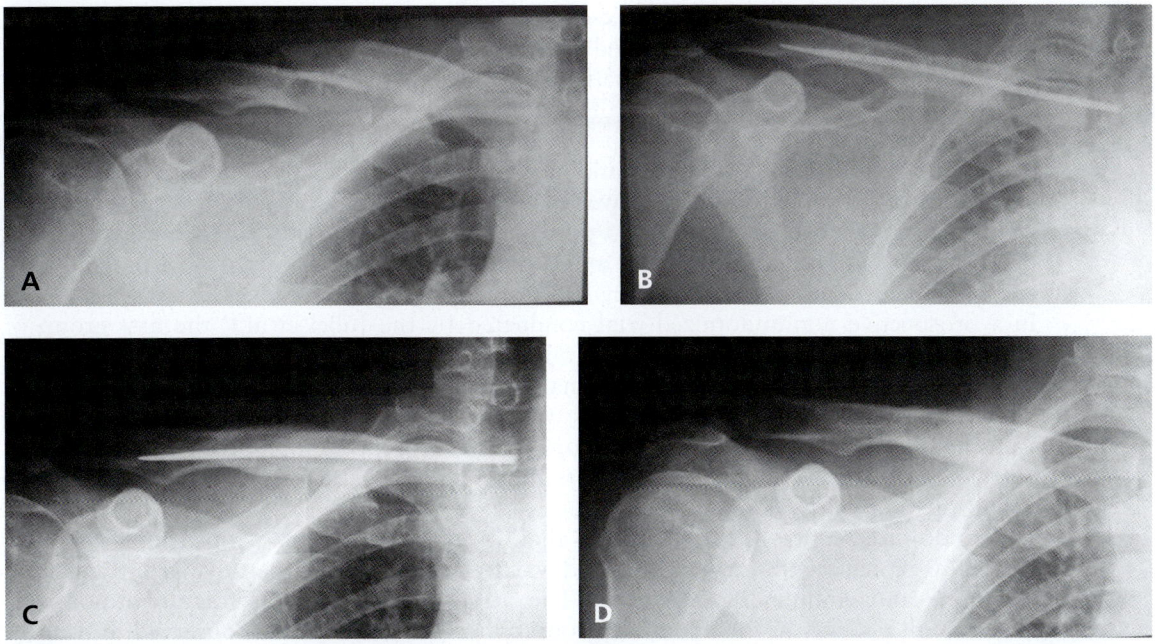

Figure 7.9 Anteroposterior view of a fractured clavicle in a 27-year-old man after a bicycle fall who sustained a simple midclavicular fracture **(A)**. Excellent reduction was achieved and intramedullary nailing was performed **(B)**. Six months postoperatively he had healed completely **(C)**. The nail was removed at 7 months postoperatively **(D)**, and he returned to full function.

avoided for 3 to 4 weeks. In the presence of midclavicular fractures with a butterfly fragment (OTA type B), active abduction and forward flexion of the arm is limited to 90 degrees for the first 6 weeks postoperatively to prevent rotation of the fragments. In patients with additional injuries of the lower limb, the use of forearm crutches is safe.

NAIL REMOVAL

Postoperative radiographs should be taken at 6 weeks, 3 months, and 6 months. In the absence of nail-related symptoms, the implant should not be removed before 6 months. When the patient requests nail removal, the implant can be removed in an ambulatory surgery setting after fracture healing (Fig. 7.9). Typically general anesthesia is used. Experience has shown that local anesthesia is too painful. The patient is placed in the supine position. The incision is made in the scar at the medial end of the clavicle. Generally the palpable end of the nail is covered by a bursa that should be excised. To remove the nail, extraction pliers with a ratchet lock specifically designed to grasp the nail facilitates removal.

OUTCOME

Outcome of ESIN in clavicle fractures has recently been reported by several authors.[6,12–15,19–28] Rehm et al.[7] reported a series of 132 patients with 136 clavicle fractures. There were 89 men and 43 women with an average age of 32.9 years. An open reduction was necessary in 54 fractures (41%). In most instances, a 3-mm nail was used. The average duration of fluoroscopy was 2.9 minutes. A significant reduction in pain was reported postoperatively. Before surgery the patients assessed their pain as being 72.4 ± 15 on a visual analog scale. On day 3, the level of pain had decreased to 18.9 ± 10 points. Simultaneously, a marked improvement in shoulder function could be observed. The abduction improved from 42 degrees preoperatively to 121 degrees postoperatively ($p < 0.001$). Nail removal was performed at an average of 7.6 months after surgery. In 106 patients, the shoulder function and the clinical result 12 months after implant removal using the Constant-Murley score were evaluated. The average score was 97.1 ± 3.5 points. In eight patients (6%), shortening of the nail at the insertion site was necessary 1 to 33 weeks after the index operation due to local pain and skin irritation. In three patients (2%) with a comminuted fracture, secondary shortening of the clavicle of 1.5 ± 0.5 cm was observed. In five patients, cortical perforation of the lateral fragment occurred. In one of these patients, nail migration into the lateral soft tissues was seen 2 months after surgery necessitating a premature removal of the nail through a lateral incision. Transient paresthesias of the arm and hand occurred in three patients. In this series one nonunion in a polytraumatized patient was observed.

Kettler et al.[22] reported a series of 95 patients. An open reduction was required in 56%. They observed a nonunion rate of 2% and a malunion rate of 8%. In 4% of patients, pin migration occurred and 5% required revision surgery.

In a prospective nonrandomized trial conducted by the Jubel et al.[15] the first group of 27 patients was treated nonoperatively, and the second group underwent intramedullary fixation with a titanium pin using a minimally invasive technique. At each follow-up time point, significantly ($p < 0.05$) better results were observed in the group of operated patients concerning shoulder function, Constant score, DASH score, personal satisfaction, pain, and cosmetic result. In the group treated with titanium nailing, return to work occurred in less than half the time of the nonoperative group.

In a randomized controlled trial, Smekal et al.[26] treated 30 patients with a simple shoulder sling and 30 patients with ESIN within 3 days after trauma. The operative group included both simple and comminuted fractures. The authors reported that fracture union was achieved in all patients in the operative group, whereas nonunion was observed in 3 of 30 patients (10%) of the nonoperative group. Two symptomatic malunions required corrective osteotomy in the nonoperative group. Medial nail protrusion was observed in seven cases in the operative group. Implant failure with revision surgery was necessary in two patients after additional trauma. DASH scores were lower in the operative group throughout the first 6 months and 2 years after the injury, with a significant difference during the first 18 weeks. Constant scores were significantly higher after 6 months and 2 years after intramedullary stabilization. Patients in the operative group showed a significant improvement of post-traumatic clavicular shortening; they were also more satisfied with cosmetic appearance and overall outcome.

Jubel et al.[13] conducted a prospective clinical trial to assess healing, clinical outcomes, and complications after intramedullary nailing of midshaft clavicular nonunions in 14 patients. Exclusion criteria were pathologic fractures, bony defects, previous operative treatment, atrophic and infected nonunions, and patients age <18 or >70 years. Results were evaluated after 3, 6, 12, and 18 months. At 3 months after surgery, pain, subjective satisfaction, Constant score, and DASH Score were significantly better than preoperatively ($p < 0.001$). There were no infections, no implant displacements or refractures. Based on these results, intramedullary fixation of midshaft clavicular nonunions after careful and critical patient selection is a safe minimally invasive surgical technique, producing excellent functional and cosmetic results without additional bone grafting.

REFERENCES

1. Allman FL Jr. Fractures and ligamentous injuries of the clavicle and its articulation. *J Bone Joint Surg Am.* 1967;49:774.
2. McKee MD, Pedersen EM, Jones C, et al. Deficits following nonoperative treatment of displaced midshaft clavicular fractures. *J Bone Joint Surg Am.* 2006;88:35.
3. Nowak J, Holgersson M, Larsson S. Sequelae from clavicular fractures are common: A prospective study of 222 patients. *Acta Orthop.* 2005;76:496.
4. Robinson CM, Court-Brown CM, McQueen MM, et al. Estimating the risk of nonunion following nonoperative treatment of a clavicular fracture. *J Bone Joint Surg Am.* 2004;86-A:1359.
5. Zlowodzki M, Zelle BA, Cole PA, et al. Treatment of acute midshaft clavicle fractures: Systematic review of 2144 fractures: On behalf of the Evidence-Based Orthopaedic Trauma Working Group. *J Orthop Trauma.* 2005;19:504.
6. Jubel A, Andermahr J, Schiffer G, et al. Elastic stable intramedullary nailing of midclavicular fractures with a titanium nail. *Clin Orthop Relat Res.* 2003;408:279.
7. Rehm KE, Andemahr J, Jubel A. Intramedullary nailing of midclavicular fractures with an elastic titanium nail. *Operat Orthop Traumatol.* 2004;16:365.

8. Schiffer G, Faymonville C, Skouras E, et al. Midclavicular fracture: Not just a trivial injury: Current treatment options. *Dtsch Arztebl Int.* 2010;107:711.
9. Marsh JL, Slongo TF, Agel J, et al. Fracture and dislocation classification compendium—2007: Orthopaedic Trauma Association classification, database and outcomes committee. *J Orthop Trauma.* 2007;21:S1.
10. Marsh JL. OTA fracture classification. *J Orthop Trauma.* 2009;23:551.
11. Robinson CM. Fractures of the clavicle in the adult. Epidemiology and classification. *J Bone Joint Surg Br.* 1998;80:476.
12. Jubel A, Andemahr J, Bergmann H, et al. Elastic stable intramedullary nailing of midclavicular fractures in athletes. *Br J Sports Med.* 2003;37:480.
13. Jubel A, Andermahr J, Weisshaar G, et al. [Intramedullary nailing (ESIN) in clavicular pseudoarthroses. Results of a prospective clinical trial]. *Unfallchirurg.* 2005;108:544.
14. Millett PJ, Hurst JM, Horan MP, et al. Complications of clavicle fractures treated with intramedullary fixation. *J Shoulder Elbow Surg.* 2011;20:86.
15. Jubel A, Andermahr J, Prokop A, et al. [Treatment of mid-clavicular fractures in adults. Early results after rucksack bandage or elastic stable intramedullary nailing]. *Unfallchirurg.* 2005;108:707.
16. Jubel A, Andemahr J, Rehm KE. Elastic stable intramedullary nailing of clavicle fractures. *Trauma und Berufskrankheit.* 2008;10:47.
17. Reissner L, Rillmann P, Ryf C, et al. [Treatment of clavicular mid-shaft fractures with TEN and end cap—reduced complications by careful operative technique and limited range of motion]. *Sport-Orthopädie Sport Traumatologie—Sports Orthopaedics and Traumatology.* 2010;4:247–253.
18. Frigg A, Rillmann P, Perren T, et al. Intramedullary nailing of clavicular midshaft fractures with the titanium elastic nail: Problems and complications. *Am J Sports Med.* 2009;37:352.
19. Jubel A, Andermahr J, Faymonville C, et al. [Reconstruction of shoulder-girdle symmetry after midclavicular fractures. Stable, elastic intramedullary pinning versus rucksack bandage]. *Chirurg.* 2002;73:978.
20. Jubel A, Andermahr J, Schiffer G, et al. [Technique of intramedullary osteosynthesis of the clavicle with elastic titanium nails]. *Unfallchirurg.* 2002;105:511.
21. Jubel A, Prokop A, Kress J, et al. Die elastisch stabile Marknagelung der Klavikulafraktur im mittleren Drittel. *Hefte zu der Unfallchirurg.* 1998;272:738.
22. Kettler M, Schieker M, Braunstein V, et al. Flexible intramedullary nailing for stabilization of displaced midshaft clavicle fractures: Technique and results in 87 patients. *Acta Orthop.* 2007;78:424.
23. Liu PC, Chien SH, Chen JC, et al. Minimally invasive fixation of displaced midclavicular fractures with titanium elastic nails. *J Orthop Trauma.* 2010;24:217.
24. Mueller M, Burger C, Florczyk A, et al. Elastic stable intramedullary nailing of midclavicular fractures in adults: 32 patients followed for 1-5 years. *Acta Orthop.* 2007;78:421.
25. Mueller M, Rangger C, Striepens N, et al. Minimally invasive intramedullary nailing of midshaft clavicular fractures using titanium elastic nails. *J Trauma.* 2008;64:1528.
26. Smekal V, Irenberger A, Struve P, et al. Elastic stable intramedullary nailing versus nonoperative treatment of displaced midshaft clavicular fractures-a randomized, controlled, clinical trial. *J Orthop Trauma.* 2009;23:106.
27. Walz M, Kolbow B, Auerbach F. [Elastic, stable intramedullary nailing in midclavicular fractures–a change in treatment strategies?]. *Unfallchirurg.* 2006;109:200.
28. Köstler W, Strohm PC, Jäger M, et al. Intramedullary stabilization of clavicle fractures. *Akt Traumatol.* 2006;35:308.

CHAPTER 8

Percutaneous Pelvic Ring Fixation

Jason M. Evans

INDICATIONS

Management of injured patients with pelvic ring disruptions is driven by both deformity and the treating physician's interpretation of pelvic stability. As such, the goals of operative intervention for pelvic fractures are based on reducing deformity and providing enough stability to the injured pelvis to allow for patient mobilization. Any discussion regarding the utility of minimally invasive stabilization must be made with respect to the necessity of obtaining a reduction. If the deformity cannot be corrected through minimally invasive techniques, then a formal open reduction should be utilized. This will frequently carry additional surgical morbidity, including the potential for increased blood loss and deep infection or wound dehiscence. Therefore, even when planning a percutaneous procedure, discussion should be had with the patient regarding the potential need to convert to an open procedure, and consent should be obtained for both options. In addition, patients with pelvic ring disruptions frequently have injuries to other organ systems. The coordinating intensive care service, typically the general trauma surgeons should also be made aware of the potential need to convert to an open procedure. In the common scenario of ongoing resuscitation or incomplete resuscitation, they may feel that a patient may be able to tolerate only a percutaneous procedure, and open discussion should then proceed regarding what may be the optimal timing for the procedure. Generally speaking, minimally invasive techniques can be considered for both anterior and posterior ring pathology, including both ligamentous injuries (symphysis and sacroiliac disruptions) and fractures (sacral fractures, posterior iliac fractures, pubic ramus fractures).

Pelvic ring disruptions with minimal displacement are frequently managed nonsurgically; however, some demonstrate considerable instability to stress under anesthesia.[1] These patterns are particularly well suited for percutaneous management. While displacement is not a contraindication to definitive minimally invasive treatment, the surgeon should acknowledge that as the displacement becomes more dramatic, reductions do become more difficult to obtain by closed or limited open means. This is potentially due to a number of factors, including interposed periosteum, fascia, or nerves.

Severely displaced pelvic ring disruptions frequently involve injury to the symphysis, and patients with these types of high-energy pelvic ring disruptions commonly present in hemorrhagic shock. Rapid angiographic embolization of arterial bleeding is employed at many trauma centers and plays a key role in resuscitation. Venous bleeding, however, is much more common and can result in significant loss of blood volume. Minimally invasive means of diminishing pelvic volume with the use of circumferential sheeting, percutaneous "C-clamp," or percutaneous application of an external fixator are effective at minimizing ongoing bleeding and are theorized to provide enough stability to allow clotting to occur to tamponade the bleeding.

Application of an external fixation frame to the pelvis in an attempt to manage the physiologically unstable patient by controlling pelvic volume and stabilizing clot has historically been the most common application of minimally invasive techniques for managing pelvic fractures. Technologic advances such as therapeutic embolization, and application of 'low-tech' circumferential wraps using either hospital linens or commercial binders, have increasingly limited the use of a "resuscitative" anterior pelvic external fixator or the closely related posterior pelvic "C-clamp." Drawbacks to anterior pelvic external fixation are many, and include: Improperly positioned pins, interference with future operative approaches, pin tract infections, potential for septic seeding of joints, and negative impact on patient positioning.

These have led to an increasing utilization of percutaneous insertion of internal fixation. In addition to minimizing the potential complications of external fixation, internal fixation adds superior biomechanics to the definitive construct.[2–5] Recently a technique for rapid stabilization of an unstable patient with a pelvic ring disruption has been described, utilizing a "damage-control iliosacral screw," demonstrating the expanding indications for minimally invasive stabilization of the injured pelvis.[6]

Specific indications for minimally invasive pelvic surgery vary based on surgeon experience and technical ability. In addition, hospital resources, such as appropriate preoperative and intraoperative imaging capabilities, play a substantial role. As patient anatomy is variable, it is vital to have imaging information that can be properly interpreted with regard to various feasible pathways for fixation. Inability to safely place an implant, either due to inaccurate reduction, inadequate imaging, or incompatible patient anatomy, is an absolute contraindication to percutaneous surgery.

PATIENT POSITIONING

Patients with pelvic ring injuries frequently will have multiple associated injuries that may complicate patient transfer and intraoperative positioning.[7] Perhaps the most inconvenient of these is associated unstable spine injuries; however, nonskeletal injuries can also pose a problem when planning percutaneous surgery. Placement of chest tubes, cystostomy tubes, and ostomies can pose difficulties in both positioning and creating and maintaining a sterile surgical field.

The supine position is appropriate for most percutaneous intervention, but prone positioning is occasionally preferred for fracture patterns involving the posterior ilium, or if a retrograde posterior column screw is planned. The lateral position carries multiple disadvantages to percutaneous surgery, including greatly increased difficulty in obtaining necessary imaging, potential obstruction of hand position necessary for proper screw trajectory, accentuation of rotational deformity due to gravity forces, and limited or no access to contralateral hemipelvis. While the lateral position is familiar to surgeons, operating room personnel, and occasionally preferred by the anesthesia team, it should be avoided for most minimally invasive pelvic fixation procedures.

A fully radiolucent table is important to provide consistent and reproducible high-quality imaging. A close working relationship with the fluoroscopy technician can eliminate many of the potential frustrations during minimally invasive surgery, and is facilitated by utilizing a consistent set of terminology to describe c-arm positions. When planning percutaneous iliosacral screw insertion, elevating the patient on several folded blankets placed midline from the lumbar region and distal will permit proper trajectory when oblique screw orientation is called for, such as sacroiliac joint disruptions and patients with sacral dysmorphism. Without this moderate elevation on the table, the wire, drill, or screwdriver may abut the table, making proper insertion difficult or impossible (Fig. 8.1).

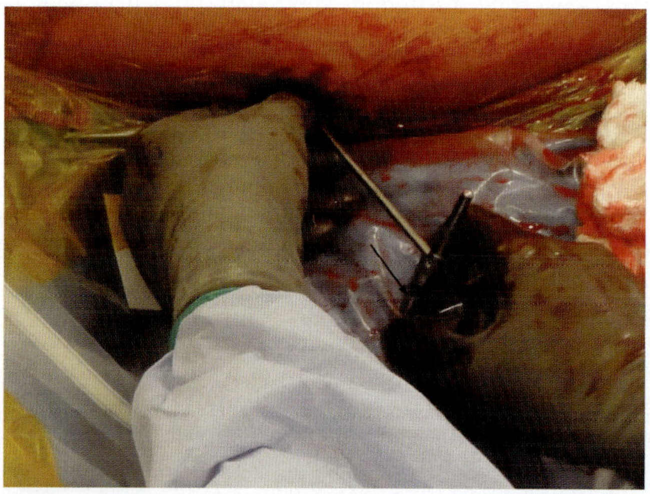

Figure 8.1 Due to posterior-to-anterior trajectory necessary for safe screw entry, the instruments may abut the edge of the radiolucent table. Here, the black *arrow* highlights the handle of the tap impinging on the edge of the table and drapes. Elevation of the patient can minimize this occurrence.

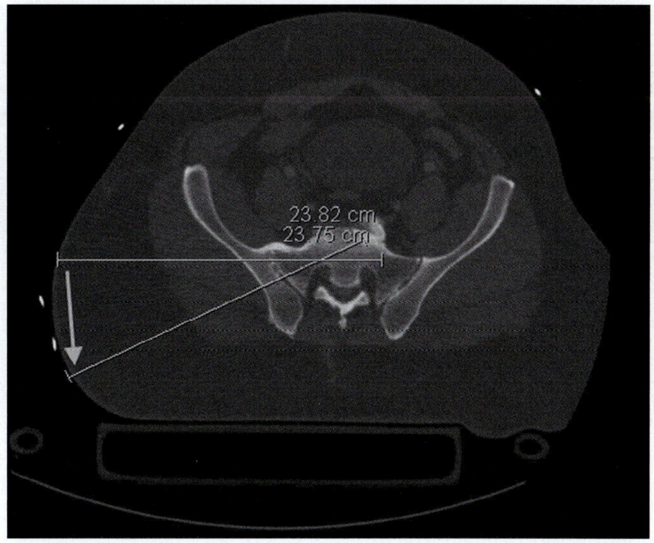

Figure 8.2 Potential screw trajectories in the upper sacral segment are drawn in white. The resultant starting point on the skin is dramatically altered, as shown by gray *arrow.*

SURGICAL APPROACHES

Palpable bony landmarks can be used to orient and provide regional safe zones for incision placement. Virtual quadrants can be drawn on the flank, for example, when preparing for iliosacral screw insertion, using a line drawn parallel to the axis of the femoral shaft and another drawn straight posterior from the anterior superior iliac spine. The majority of safe screw insertions are placed in the posterosuperior quadrant. It is critical to recall that screw trajectory within the sacrum will dramatically alter the location of the correct skin incision. This is perhaps most clearly depicted when placing fixation in each of the two upper sacral segments in a dysmorphic sacrum. The caudal-to-cranial and posterior-to-anterior trajectory of the upper screw will have a skin incision that is more distal and posterior on the skin than the more horizontally inserted second sacral screw (Fig. 8.2).

Incision placements for Schanz pins are based in relation to subcutaneous landmarks. Incisions for screws placed down the gluteus medius pillar are placed using the palpable iliac crest as a guide. Although incisions may initially start very small, if the pelvic displacement is dramatic, then correction of displacement does not uncommonly require the incision to be extended quite a bit. This should be considered when making the incision and critical assessment should be made to determine the orientation of the incision as well. This wound extension may interfere with surgical incisions if open reduction is planned for definitive management. When utilizing the supraacetabular pin location, an incision approximately 2 cm distal to the ASIS is a good starting point, but given that appropriate trajectory can be dramatically influenced by existing displacement, it is again helpful to obtain a precise starting point on the AIIS with fluoroscopic guidance and a small diameter wire placed percutaneously prior to definitive incision.

For retrograde ramus screws, the incision is typically a centimeter or so across the midline on the contralateral side of the body from the fractured ramus. Variations in anatomy can make this insertion technique impossible. Varying pelvic obliquity, or relative flexion and extension of the pelvis, which may result in a symphysis that "sits low," combined with the perineal structures in both males and females, can prevent safe creation of incisions that allow for the necessary screw trajectory. Special attention to prepping in a large surgical field and isolation of the perineum with adhesive drapes can help assure that the appropriate start point is not "prepped-out." Taking advantage of the relative mobility of the skin and soft tissues in this region by drawing the skin distally with the opposite hand can help with this approach. Relaxation of this tension following screw insertion allows the incision to "retract" cranially.

There is no fracture exposure utilized and the procedures are performed through 1.5- to 2-cm "stab" incisions. A common error is to try to make these incisions too small, precluding the insertion of the surgeon's finger along with the screw. This is frequently helpful to "guide" the screw through the occasionally deep soft tissue envelope. The deep investing

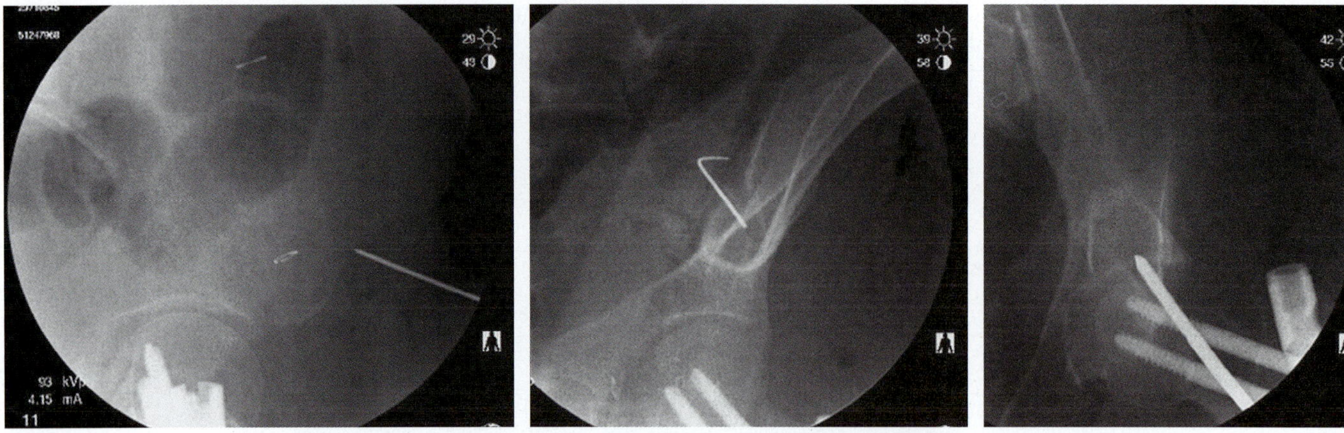

Figure 8.3 Intraoperative imaging to insertion of supraacetabular instrumentation. From left to right. Iliac oblique view highlighting profile of anterior inferior iliac spine. Obturator-outlet "tee-pee" view. Inlet view highlighting the widest available corridor of supraacetabular bone from anterior to posterior. This view is especially helpful to assist with trajectory during pin insertion, avoiding medial and lateral cortical breach.

muscle fascia can impede the precise adjustments in positioning, and special attention should be paid to incising this deep fascia with the blade to provide improved control of wires and drill bits passing through a single soft tissue "tunnel." Specialized cannulated instrumentation is also available to facilitate instrument and implant placement.

Frequently, the percutaneous incisions utilized for minimally invasive fracture fixation in the extremities are planned along the line of a traditional exposure, and can easily be incorporated into the full approach in the event that it is deemed necessary intraoperatively. The limited available pathways for fixation in the pelvis necessitate precise trajectory, placing the stab incisions fairly remote from traditional approaches to the pelvis. It should be noted, however, that traditional exposures could still be safely used, without need for modification, should minimally invasive techniques be abandoned intraoperatively.

Imprecise placement of the stab incisions can be frustrating, as the surgeon needs to "fight" the interfering tissues. A small diameter long smooth K-wire or Steinmann pin can be used percutaneously prior to incision to more accurately position the surgical incision. This can be used with fluoroscopy to find the desired starting position on the bone, and is easily withdrawn and repositioned several times with very minimal insult to skin and soft tissue.

IMAGING

As previously stated, adequate intraoperative imaging is critical to the success of any minimally invasive stabilization procedure for pelvic disruptions. Several reproducible fluoroscopic images are routinely used during these procedures. In addition to AP hip and pelvis, inlet and outlet views, and traditional Judet oblique views, merging these views to provide an "obturator-outlet," or "tee-pee" view helps to guide implants into the columns of bone available for fixation (Fig. 8.3). Making subtle modifications to these images is typically used to most accurately represent the patient's anatomy.[8] For example, the inlet view can be modified slightly to enhance the anterior cortical border of different sacral segments, and adding varying obliquity to the outlet view can bring the posterior iliac lateral cortex into profile, which can be particularly helpful to avoid washer cortical intrusion during iliosacral screw insertion (Fig. 8.4), and slight outlet tilt on an oblique view can enhance the cortical projection of the anterior column.

REDUCTION TECHNIQUES

Disruptions of the pelvic ring produce several recognizable and reproducible patterns of fracture, dislocation, and displacement. These patterns have been well described and studied.[9–11] Closed reduction techniques are utilized in relation to these concepts, and utilize large

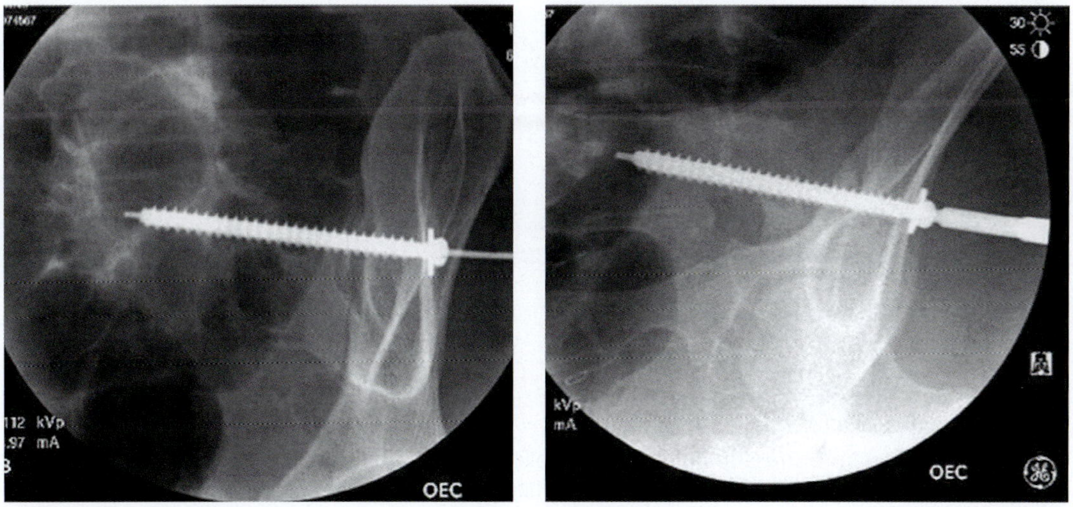

Figure 8.4 Adding obliques to the intraoperative inlet **(left)** and outlet **(right)** views by rolling the image intensifier "over the top" can put the lateral cortex of the posterior ilium on profile, improving visualization for final seating of the washer.

diameter Schanz pins placed strategically into each hemipelvis. These screws function as "joysticks" for reduction maneuvers, and can easily be removed or incorporated into an external fixator as part of definitive fixation.

Resuscitative external fixation frames have taken many forms over the years. Attempts to improve the stability imparted to the posterior pelvic ring have resulted in some fairly complex configurations, none of which ultimately reliably control the posterior ring, or have proven more effective than a simple, two-pin design.[12,13] While acknowledging the shortcomings of this type of fixation, it can still play a role in temporary stabilization of the unstable patient and pelvis, although far less frequently at major trauma centers today than in the past.

While external fixation lacks ideal biomechanics,[14] it is very effective as a manipulative device for mobilizing both hemipelves.[13] For widely displaced pelvic fractures, long Schanz pins act as joysticks to grossly realign the pelvic ring and decrease overall pelvic volume. Historically, these Schanz pins have been placed from the subcutaneous iliac crest directed down the column of bone referred to anatomically as the gluteus medius pillar. One, two, or three pins can be placed between the cortical "tables" on each ilium, distributing the forces over a greater portion of the iliac bone. This technique can be used without fluoroscopy if necessary, by using smooth K-wires slid extraosseously on the medial and lateral cortex of the ilium to guide the Schanz pins. This increases the likelihood of a pin obtaining solid purchase in bone without cortical extrusion. This scenario should be unusual, however, as c-arm imaging should be routinely available.

Another two-pin technique involves placing Schanz pins into the dense supraacetabular bone with a trajectory from the AIIS toward the PSIS, or slightly more caudally directed toward the sciatic notch. This technique is slightly more technically demanding, and is safest with good imaging, since the entry point is not palpable subcutaneously, and carries a risk of inadvertent violation of the hip joint. Frames constructed in this manner are particularly effective at closing pelvic volume when some posterior stabilizing structures remain functional, minimizing vertical instability.

For widely displaced pelvic fractures with both vertical and rotational displacement, combining external fixation with skeletal traction to the limb ipsilateral to the posterior ring injury can dramatically improve alignment and allows patient to be further resuscitated until stable for definitive pelvic fixation can be safely performed. One benefit over a circumferential sheet is the unobstructed access to abdomen, which can be helpful when patients have undergone exploratory laparotomy.

Reduction of pelvic disruptions is focused on restoration of its ring-like architecture, more than anatomical repositioning of fracture fragments. Sometimes restoring the ring mandates anatomical reduction of fractures, but fractures throughout the cancellous bone of the

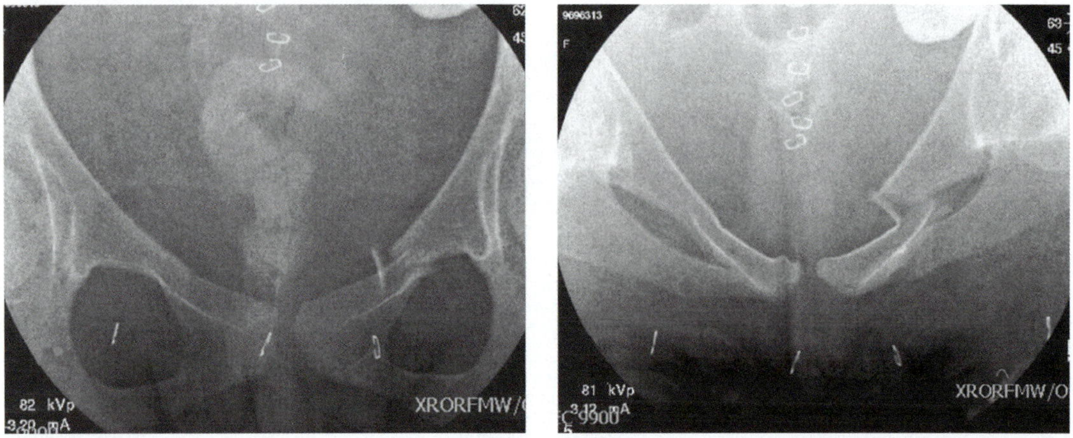

Figure 8.5 Dynamic stress imaging with application of internal rotation displacing force can demonstrate supraphysiologic motion. This is particularly evident when imaging the anterior aspect of the pelvic ring, since the "pivot-point" of displacement typically remains near the posterior structures. Image on left is static, with no force applied; image on right, with manual lateral compressive force applied through iliac crests, demonstrates inability to maintain ring structure.

sacrum generally tolerate minor residual displacements with reliable healing provided gaps can be eliminated and stable fixation can be achieved.

Many sacral fractures present minimally displaced, and are best characterized on CT scanning. While the exact indications for operative fixation of these injuries remain a topic of considerable controversy among surgeons, most agree that complete vertical fractures through the sacrum have some intrinsic potential to displace as patients mobilize. Addition of an examination under anesthesia to radiographic interpretation of stability found occult instability warranting internal fixation in 35% of ring disruptions from lateral compressive mechanisms which were initially classified as stable based on radiographs and computed tomography alone.[1] While the decision to operate should be individualized based on a critical analysis of the fracture characteristics and clinical examination, minimally invasive techniques are particularly useful if operative treatment is deemed proper (Fig. 8.5).

Impacted sacral fractures commonly occurring from lateral impact will occasionally be associated with an internal rotation deformity of the entire affected hemipelvis. Often this is well visualized on an inlet view, but critical assessment of the outlet view may better characterize the deformity. This deformity can be rather dramatic, often with little measurable sacral fracture displacement. This pattern can be effectively reduced with Schanz screws. These are placed percutaneously in various positions, but are effective and unobtrusive to posterior ring fixation when placed from the region of the AIIS toward the PSIS or slightly more caudal toward the region of the greater sciatic notch. This can be used to manipulate the hemipelvis, but is a much more powerful instrument when combined with an additional Schanz screw in the contralateral hemipelvis and incorporated into an external fixator or used with a universal distractor, which adds the ability to compress or distract in an angular stable manner. Additional injury to the contralateral hemipelvis, sometimes occult, can diminish the effectiveness of this technique and should be aggressively sought out, as the surgeon would no longer have a "stable segment" to provide a counterforce. A purely external rotational force can be very efficiently applied via these pins and has the additional benefit of being incorporated into a two-pin "distracting frame" to provide maintenance of reduction during implant insertion without obstructing necessary imaging. More dramatic internal rotation deformities occur in conjunction with other planes of displacement, commonly flexion of the hemipelvis. This pattern of displacement is effectively reduced by altering the pin position with the pin in the stable hemipelvis being inserted from the iliac crest down the gluteus medius pillar bone (Fig. 8.6). Distraction along the trajectory created by connecting this pin to the AIIS pin either with a universal distractor or external fixation bar generates a combined extension-external rotation moment for reduction. Some also advocate the use of a table-skeletal fixation apparatus that can effectively stabilize the hemipelvis to the operating table and assist in reduction of the ring displacement.[15]

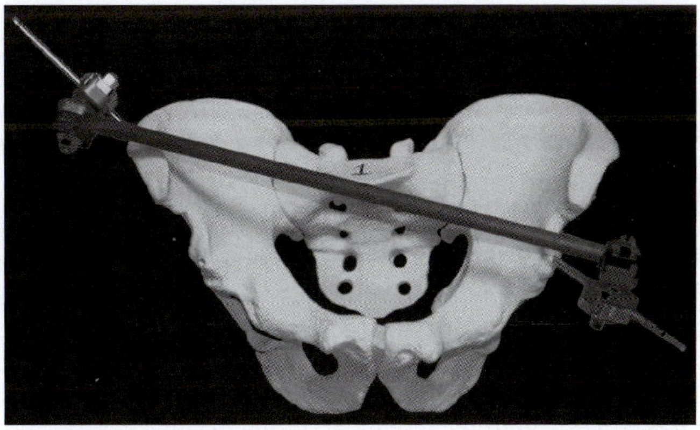

Figure 8.6 Asymmetric pin placement in each hemipelvis can enhance ability to apply a reduction vector that can effectively counteract displacement. This model shows a gluteus pillar pin placement in the right hemipelvis with a supraacetabular pin in the left hemipelvis. This is helpful with very common combined internal rotation deformities with a hemipelvic flexion component.

Sacral fractures presenting with more displacement, typically posterior and cranial to varying degrees, can also be managed by minimally invasive techniques. In these circumstances, skeletal traction plays an important role. Initiated soon after injury, a moderate amount of weight, generally not more than 6.8 to 9.07 kg (15 to 20 lb) provides a reducing force along a vector that not uncommonly results in rather dramatic improvement in the alignment of the displaced posterior pelvic ring. This initial intervention provides both a gross reduction and minimal stability while not interfering with other procedures or imaging often necessary in injured patients with pelvic fractures. Traction alone does not correct external rotation deformity, and if this is present, addition of a circumferential sheet approximately the width matching distance between the patient's iliac crests to greater trochanters should be applied and secured with clamps. A properly applied, smooth circumferential sheet can assist in minimizing pelvic volume, and stabilizing venous bleeding[16,17] (Fig. 8.7). Occasionally, the reduction of the pelvis disruption obtained following application of the circumferential sheet is adequate to allow it to be utilized as provisional fixation in the operating room while definitive fixation of the pelvis is obtained through "working portals" cut into the sheet, as recently described by Gardner et al.[18]

It should be noted that timing of reduction could have an impact on the ability to accurately reduce the pelvic ring using closed methods. Organization of clot, retention of resuscitative fluids in the third space, and muscular contraction may begin to impact closed manipulative ability as soon as 48 hours. It is helpful to reduce and stabilize the ring injury as soon as feasible to minimize this difficulty and avoid necessitation open reduction. While the exact duration is unclear beyond which closed manipulation would not be possible, if weeks have passed since injury before patient is appropriately stabilized for surgical management, the

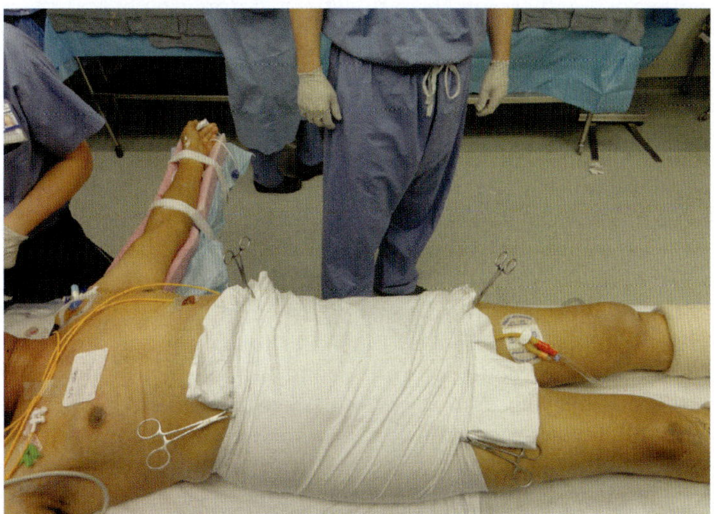

Figure 8.7 Image depicting applied circumferential sheet. Note the peripheral clamp position to minimize interference with imaging.

surgeon should be prepared to utilize open reduction, especially for fractures, which tend to have large cancellous surfaces that may begin to consolidate with soft callus rather quickly.

IMPLANTS/FIXATION

Percutaneous Anterior Ring

While Schanz pins and external fixators are the most efficient devices for reduction of displacement, internal fixation provides superior biomechanical properties and is better suited for definitive management.[2] Disruptions of the anterior ring generally fall into symphysis disruptions and fractures of the superior or inferior ramus. Classically, these injuries are either managed without fixation, or with a formal approach and plating. Laparotomy incisions, incisions for bladder repair, previous hernia repairs, suprapubic cystostomy tubes, and open wounds can complicate management via formal ORIF, and may represent relative indications for minimally invasive stabilization. Simple anterior external fixation has been used with success for symphysis injuries, especially when part of a constellation of anterior ring injury that includes bilateral superior and inferior ramus fractures.

More recently, a subcutaneous modification of an anterior internal fixator (INFIX) using spinal instrumentation has been described with promising results when combined with posterior iliosacral screw fixation.[19] Large diameter pedicle screws (7 to 8 mm) from spinal instrumentation are placed in a supraacetabular location, and then connected using a 6-mm titanium rod that is tunneled subcutaneously. Routine removal under anesthesia has been recommended 3 months postoperatively. This is currently an off-label use of the spinal instrumentation.

ILIOSACRAL SCREWS

Stabilization of posterior pelvic ring injuries, sacroiliac joint dislocations, and sacral fractures, with the use of percutaneous means, has dramatically reduced the reported deep infection and wound complication rates associated with open reduction and internal fixation.[20,21] Wound complications of up to 25% were reported when operative procedures were performed through severely injured posterior soft tissues on critically ill patients.[22] Both prone and supine insertion has been advocated.[21] Prone position may be particularly beneficial in instances of displaced transforaminal sacral fractures associated with neurologic deficits where an open decompression of nerve roots with removal of incarcerated bony fragments can be performed through a vertical paramedian approach. This decompression and open reduction can then be stabilized with a percutaneously inserted iliosacral screw or screws.

Supine positioning offers several advantages. It allows unrestricted access to anterior ring pathology for closed manipulation and eliminates the potential worsening of deformity that can occasionally result from the effect of gravity while in the prone position. Supine positioning is also simpler in the multiply injured patient. Frequently, open reduction of the anterior ring injuries will assist with the reduction of the posterior ring. This is most commonly encountered with symphysis disruptions and associated incomplete sacroiliac joint injuries. Formal ORIF of the symphysis will frequently reduce the sacroiliac joint to a nearly anatomic position utilizing the intact posterior ligamentous structures as a hinge. An iliosacral screw can then be safely inserted percutaneously, allowing final "fine-tuning" of the reduction to be accomplished with a partially threaded screw, placed perpendicular to the sacroiliac joint. Compression generated in this vector will close a residual gap at the joint. Cannulated screws have simplified percutaneous iliosacral screw technique, but a thorough and complete understanding of three-dimensional neural, vascular, and sacral anatomy and its variability is an absolute prerequisite to this fixation technique. Precise placement can generally be performed in both the upper and second sacral segments, but critical analysis of the fine-cut CT provides objective data regarding space available for fixation.[23] Specific insertion techniques vary. While the differences may be a matter of surgeon preference, it is important that the technique allows accurate, precise, and reproducible results. Routt described an efficient technique for iliosacral screw insertion in the supine position.[24] A small caliber smooth wire can be used percutaneously to obtain an appropriate starting point on the lateral ilium before making skin

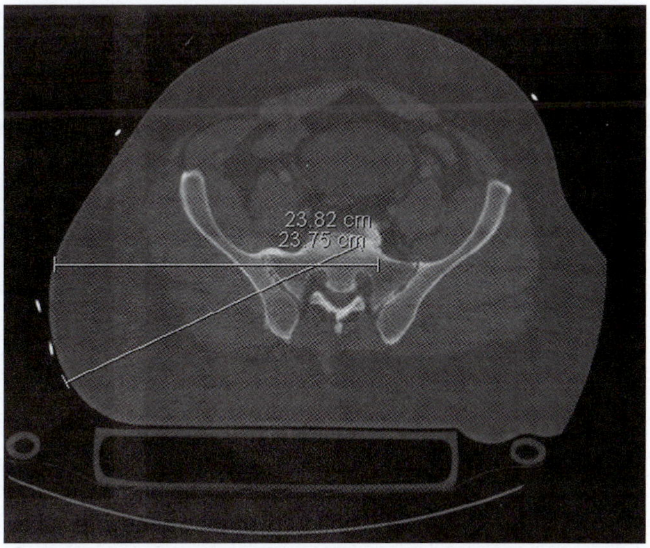

Figure 8.8 Axial CT cut depicting the change in location of skin incision with varying iliosacral screw insertion trajectories. Clinically, this anterior-to-posterior change is frequently accompanied by a corresponding change in cranial to caudal location as well.

incision. This minimizes inaccuracies that can result in multiple incisions or unnecessary extension. Presence of sacral dysmorphism and its implication on sacral alar slope impact safe screw trajectory and can dramatically alter the location of the skin incision (Fig. 8.8). Once the starting point on the ilium is confirmed as being slightly posterior to the superimposed anterior cortical surfaces of the sacrum when viewed from the inlet fluoroscopic projection, and slightly cranial to the superior cortical edge of the sacral neural foramen on the outlet projection, a skin incision can be made over the wire. It is helpful to incise to the deep fascia along this wire to ease the insertion of a guidewire sleeve. This sleeve is then firmly held against the lateral ilium, and the smooth wire is then exchanged for guidewire for the cannulated screw system. The wire sleeve can then be used to precisely direct the wire as it is advanced through the ilium and into the sacral alar region. As part of cannulated screw systems, the guidewires are fairly flexible, making minor adjustments to wire trajectory difficult. This is especially true once the wire has penetrated both the lateral and medial cortices of the ilium, creating two fixed points on the wire, effectively locking its direction. If additional adjustments are desired for accurate position, the cannulated drill can then be inserted over the wire and advanced. The drill is more rigid, allowing minor adjustments even as it is advanced well into the sacral body. When utilizing this technique, the drill should be used in oscillating mode until the wire is "swallowed" by the drill, so as not to inadvertently advance the threaded tip of the wire. No trajectory adjustments should be made until the wire is covered; otherwise there is risk that the drill will break off the tip of the wire. As the drill is advanced, continue the use of oscillation mode. This helps prevent cortical breech, as the drill bit will "bounce" off the denser cortex of the anterior sacrum or the neural tunnel and stay in the cancellous bone. Oscillation can also theoretically minimize risk to nerve roots when stabilizing comminuted transforaminal fractures, limiting the risk of "wrapping-up" the nerve that may occur if the drill bit was spinning. Oscillation torque destabilizes the drill in the surgeon's hands, making precise advancement difficult. It is helpful to create a stable platform with the nondrilling arm utilizing the table as a fixed point to minimize unintended instrument movements.

Biplanar fluoroscopy confirms position of the guidewire or drill with frequent switching between an inlet view that best superimposes the anterior cortical borders of the upper two sacral segments, and the outlet view, obtained by superimposing the superior aspect of the symphysis or pubic tubercles on the body of the second sacral body. Either lateral "scout" image from the CT scan, or a midline sagittal slice through the sacrum with patient in supine position can provide a guide to initial c-arm positions necessary to obtain biplanar images of the sacrum, by providing insight into the sacrum's relative kyphosis or lordosis.

In most nondysmorphic sacra, the lateral anterior sacral alar border aligns with the pelvic brim, represented by iliac cortical densities on the lateral sacral fluoroscopic image.[23] This image is critical to safe screw placement and should routinely be obtained once the guidewire or drill has been advanced into the lateral sacrum up to, but not more medial than, the lateral border of

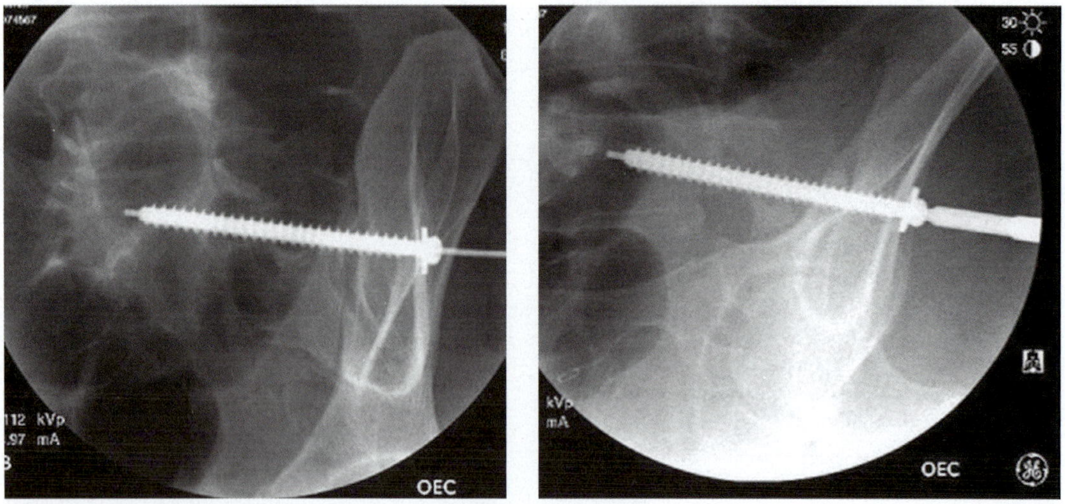

Figure 8.9 Altering the obliquity of the image intensifier to enhance the projection of the lateral posterior iliac cortex provides intraoperative confirmation of a fully seated washer.

the bony neural tunnel of the upper sacral nerve root. Visualization of the tip of the wire posterior to the iliac cortical densities and cranial to the neural tunnel confirms safe positioning when combined with the inlet and outlet views. Effort should be taken to achieve this image with the greater sciatic notches, femoral heads, and iliac cortical densities superimposed on the contralateral structure. This confirms reduction of ring deformity as well. The wire can then be advanced medially, staying cranial to the neural foramen on the outlet image and posterior to the anterior cortical border on the inlet image. Remember that crossing the midline of the sacrum places contralateral neural structures at risk, and screws that are too long may violate the anterior cortex of the sacrum as it curves posteriorly, posing a risk to the contralateral vascular structures lying anterior to the sacrum. Upon final seating of the screw, confirm that the washer is fully seated on the lateral ilium with an oblique view on the outlet or inlet. When seated, the washer should tilt slightly, with the anterosuperior aspect positioned more lateral than the inferior aspect (Fig. 8.9). This is due to the normal contour of the posterior ilium. If the obliquity is not present, or is tilted the opposite way, this is a clue that there may be washer intrusion.

Screw trajectory impacts the ultimate screw length able to be utilized. While the densest cancellous bone is in the sacral body, obtaining purchase with as many threads as possible may be beneficial, particularly in sacral fractures closer to the midline. A slightly more anterior starting point with a horizontal screw trajectory may allow for screw placement all the way to the contralateral sacroiliac joint, and in some cases, through the contralateral joint to obtain transiliac–transsacral–transiliac fixation.[25] This fixation provides up to six cortices of purchase and may have superior biomechanical qualities to unilateral iliosacral screws. Presence of dysmorphism generally makes this type of fixation impossible in the upper segment, but may actually increase the safe zone for this fixation in the second sacral segment.[26]

RAMUS SCREWS

Overall construct stiffness is improved by adding fixation at additional points of instability.[5] While ramus fractures tend to heal with abundant callus formation when managed without internal fixation, intramedullary screws can be effectively used to add additional stability to pelvic ring disruptions treated with iliosacral screws, or other form of posterior pelvic ring fixation. This improved stability may improve patient comfort with early mobilization, and potentially prevent late recurrence of deformity, particularly internal rotation.

Intramedullary screws can be inserted both retrograde and antegrade, using the same fluoroscopic images. An inlet image centered on the symphysis provides visualization of the anterior and posterior borders of the superior ramus, guiding appropriate trajectory in that plane. The oblique outlet image, also referred to as the obturator-outlet, or tee-pee view enhances visualization of the superior and inferior cortices of the superior ramus as well as the anteromedial acetabular subchondral surface. This view is critical to avoid errant screw penetration into the hip joint as it advanced superior to the joint across the supraacetabular corridor and into the lateral ilium. As the fixation is on the convex surface of the hip joint, the surgeon must confirm that the implant does not cross the subchondral line on one view to confirm safe placement. This is in contrast to fixation in the femoral head, which requires an infinite number of images to absolutely confirm safe placement.

The starting point for retrograde insertion can be either at the symphysis or at the pubic tubercle. A small caliber wire is inserted to bone percutaneously with the surgeon on the opposite side of the table as the c-arm. The ideal starting position is at the anteromedial most point of the ramus at the symphysis, parallel to an imaginary line drawn along the axis of the ramus on the inlet view, and at the cranial/caudal midpoint of the pubic body on the obturator-outlet view. The starting point on this view is ideally in line with an imaginary straight line drawn along the axis of the superior ramus, running cranial to the anteromedial acetabular subchondral arc, exiting the lateral ilium (Fig. 8.10). The wire is tapped into position to

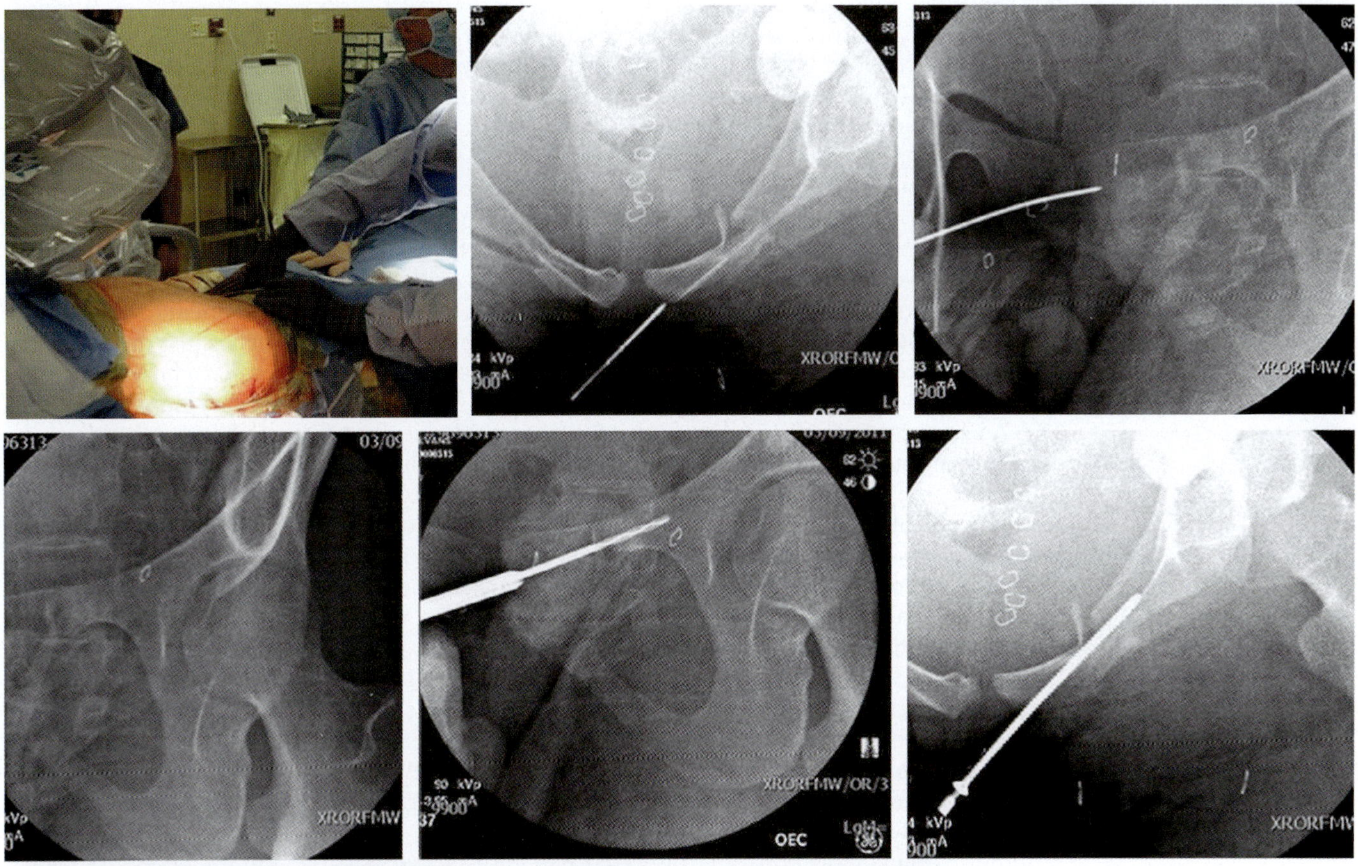

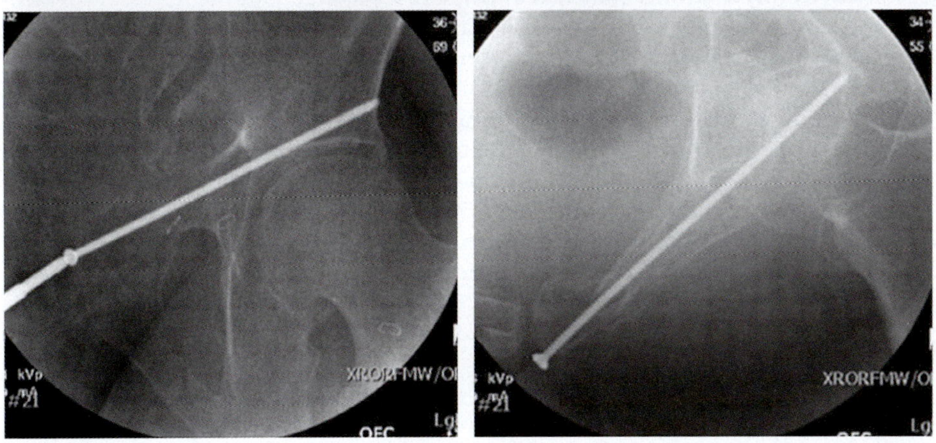

Figure 8.10 Sequence of images from top left to bottom right depicts insertion of retrograde small fragment cortex screw to stablilize a left-side mid ramus fracture. The inlet view highlights the anterior and posterior margins at their widest, while the obturator-outlet view confirms extra-articular positioning and lateral cortical penetration.

stabilize it and a percutaneous incision is made over the wire to release the soft tissues. If planning 6.5- or 7-mm cannulated screws for fixation, a wire sleeve is then advanced over the wire and the guidewire exchanged, and advanced into the parasymphyseal ramus, using frequent images to guide advancement to the lateral ilium. Alternatively, a 3.5- or 4.5-mm drill may be used through the corresponding sleeve and advanced through the parasymphyseal portion to create a glide hole in the distal segment of the fracture. This is then exchanged through the drill sleeve for a long calibrated 2.5-mm drill bit, which is then advanced to the lateral ilium, if anatomically possible. This can be advanced using oscillation mode to stay intraosseous and minimize risk of inadvertent cortical perforation. The pectineal gutter portion of the superior ramus, at the midportion of the lateral third of the ramus, is not well visualized on the two fluoroscopic images available. This is a shallow groove area from which the pectineus originates from the pelvis. The anterior portion of the ramus at this level is narrower, and the safest path through this region is slightly more posterior and central. Frequent imaging can help to identify an extraosseous position by highlighting subtle angulations at the tip of the drill bit or wire. If the tip bounces anterior and cranial at this region, this should be interpreted as highly suspicious for incorrect placement.

Retrograde insertion is particularly useful in parasymphyseal fractures. Often, displacement can be reduced without direct fragment manipulation. For ramus fractures associated with a lateral compressive force mechanism and resultant internal rotation deformity, simply reducing the internal rotation with a Schanz pin in one hemipelvis will grossly realign the ramus. When additional manipulation is necessary to align the medullary canal, a small incision can be made near midline, just superior to the symphysis to allow passage of a bone hook or joker elevator. This can be used along the posterior-superior aspect of the ramus to gently reduce the unstable fragment. Caution should be used when considering this technique, as fracture displacement and hematoma associated with pelvic ring disruptions frequently displace structures from their typical location. When feasible, blunt instruments are preferred to minimize risk to the bladder or vascular structures as they exit the pelvis just medial to the iliopectineal fascia. When the medial fragment is displaced, it may be able to be manipulated via the intramedullary drill once it has been used to get access to the parasymphyseal ramus. The 2.5-mm calibrated drill bit or the 2.8-mm guidewire are frequently too flexible to be used as manipulative instruments. The 3.5- or 4.5-mm drill are more stout and can be used to joystick the ramus into position, and allow temporary stabilization with a wire placed remote from planned screw position. Alternatively, it is occasionally helpful to overdrill the near medullary canal with a cannulated drill, use it to reduce the ramus, and then advance the guidewire by tapping through the drill into the far fragment. The drill can then be removed, the wire left in place, and the cannulated screw inserted over the guidewire. This technique requires that the patient anatomy can accommodate a large caliber cannulated screw.

There is considerable variability in the morphology of the anterior pelvis. Some rami are narrow, or tortuous, and will not accommodate safe screw insertion. Implants should be adjusted for patient anatomy. When a 6.5 mm or larger cannulated screw is not feasible, a 4.5- or 3.5-mm cortical screw can be used, as these screws will often flex and bend to pass the narrow, curved intraosseous, extra-articular corridor that exists between the symphysis and the lateral ilium.

Other patients have bony anatomy that will allow screw passage, but the necessary trajectory for retrograde insertion may not be anatomically possible. This can be due to several factors, including the relative extension or flexion of the pelvis in the body or large thighs. Antegrade insertion should be considered in these instances. It is helpful to be proficient at each technique, as it is not uncommon to use intramedullary stabilization bilaterally, and placing one screw retrograde, and the other antegrade can eliminate the need for routine c-arm repositioning to the opposite side of the bed, which risks compromising sterility. Repositioning is necessary because the c-arm arc interferes with the surgeon when obtaining the inlet view for antegrade insertion and when obtaining the obturator-outlet view for retrograde insertion, if the surgeon is on the same side of the table as the c-arm machine.

Complications

Percutaneous and minimally invasive techniques place tremendous importance on intraoperative imaging. Many potential complications occur in association with inadequate imaging, or

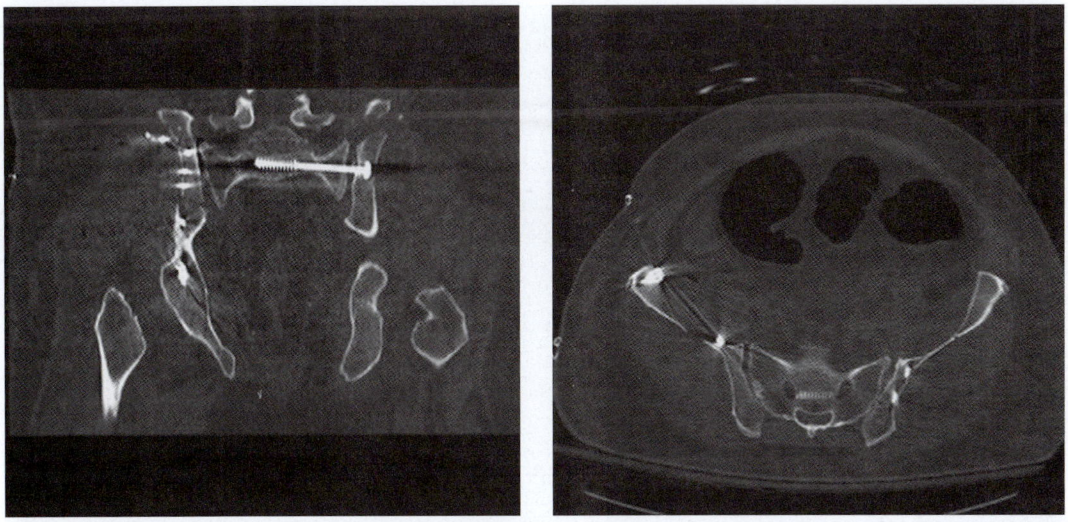

Figure 8.11 Postoperative images confirming complete cortical intrusion of the washer. The impact of this complication on stability is unknown.

inaccurate interpretation of an image. The importance of preoperative planning and three-dimensional understanding of the complex, and often variable, pelvic anatomy cannot be overemphasized. Templeman et al.[27] showed that a change in hand position of only four degrees could result in nerve damage. Several publications have characterized the upper sacral safe zones for screw placement and anatomy of the nerve conduits of the sacrum.[28,29]

Multiple publications document complications of percutaneous stabilization of posterior pelvic ring disruptions.[30–33] Cadaveric and CT-based studies describe relations of implants to "at risk" structures.[27,34] Damage to the superior gluteal artery during iliosacral screw insertion can occur and may require urgent embolization to control hemorrhage.[35–37] More subtle complications, such as screw head or washer cortical intrusion on the lateral ilium can have clinically relevant implications resulting from less than optimal fixation (Fig. 8.11).

Screw malposition has been reported as an infrequent complication in experienced hands, but is a complication that must be avoided due to potentially devastating impact.[20] A screw that is placed too posteriorly in the sacrum may violate the spinal canal. One placed too caudal and posterior may violate the nerve root exit tunnel, and one placed too cranial and anterior may breach the anterior/superior cortex of the sacrum, potentially injuring a nerve or iliac vessels (Fig. 8.12). The surgeon should be acutely aware of these surgical missteps, especially if advancing the screw, or guidewire, beyond midline. Even in the situation that a malpositioned screw does not cause a postoperative deficit, consideration should be given to return for accurate repositioning.

Appropriately positioned partially threaded iliosacral screws can result in iatrogenic injury to sacral nerve roots when utilized in comminuted fractures involving the upper sacral neural foramina. Attempts to gain stability through interfragmentary compression can potentially narrow the available space for the exiting nerve root and result in neurologic deficit postoperatively. Occasionally, this can be effectively managed by backing off on the screw a few threads, but more routinely would present an indication for an open decompression. Similarly, cortical fragments may be pushed into the tunnel during screw insertion, occasionally with identical result.

The nature of percutaneous fixation, specifically the inability to directly visualize structures at the injury site, also places a theoretical risk to adjacent structures due to the potential for them to be displaced from their typical anatomic location by clot. The fifth lumbar nerve root's relation to the sacral alar region is one such structure that could potentially be displaced by the injury, then entrapped during closed reduction, resulting in postoperative nerve deficit despite appropriate radiographic reduction and implant placement. Small bowel entrapment in a percutaneously reduced and stabilized sacral fracture has also been reported.[38]

Complications related to external fixation of the pelvis are not rare. Inaccurate placement of Schanz pins can diminish the effectiveness of the construct. Even appropriately positioned

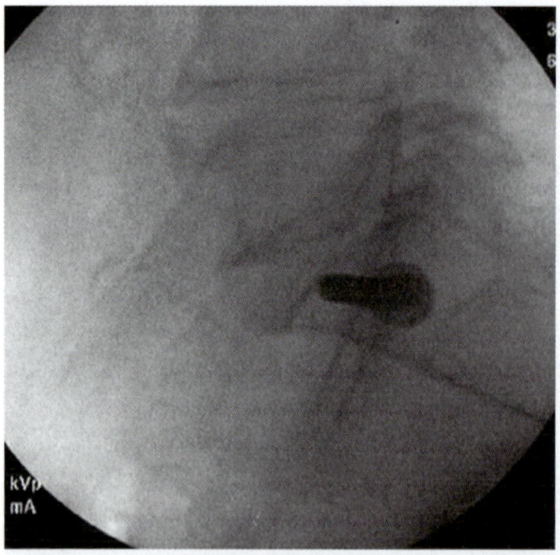

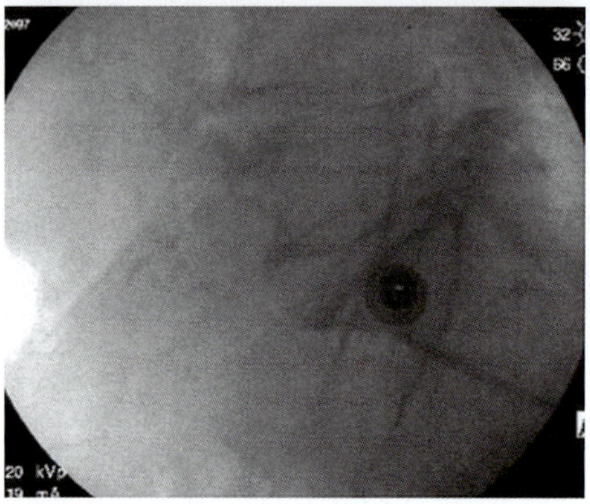

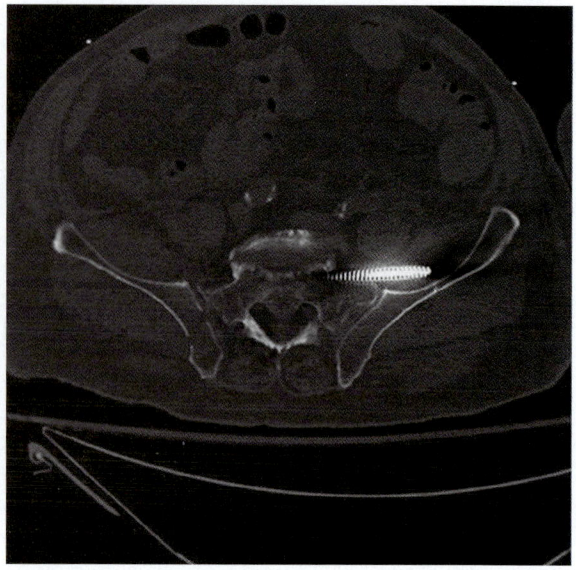

Figure 8.12 Fluoroscopic image (top left) demonstrating extraosseous screw positioning. CT image shows in detail the path and structures at risk. Note that the top left fluoroscopic image is diagnostic because this is a transiliac–transsacral screw. The entire implant must be posterior to both iliac cortical densities in this case.

pins can be incorporated into a construct that may actually increase the pelvic deformity, as shown by Dickson and Matta[39] in a retrospective review of transferred patients. While all external fixator pins can become colonized and secondarily infected, pelvic external fixator pins are especially prone to infection due to several factors, including frequently being inserted through the "zone of injury," a fairly thick soft tissue tract, severely injured patients with diminished ability to fight infection, and location in an ICU setting. Supraacetabular pin position is more commonly used in trauma centers and is associated with complications specific to that configuration. Damage to the lateral femoral cutaneous nerve can occur during placement. Supraacetabular pin position can be counterproductive to early patient mobilization by blocking hip flexion necessary to sit upright. This potential drawback and its impact on adequate pulmonary toilet should not be overlooked. Development of an acutely septic hip joint can also occur in patients treated with a supraacetabular frame, with potentially devastating consequences.[40]

REHABILITATION PROTOCOL

Rehabilitation following minimally invasive fixation of pelvic ring disruptions generally follows a similar sequence as following open procedures. One of the important principles guiding surgical management of pelvic ring disruptions is to allow early, meaningful patient mobilization. Weight-bearing precautions generally relate to the side of the involved posterior ring disruption. Following stabilization, mobilization using weight-of-leg weight-bearing on the side with the posterior ring injury and unrestricted, as-tolerated weight-bearing on the opposite leg can be initiated under the supervision of a physical therapist. For the first 6 weeks, the emphasis is on overall mobility and strength. If radiographs at 6 weeks show early consolidation and no evidence of loss of fixation or reduction, a compliant patient can then begin a progressive weight-bearing protocol, under therapist guidance. Generally, this can be safely accomplished with weekly advancement of weight-bearing, based on percentage of body weight, with most patients able to "graduate" to full weight-bearing over the course of the next 6 weeks. This protocol is often used as a guideline, with adjustments made relative to specific patient and injury factors. Morbidly obese patients, for example, may not progress to full weight-bearing as rapidly, and patients with bilateral posterior ring injuries and upper extremity injuries may be relegated to bed-to-chair exercises for longer periods to avoid catastrophic failure.

OUTCOMES

Early fixation of pelvic ring disruptions has been shown to reduce hospital stay, diminish long-term disability, improve survival, decrease blood loss, and may decrease complications.[7,10] Smaller surgical incisions, limited dissection, and shorter intensive care unit stays can help to minimize nosocomial infections. Reduction of ring displacement must still be emphasized over simple insertion of fixation, as outcomes may be related to residual deformity. In one study, 82% of patients with no residual deformity reported normal function at 5 years, while only 30% of those with greater than 1 cm residual posterior displacement reported normal function.[41] A retrospective review of over 200 pelvic ring injuries including both rotationally unstable and completely unstable patterns found that function was good or excellent in up to 92% of rotationally unstable injuries, but only 71% of completely unstable patterns.[42] Anatomic reduction was obtained in 75% or more of rotationally unstable patterns and only 62% of completely unstable patterns. Others have shown no direct correlation between reduction and functional outcome, indicating that the combination of the injury to the pelvic soft tissues as well as associated nonpelvic injuries may play an important role in final outcome.[43]

Percutaneous techniques have evolved to make obtaining optimal biomechanics with internal fixation feasible in the early postinjury period for polytrauma patients, largely due to minimal blood loss, and short procedure duration. Minimally invasive reduction and stabilization techniques represent a true advancement in treatment of the polytraumatized patient with pelvic ring disruption, and represent a critical skill set for orthopaedic surgeons charged with their care.

REFERENCES

1. Sagi HC, Coniglione FM, Stanford JH. Examination under anesthetic for occult pelvic ring instability. *J Orthop Trauma.* 2011;25(9):529–536.
2. Simonian PT, Routt ML. Biomechanics of pelvic fixation. *Orthop Clin North Am.* 1997;28(3):351–367.
3. Simonian PT, Routt ML, Harrington RM, et al. Anterior versus posterior provisional fixation in the unstable pelvis. A biomechanical comparison. *Clin Orthop Relat Res.* 1995;(310):245–251.
4. Mears DC, Rubash HE. External and internal fixation of the pelvic ring. *Instr Course Lect.* 1984; 33:144–158.
5. Simonian PT, Routt ML, Harrington RM, et al. Internal fixation of the unstable anterior pelvic ring: A biomechanical comparison of standard plating techniques and the retrograde medullary superior pubic ramus screw. *J Orthop Trauma.* 1994;8(6):476–482.
6. Gardner MJ, Chip Routt ML. The antishock iliosacral screw. *J Orthop Trauma.* 2010;24(10):e86–e89.
7. Latenser BA, Gentilello LM, Tarver AA, et al. Improved outcome with early fixation of skeletally unstable pelvic fractures. *J Trauma.* 1991;31(1):28–31.
8. Ziran BH, Wasan AD, Marks DM, et al. Fluoroscopic imaging guides of the posterior pelvis pertaining to iliosacral screw placement. *J Trauma.* 2007;62(2):347–356; discussion 356.
9. Tile M. Pelvic ring fractures: Should they be fixed? *J Bone Joint Surg Br.* 1988;70(1):1–12.
10. Burgess AR, Eastridge BJ, Young JW, et al. Pelvic ring disruptions: Effective classification system and treatment protocols. *J Trauma.* 1990;30(7):848–856.
11. Pennal GF, Tile M, Waddell JP, et al. Pelvic disruption: Assessment and classification. *Clin Orthop Relat Res.* 1980;(151):12–21.
12. Kim WY, Hearn TC, Seleem O, et al. Effect of pin location on stability of pelvic external fixation. *Clin Orthop Relat Res.* 1999;(361):237–244.
13. Tucker MC, Nork SE, Simonian PT, et al. Simple anterior pelvic external fixation. *J Trauma.* 2000; 49(6):989.
14. Rubash HE, Mears DC. External fixation of the pelvis. *Instr Course Lect.* 1983;32:329–348.

15. Matta JM, Yerasimides JG. Table-skeletal fixation as an adjunct to pelvic ring reduction. *J Orthop Trauma*. 2007;21(9):647–656.
16. Krieg JC, Mohr M, Ellis TJ, et al. Emergent stabilization of pelvic ring injuries by controlled circumferential compression: A clinical trial. *J Trauma*. 2005;59(3):659–664.
17. Routt ML Jr, Falicov A, Woodhouse E, et al. Circumferential pelvic antishock sheeting: A temporary resuscitation aid. *J Orthop Trauma*. 2006;20(1 Suppl):S3–S6.
18. Gardner MJ, Osgood G, Molnar R, et al. Percutaneous pelvic fixation using working portals in a circumferential pelvic antishock sheet. *J Orthop Trauma*. 2009;23(9):668–674.
19. Vaidya RM, Tonnos FD, Colen RD, et al. Minimally invasive treatment of unstable pelvic ring injuries with an internal anterior fixator (INFIX) and posterior iliosacral screws. In: *Annual Meeting of the Orthopaedic Trauma Association 10/8/9002*. San Diego, CA.
20. Routt ML, Kregor PJ, Simonian PT, et al. Early results of percutaneous iliosacral screws placed with the patient in the supine position. *J Orthop Trauma*. 1995;9(3):207–214.
21. Routt ML, Simonian PT, Inaba J. Iliosacral Screw Fixation of the Disrupted Sacroiliac Joint. *Techniques in Orthopaedics*. 1994;9:300.
22. Kellam JF, McMurtry RY, Paley D, et al. The unstable pelvic fracture. Operative treatment. *Orthop Clin North Am*. 1987;18(1):25–41.
23. Routt ML, Simonian PT, Agnew SG, et al. Radiographic recognition of the sacral alar slope for optimal placement of iliosacral screws: A cadaveric and clinical study. *J Orthop Trauma*. 1996; 10(3):171–177.
24. Chip Routt Jr ML, Meier MC, Kregor PJ, et al. Percutaneous iliosacral screws with the patient supine technique. *Oper Tech Orthop*. 1993;3(1):35–45.
25. Gardner MJ, Routt ML Jr. Transiliac–transsacral screws for posterior pelvic stabilization. *J Orthop Trauma*. 2011;25(6):378–384.
26. Conflitti JM, Graves ML, Chip Routt ML Jr. Radiographic quantification and analysis of dysmorphic upper sacral osseous anatomy and associated iliosacral screw insertions. *J Orthop Trauma*. 2010; 24(10):630–636.
27. Templeman D, Schmidt A, Freese J, et al. Proximity of iliosacral screws to neurovascular structures after internal fixation. *Clin Orthop Relat Res*. 1996;(329):194–198.
28. Farrell ED, Gardner MJ, Krieg JC, et al. The upper sacral nerve root tunnel: An anatomic and clinical study. *J Orthop Trauma*. 2009;23(5):333–339.
29. Noojin FK, Malkani AL, Haikal L, et al. Cross-sectional geometry of the sacral ala for safe insertion of iliosacral lag screws: A computed tomography model. *J Orthop Trauma*. 2000;14(1):31–35.
30. Ricci WM, Padberg AM, Borrelli J. The significance of anode location for stimulus-evoked electromyography during iliosacral screw placement. *J Orthop Trauma*. 2003;17(2):95–99.
31. Webb LX, de Araujo W, Donofrio P, et al. Electromyography monitoring for percutaneous placement of iliosacral screws. *J Orthop Trauma*. 2000;14(4):245–254.
32. Keating JF, Werier J, Blachut P, et al. Early fixation of the vertically unstable pelvis: The role of iliosacral screw fixation of the posterior lesion. *J Orthop Trauma*. 1999;13(2):107–113.
33. van den Bosch EW, van Zwienen CM, van Vugt AB. Fluoroscopic positioning of sacroiliac screws in 88 patients. *J Trauma*. 2002;53(1):44–48.
34. Collinge C, Coons D, Aschenbrenner J. Risks to the superior gluteal neurovascular bundle during percutaneous iliosacral screw insertion: An anatomical cadaver study. *J Orthop Trauma*. 2005; 19(2):96–101.
35. Altman DT, Jones CB, Routt ML. Superior gluteal artery injury during iliosacral screw placement. *J Orthop Trauma*. 1999;13(3):220–227.
36. Marmor M, Lynch T, Matityahu A. Superior gluteal artery injury during iliosacral screw placement due to aberrant anatomy. *Orthopedics*. 2010;33(2):117–120.
37. Maled I, Velez R, Lopez R, et al. Pseudoaneurysm of the superior gluteal artery during iliosacral screw fixation. *Acta Orthop Belg*. 2007;73(4):544–547.
38. Bushnell BD, Dirschl DR. Small bowel obstruction from entrapment in a sacral fracture stabilized with iliosacral screws: Case report and review of the literature. *J Trauma*. 2008;65(4):933–937.
39. Dickson KF, Matta JM. Skeletal deformity after anterior external fixation of the pelvis. *J Orthop Trauma*. 2009;23(5):327–332.
40. Judd KT, McKinley TO. Septic arthritis of the hip associated with supra-acetabular external fixation of unstable pelvic ring: A case report. *Iowa Orthop J*. 2009;29:124–126.
41. McLaren AC, Rorabeck CH, Halpenny J. Long-term pain and disability in relation to residual deformity after displaced pelvic ring fractures. *Can J Surg*. 1990;33(6):492–494.
42. Rommens PM, Hessmann MH. Staged reconstruction of pelvic ring disruption: Differences in morbidity, mortality, radiologic results, and functional outcomes between B1, B2/B3, and C-type lesions. *J Orthop Trauma*. 2002;16(2):92–98.
43. Suzuki T, Shindo M, Soma K, et al. Long-term functional outcome after unstable pelvic ring fracture. *J Trauma*. 2007;63(4):884–888.

CHAPTER 9

Minimally Invasive Reduction and Fixation Techniques for Acetabular Fractures

Gil R. Ortega and Hrayr G. Basmajian

INDICATIONS

Letournel and Judet[1] have demonstrated approaches to adequately open reduce and stabilize acetabular fractures. Their work as well as other authors' work has emphasized the importance of anatomical reduction and how an acetabular fracture anatomical reduction can lead to long-term satisfactory results.[2–6] Some open approaches are associated with significant risks including infection, wound healing, neurovascular injury, heterotopic ossification, femoral head avascular necrosis, and thromboembolic events.[2–5,7,8] Many of these risks are associated with the approach rather than the fixation or injury.

With the advent of improved imaging techniques including fluoroscopy and computed tomography (CT) imaging, there have been advancements in acetabular surgery reduction and internal fixation techniques. Appropriate internal fixation of acetabular fractures permits early ambulation and can significantly reduce the amount of time spent in bed.[1] Some authors agree that anatomic reduction and internal fixation are the goals of all acetabular surgery.[2,3,5,7,8] The goals when using minimally invasive techniques should include obtaining the best reduction and stable internal fixation. The following situations are described indications in the literature and also what surgeons may use when deciding between a formal open procedure and potential indications.[6,9–12]

Fracture Patterns

1. Any fracture in which an anatomic reduction can be obtained and stabilized with available methods
2. Nondisplaced (1 to 3 mm) and potentially unstable fractures
3. Minimally displaced (3 to 5 mm) with a fracture gap but no step-off
4. Transtectal fractures with medial roof-arc angle (AP radiograph) of 45 degrees or less[13]
5. Minimal comminution and no free fragments in the hip joint (Parker)[20]
6. Unstable fractures as demonstrated with validated stress examinations[15]
7. Both column fractures with acceptable secondary congruence

Patient Factors

1. Patients deemed too sick to withstand an extensive open procedure with risk of substantial blood loss
2. Obese patients at high risk of complications with open procedures[16]
3. Patients with Morel-Lavallee lesions or compromised skin around planned open procedure
4. Geriatric patients with pre-existing symptoms of arthritis

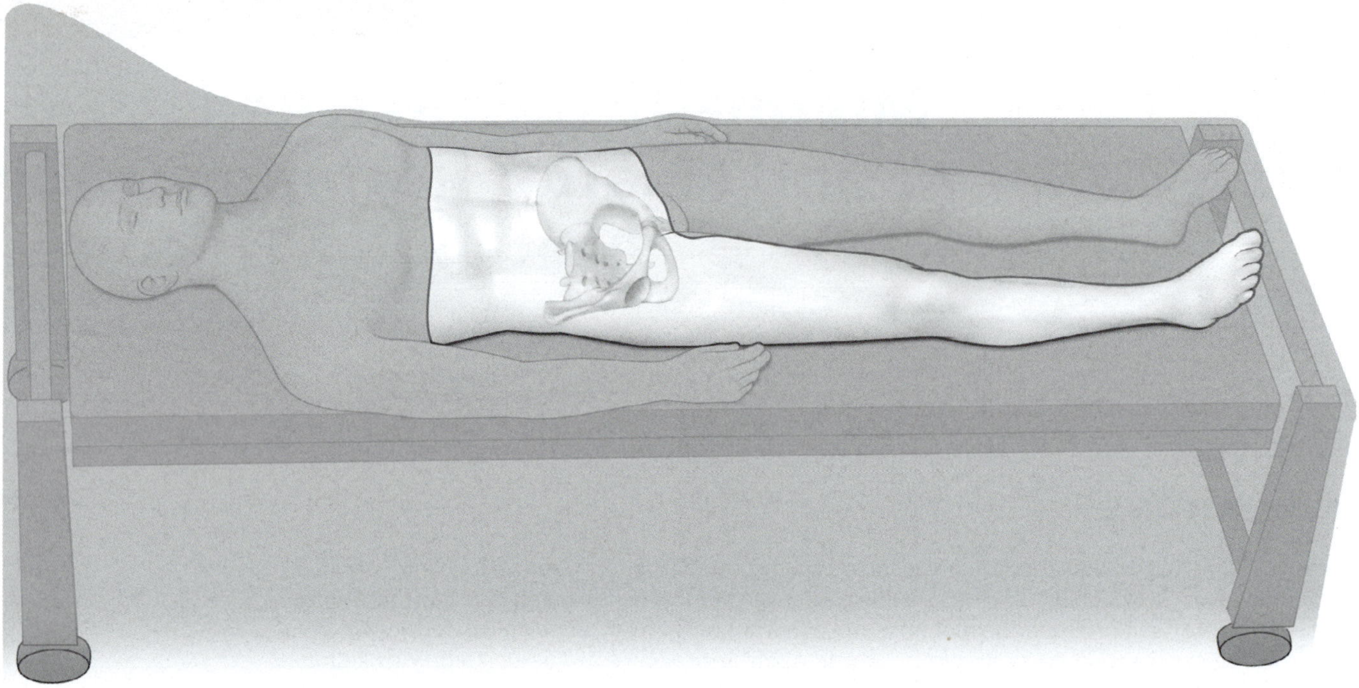

Figure 9.1 Photo demonstrating operative zone for minimally invasive acetabular surgery.

PATIENT POSITIONING

When attempting or considering minimally invasive surgery of the acetabulum, the surgeon must always be familiar and prepared to convert to an open procedure, if required. Generally, patients are positioned supine on a radiolucent operating room table. The surgeon may prepare the operating room table with traction apparatus setup in order to use skeletal traction if required. The operative zone should include the pelvis and at least the ipsilateral lower extremity (Fig. 9.1). The operative zone allows the surgeon to perform many reduction maneuvers as well as internal fixation of anterior column, posterior column, and both column fractures. We find it very important to communicate with our department of radiology and ensure that the radiology technician is familiar with the surgery and the necessary fluoroscopic views.[6] Before surgical prepping of the operative zone, the surgeon should routinely obtain practical fluoroscopic views to ensure the entire bony anatomy may be seen by fluoroscopy. The surgeon must also ensure that there is no contrast material present within the bladder that might obscure images.[12]

STRESS EXAMINATION OF ACETABULAR FRACTURES

Deciding on when not to operate on an acetabular fracture can be a difficult and sometimes an unclear decision. Most authors agree that this decision depends upon a congruent joint under the acetabular roof and a stable intact roof.[5,7,13,15,17] Matta et al.[7] first described the idea of roof arc measurements and later used CT to quantify the amount of acetabular roof recommended to be intact to treat nonoperatively.[13] Posterior wall fractures do not apply to these measurements and stability is the most crucial factor for these injuries. Studies have shown that when less than 20% of the posterior wall was fractured, hips were stable, and when the fracture involved greater than 50% of the posterior wall, they were unstable.[18,19] This leaves a fairly large gray area with room for measurement error. Tornetta[15] described the use of dynamic stress examinations to evaluate all patients they considered for nonoperative treatment. In this study, which also included patients with documented dislocations, they examined all patients under anesthesia. They described internally and externally rotating the affected hip in flexion, extension, and abduction; at each position an AP, iliac oblique, and obturator oblique image was examined for incongruence. Also, a stress "sufficient to rock the patient on the table... in the direction of displacement" was then applied. In their report, 3 of their 41 patients demonstrated a loss of congruence and were treated operatively. At a follow-up of 2.7 years, 91% of their patients had good or excellent results.

SURGICAL APPROACHES, FIXATION AND REDUCTION TECHNIQUES

For minimally invasive techniques to be successful the goals of each surgery must be considered as each fracture and patient physiology may be different. In acetabular surgery, the reduction remains the most critical aspect of any minimally invasive surgery. The inability to reduce the fracture continues to be the major critique of its opponents. It can be challenging if not impossible for surgeons to obtain an anatomic reduction using minimally invasive methods. Therefore, the surgeon must consider which fractures and patients may benefit from a minimally invasive technique or a formal open reduction and internal fixation procedure. One instance where minimally invasive techniques may be an option is in elderly patients as it has been demonstrated that elderly patients can tolerate imperfect reductions better than younger patients.[20]

For most minimally invasive acetabular procedures, surgery is best accomplished within a few days from injury.[6,10–12,14] Many times the reduction can be as straightforward as traction or rotation of the leg. Several reduction tools such as Schanz pins, ballpoint pushers, and reduction clamps are necessary for fracture reduction maneuvers (Fig. 9.2). Mini-lateral windows can assist in accessing an anterior column or posterior column fracture, and using appropriate clamps the fracture can be reduced and stabilized. At times, it may be helpful to use a universal distractor (Synthes, Paoli, PA) to help reduce and hold a fracture prior to internal fixation.

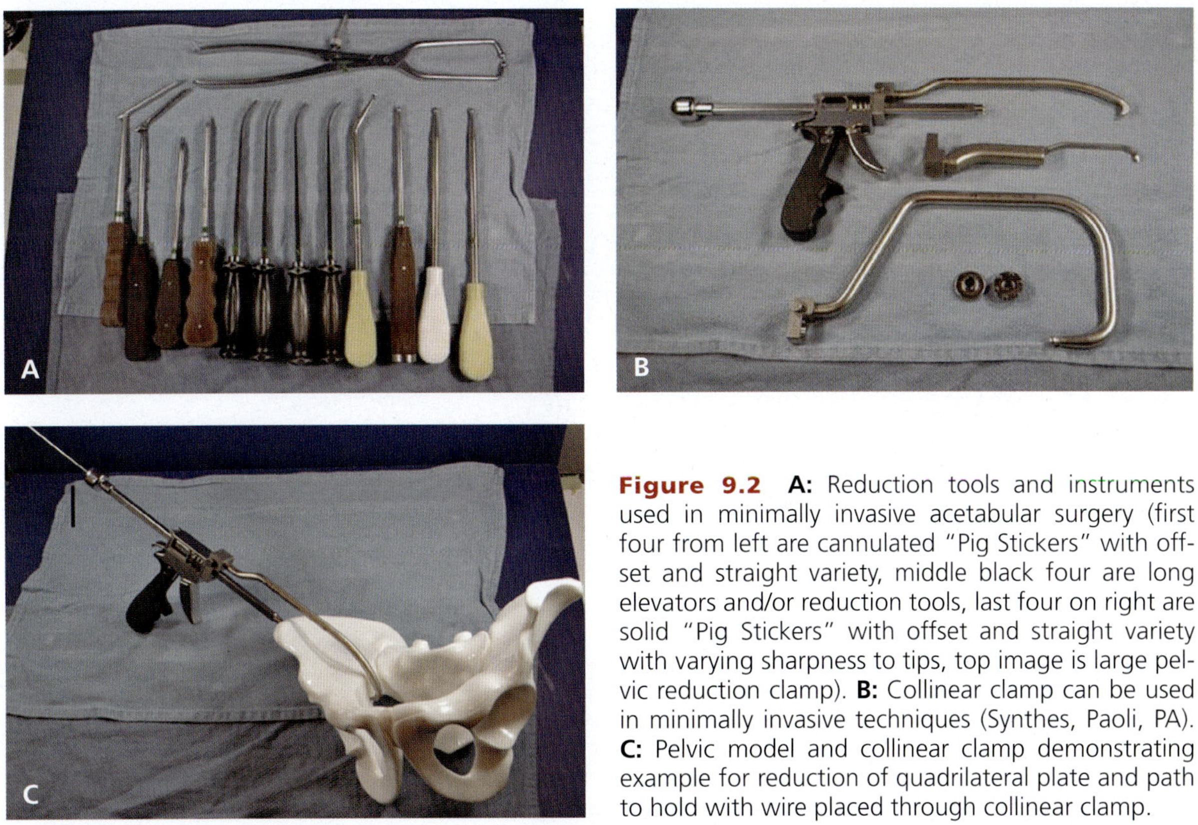

Figure 9.2 **A:** Reduction tools and instruments used in minimally invasive acetabular surgery (first four from left are cannulated "Pig Stickers" with offset and straight variety, middle black four are long elevators and/or reduction tools, last four on right are solid "Pig Stickers" with offset and straight variety with varying sharpness to tips, top image is large pelvic reduction clamp). **B:** Collinear clamp can be used in minimally invasive techniques (Synthes, Paoli, PA). **C:** Pelvic model and collinear clamp demonstrating example for reduction of quadrilateral plate and path to hold with wire placed through collinear clamp.

ANTERIOR COLUMN FRACTURE REDUCTION AND INTERNAL FIXATION

The anterior column screw can be inserted in a retrograde or antegrade fashion. An anterior column screw may be used in a majority of anterior column fractures. Routt et al.[21] first described the technique in which they used this screw in a retrograde manner after an open incision to treat pelvic ring injuries. Starr et al.[12] also demonstrated using an anterior column screw in either antegrade or retrograde fashion for anterior column fixation.

For placement of an anterior column screw, the patient is placed supine (can also be done in lateral position, but antegrade only) with a small bump under the sacrum if necessary. A small bump may be necessary to elevate the pelvis to assist hand positioning when drilling and placing an anterior column screw. For improved access, we use the fluoroscopic C-arm on the ipsilateral side as the fracture for retrograde placement and the contralateral side for antegrade placement. During the insertion of the anterior column screw, two main views are used and checked: An inlet-iliac view and an outlet-obturator view (Fig. 9.3) as described.[12,21] The former is to ensure that the wire does not perforate the inner cortex and injure the bladder or deviate anteriorly toward the vessels. The latter ensures that the wire avoids the hip joint and does not escape superiorly. These views are obtained by rotating either 20 degrees from standard inlet/outlet x-rays in a lateral oblique manner for an outlet-obturator x-ray and in a medial manner for an inlet-iliac x-ray.

The starting point for an anterior column screw is in-line from the greater trochanter to the thick part of the iliac crest, usually 4 to 5 cm posterior to the anterior-superior iliac crest in thin patients. A starting point just cephalad is used in smaller patients, whereas in obese or muscular patients, a point closer to the iliac crest is used.[12] When the surgeon uses a cannulated guide with a sharp point, he may place the drill or wire securely into bone without slipping from the highly sloped bony surface (Fig. 9.4). This cannulated guide may be used for most of the techniques described in this chapter.

The reduction techniques for anterior column fractures will be depending on the level of displacement and obliquity of the fracture pattern. For nondisplaced or minimally displaced

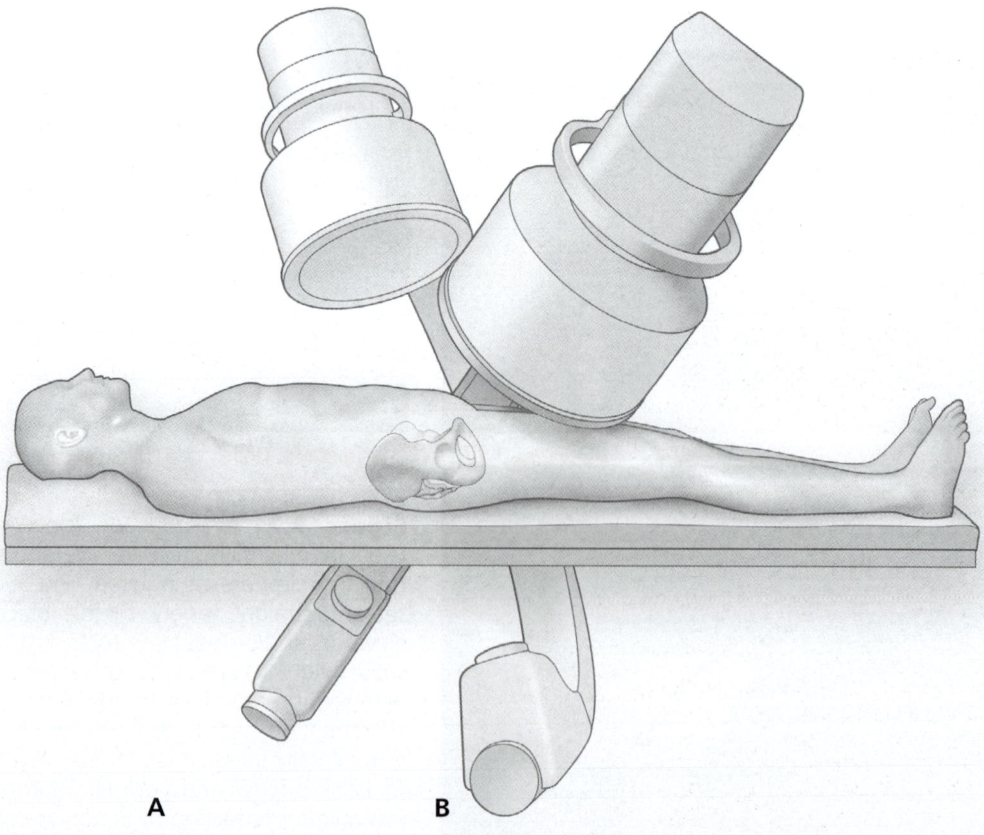

Figure 9.3 **A:** Fluoroscopic x-ray view showing outlet-obturator x-ray. **B:** Fluoroscopic x-ray view showing inlet-iliac x-ray.

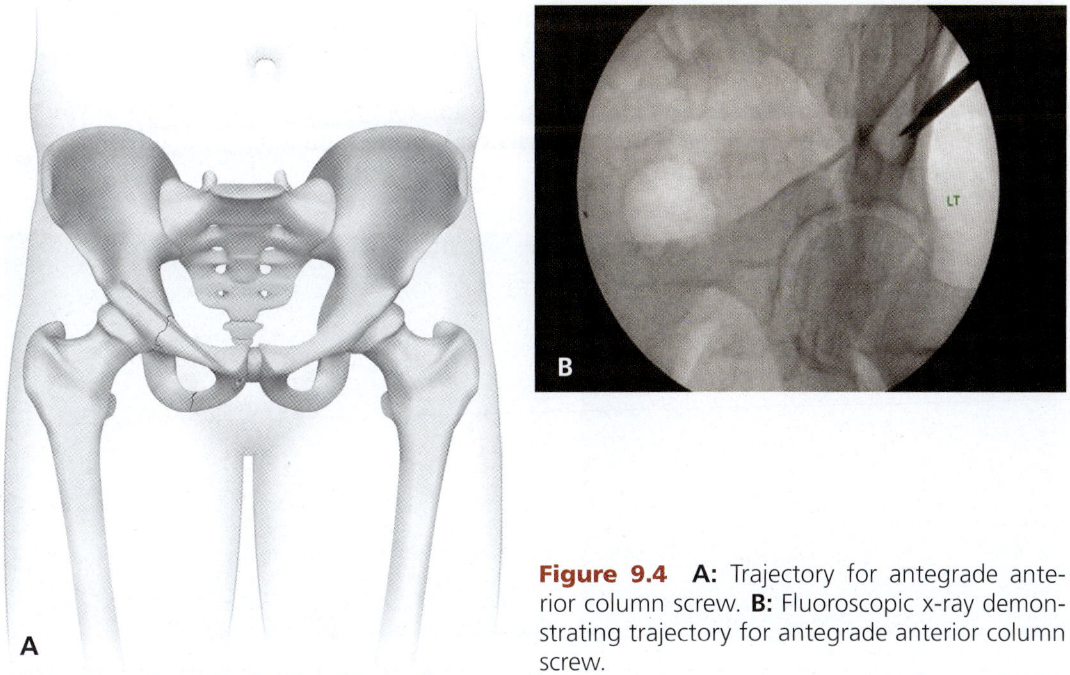

Figure 9.4 **A:** Trajectory for antegrade anterior column screw. **B:** Fluoroscopic x-ray demonstrating trajectory for antegrade anterior column screw.

fractures 2 mm or less, a reduction maneuver may not be required. For anterior column fractures that are displaced more than 2 mm, various reduction techniques may be used. In some circumstances when the fracture displacement is not in a vertical plane and is perpendicular to the screw vector, the fracture may even be reduced by using a lag effect of a screw (Fig. 9.5A, B). Percutaneous dissection may be done outside the zones of the middle window of the acetabulum in order to use a reduction tool to reduce the anterior column. For example, a percutaneous incision may be utilized in the medial (medial to femoral neurovascular bundle) or lateral windows (lateral to femoral neurovascular bundle) to use a reduction tool to help reduce the anterior column fracture while drilling and placing an anterior column screw. A ballpoint pusher, bone hook, joker, narrow bone elevator, or long hemostat may be used carefully to reduce the anterior column fracture and maintain its position while the

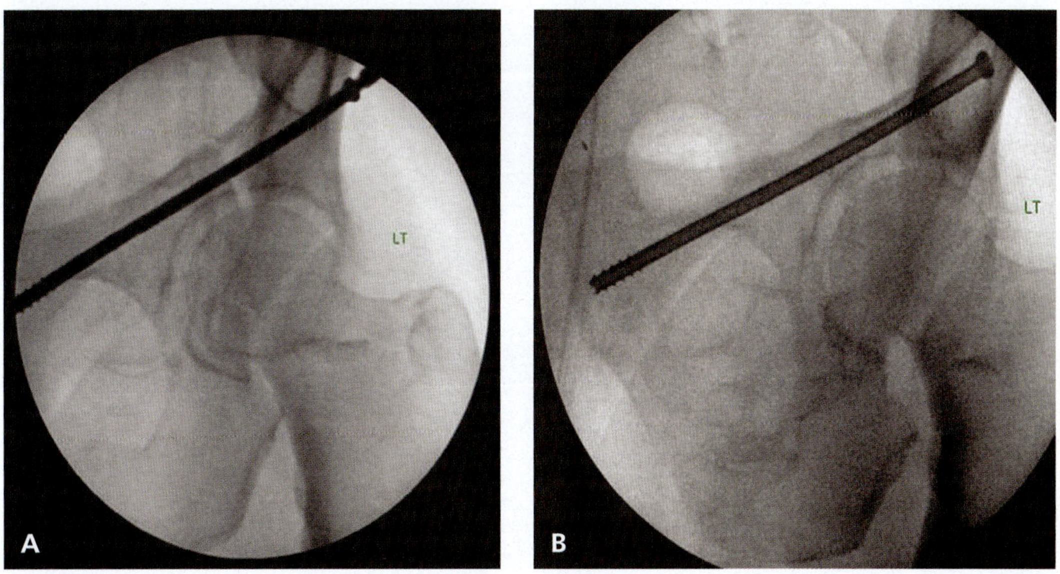

Figure 9.5 **A:** Fluoroscopic x-ray demonstrating intraoperative placement of antegrade anterior column screw with fracture displacement of 5 mm prior to final screw compression. **B:** Fluoroscopic x-ray demonstrating intraoperative placement of antegrade anterior column screw with fracture reduction after final screw compression.

drill or wire is placed. The reduction must be maintained until the final screw is placed. The long hemostat may be used to bluntly dissect down to bone in order to make a pathway for another reduction tool.

In our case example, we are using an offset reduction tool through a 2-cm lateral window incision to reduce the patient's displaced quadrilateral surface and anterior column fracture. The reduction is maintained until final screw placement (Fig. 9.6A–K). A modified pelvic

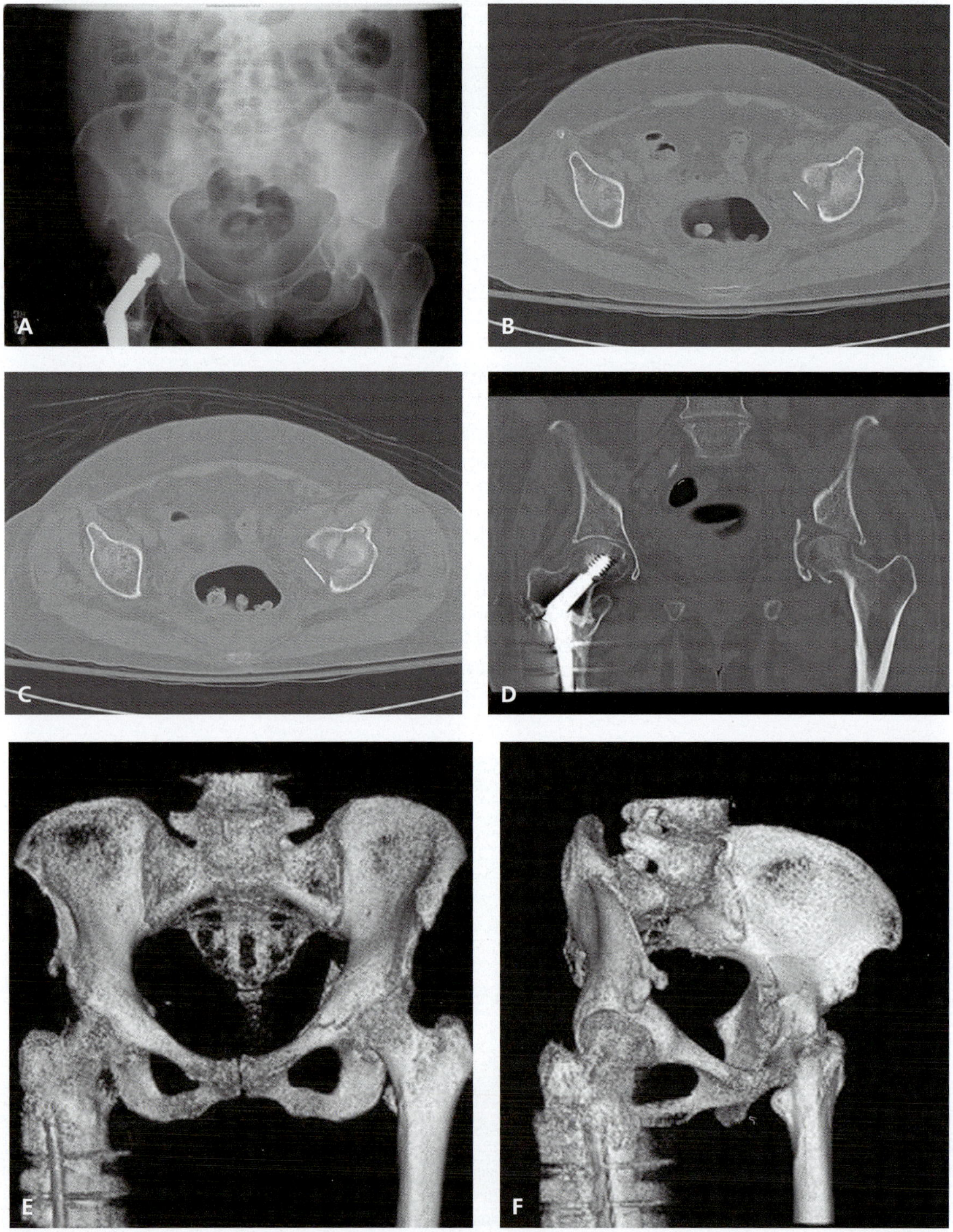

Figure 9.6 **A–G:** A 63-year-old female patient with a BMI of 50 with a left anterior column posterior hemitransverse fracture (previously injured right hip intertrochanteric fracture fixed by another surgeon). **H:** Intraoperative reduction with offset tool to reduce quadrilateral plate and anterior column fracture. **I–K:** Patient at 5-year follow-up without significant hip pain and functioning at preinjury levels.

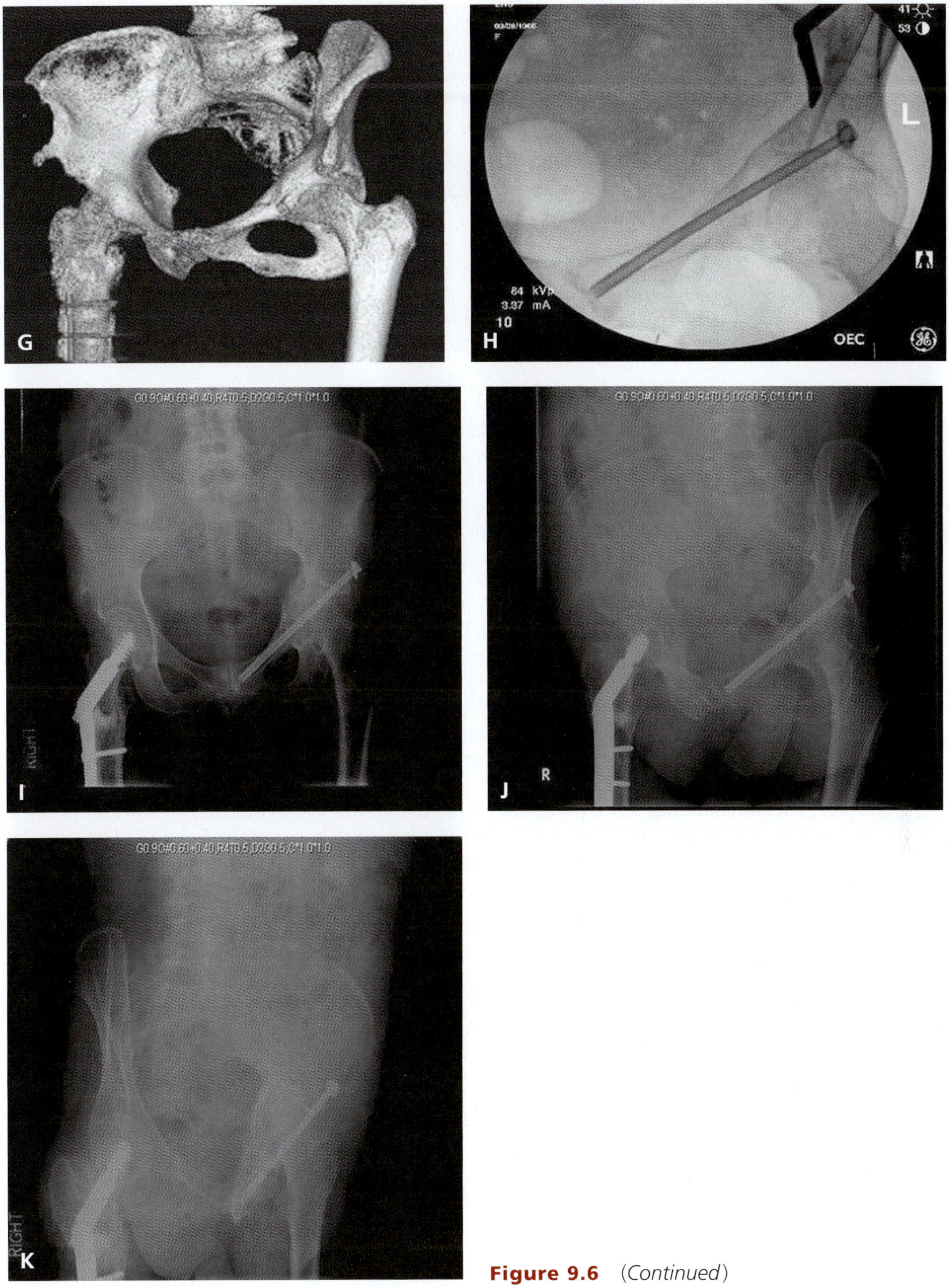

Figure 9.6 *(Continued)*

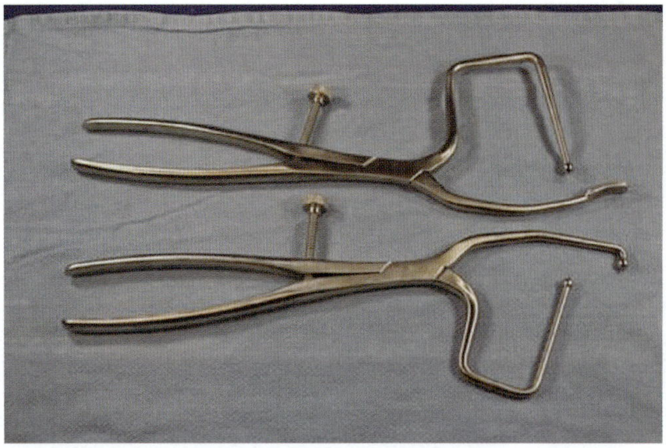

Figure 9.7 Photo displaying modified pelvic reduction clamp with built-in footplate (superior picture) and modified pelvic reduction clamp with ballpoint (inferior picture) (Reinert pelvic reduction clamps, Smith and Nephew, Memphis, TN).

reduction clamp may also be used in this manner to help reduce and maintain reduction of the quadrilateral surface. The surgeon must be aware of patients with osteoporosis as it is easy to penetrate the medial wall of the quadrilateral surface with a pointed reduction clamp. Therefore, we recommend the use of a modified pelvic reduction clamp that has a built-in footplate that may reduce the chances of medial wall penetration as well as not being lost in the true pelvis if a clamp with a modular footplate is used (Fig. 9.7).

In circumstances where the anterior column and rami have variable anatomy, the surgeon may bend the tip of the guidewire for cannulated screws by 10 to 15 degrees with the use of a pair of pliers. The bent guidewire may then be used to better allow the wire to remain intraosseously when crossing the fracture site. If the bent wire technique is used, the surgeon should gently tap the guidewire into bone as compared to using power. By tapping in the guidewire into placement, it will allow the surgeon to place the wire in its best position (Fig. 9.8).

For retrograde placement, the approach can be done through a 3-cm "mini-Pfannenstiel" incision as described by Starr et al.[12] or with a percutaneous incision at the contralateral pubic tubercle at the base of the penis or mons pubis (Fig. 9.9).[21] Drill sleeves are used to protect the surrounding tissues with all of the percutaneous methods. The starting point is just inferior to the ipsilateral pubic tubercle and lateral to the symphysis pubis. The surgeon may alternate between the described images and the drill or wire is advanced to the far cortex, measured, and then either a solid or cannulated screw is placed under fluoroscopic visualization.

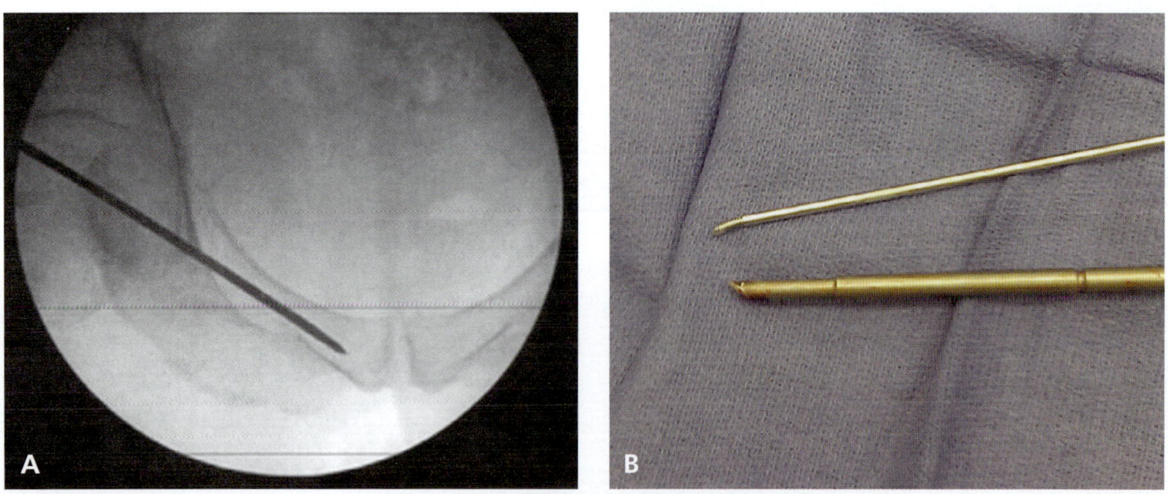

Figure 9.8 **A:** Intraoperative x-ray demonstrating 10- to 15-degree bent guidewire for enhanced placement of percutaneous screw. **B:** Photo demonstrating 10- to 15-degree bent guidewire for enhanced placement of percutaneous screw.

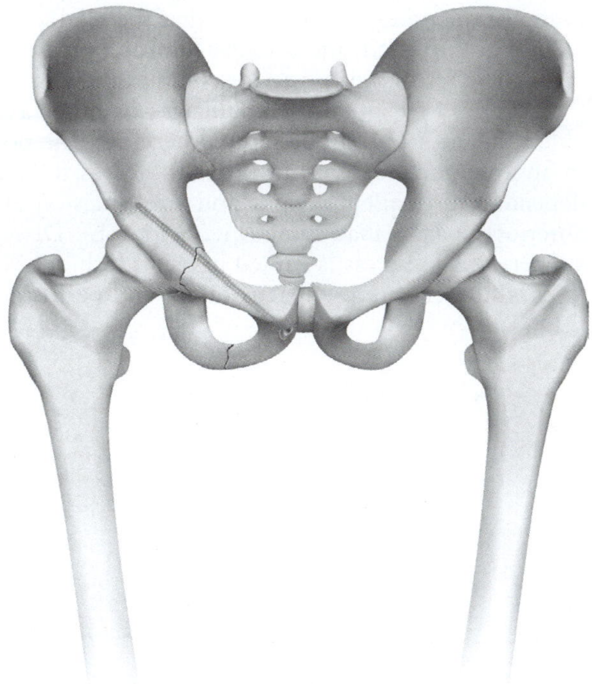

Figure 9.9 Starting point for retrograde anterior column screw.

POSTERIOR COLUMN FRACTURE REDUCTION AND INTERNAL FIXATION

When placing a posterior column screw, the C-arm machine should be positioned contralateral to the fracture and the surgeon, with the patient in the supine position. As with the anterior column screw, the posterior column screw can be placed in either antegrade or retrograde fashion. To place a retrograde screw, an assistant must hold the leg with the hip flexed and externally rotated along with the knee flexed (Fig. 9.10).[12] This position helps expose the ischial tuberosity (the start point) and also rotates the sciatic nerve further away from the start point. After palpation and dissection to the tuberosity, a drill or wire is placed in the

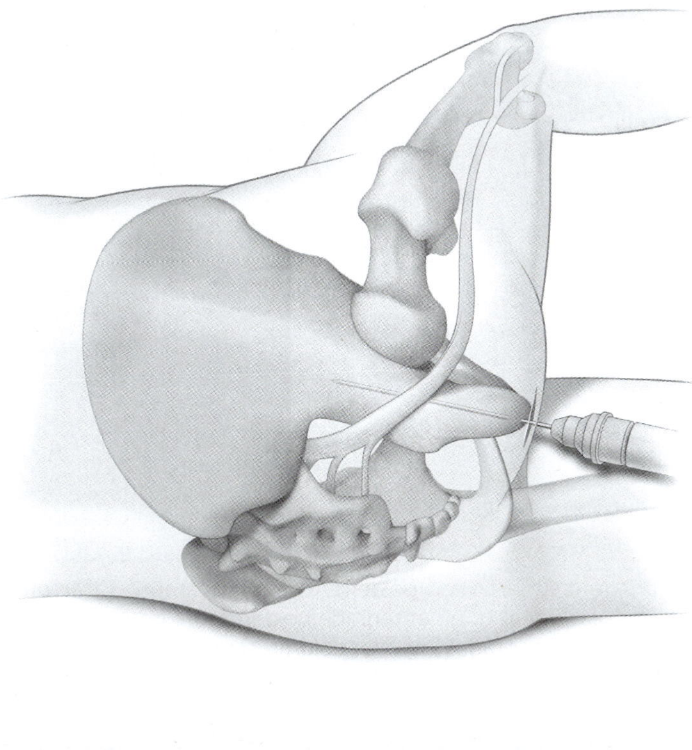

Figure 9.10 Patient positioning for placement of a retrograde posterior column screw (patient appears to be in lateral position for better illustration of start point).

center of the tuberosity, recalling that the sciatic nerve passes just lateral to this position. The guide pin is then advanced under fluoroscopic guidance using the iliac and obturator oblique views. The retrograde posterior column screw is then inserted as described before.

Secondary to soft tissue challenges or other associated injuries, the surgeon may not be able to place a retrograde screw; therefore, the posterior column screw can also be inserted in an antegrade fashion. In order to access the start point, a 3-cm (may need to be larger depending on patient weight and size) incision is made a few centimeters posterior to the anterior-superior iliac spine (Fig. 9.11A–E). Dissection is carried out to the iliac crest and subperiosteal abscess is gained in usual fashion. We use a wood handle elevator and sponge to carefully elevate the iliacus fascia and periosteum off the inner pelvic brim. A malleable

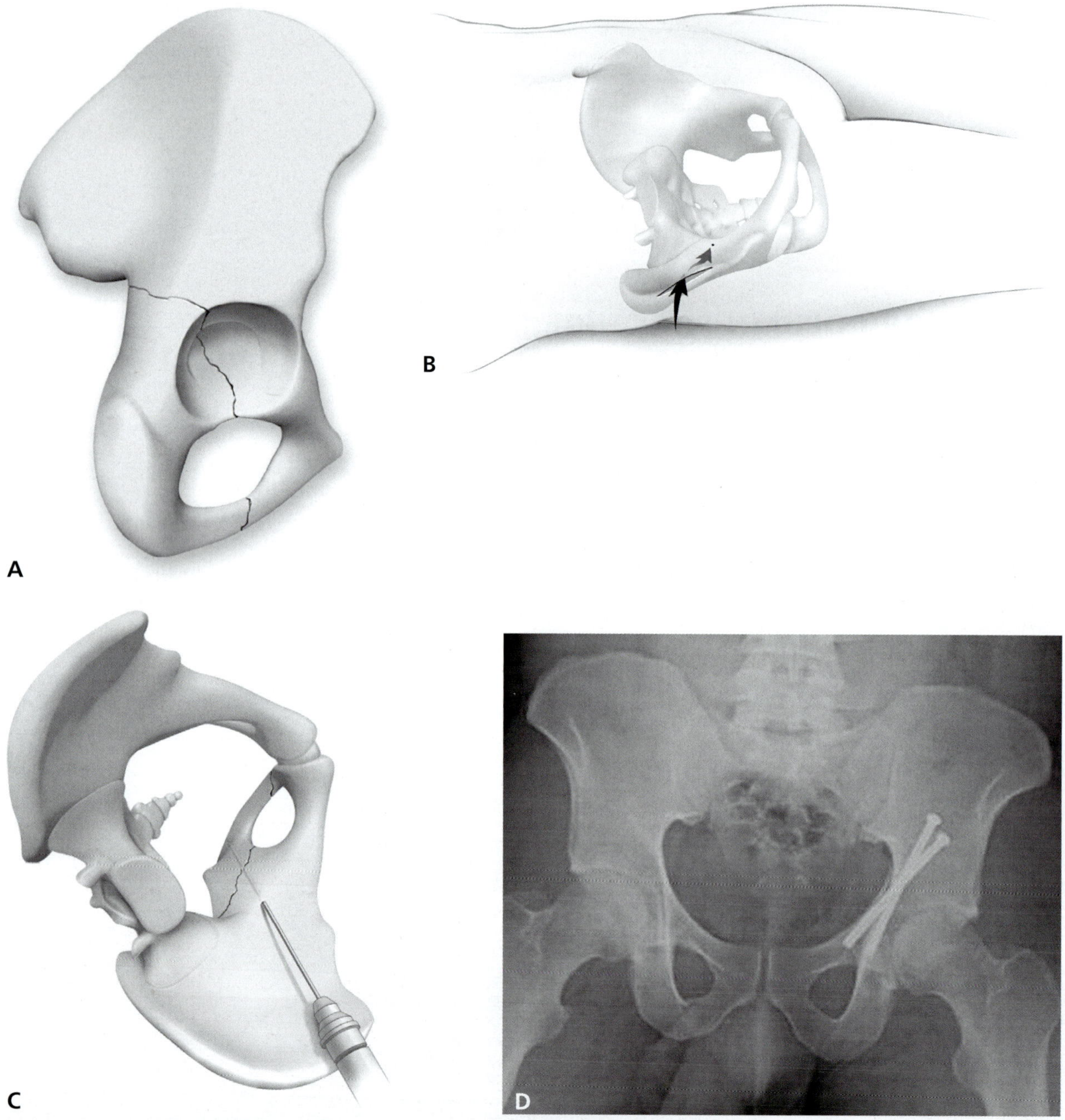

Figure 9.11 **A:** Image demonstrating posterior column acetabular fracture. **B:** Image demonstrating incision for entry into pelvis for placement of an antegrade posterior column screw. **C:** Image demonstrating appropriate placement of guidewire for antegrade posterior column screw. **D–F:** Postoperative x-rays demonstrating anterior and posterior column screw fixation. (Case courtesy of Drs. Kurtis Staples and Hrayr Basmaijan).

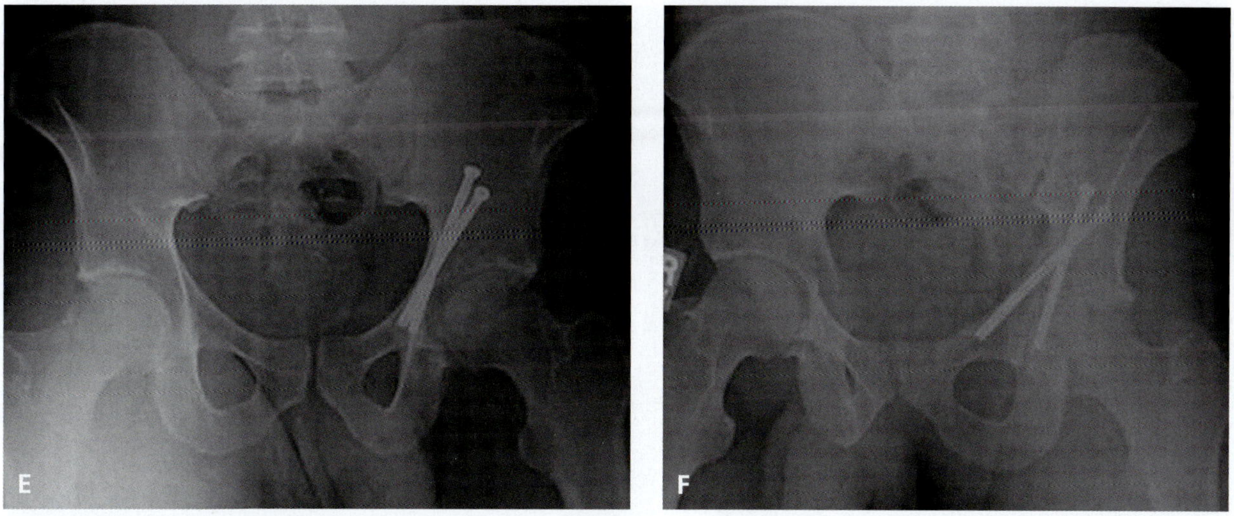

Figure 9.11 *(Continued)*

retractor is then placed over the pelvic brim. The same images are used to place an antegrade posterior column screw. The screw is placed from just proximal to the pelvic brim perpendicular to the fracture line through the posterior column.

LC II SCREW

This type of screw was first described in acetabular surgery by Gay et al.[10] and Parker and Copeland.[20] This screw is useful for coronal fracture patterns like high anterior column or both column patterns. The path of this screw is from the anterior-superior iliac spine toward the posterior–superior iliac spine in the LC II corridor.[22] The C-arm should again be positioned opposite the fracture and all of the same preparative works are needed. Its start point is usually found on an obturator oblique view, which demonstrates the percutaneous incision just above the joint (Fig. 9.12). A "teepee" view (Fig. 9.13) can be used to ensure correct

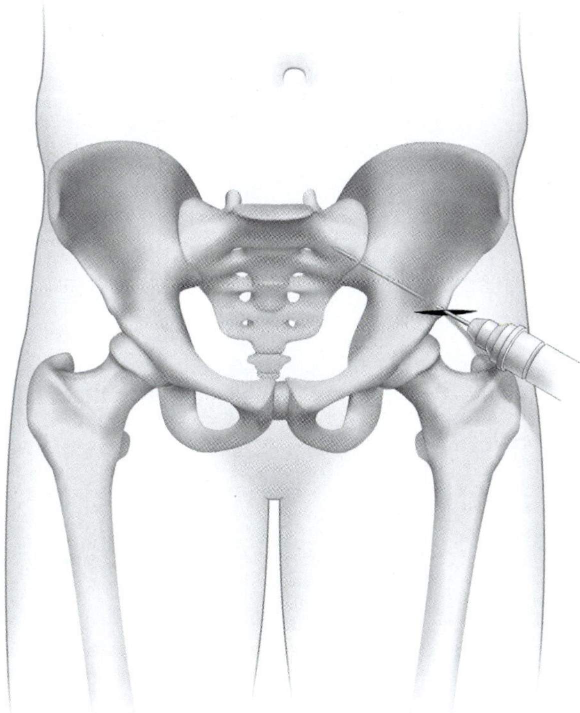

Figure 9.12 Photo demonstrating incision for placement of LC II screw.

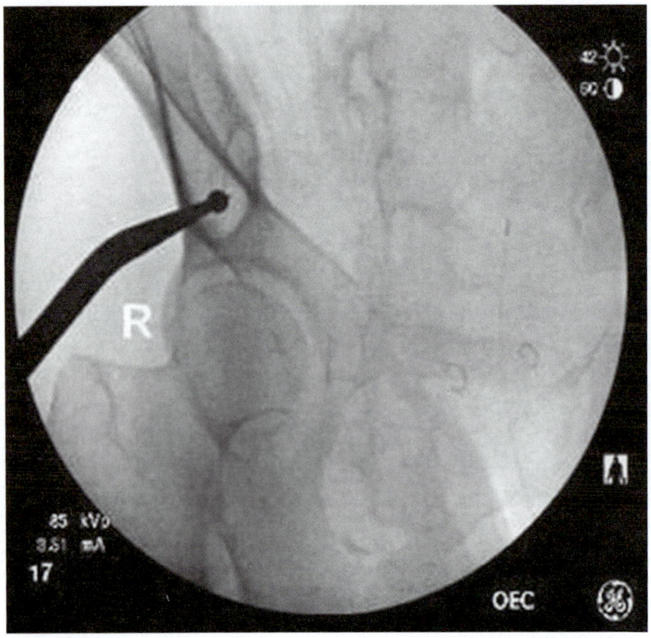

Figure 9.13 Intraoperative fluoroscopic view demonstrating teepee view.

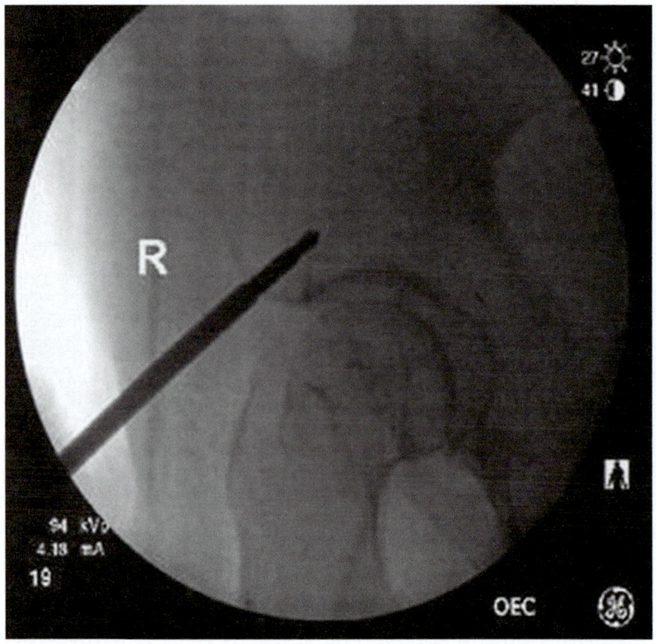

Figure 9.14 Intraoperative fluoroscopic view demonstrating iliac oblique view and entry of pin.

start point and trajectory.[22] Care must be taken to avoid injuring the nearby lateral femoral cutaneous nerve (LFCN) during dissection.[23] The iliac oblique is useful to ensure that the greater sciatic notch is not violated (Fig. 9.14). A "down the wing" view is used to visualize the corridor of bone; in order to obtain this, an inlet view is obtained with a 30- to 45-degree lateralization that allows visualization of the inner corridor of the iliac wing (Fig. 9.15). An LC II screw can be placed anterior to posterior or from the posterior to anterior (Fig. 9.16). In certain fractures that involve both the anterior column and posterior column or both

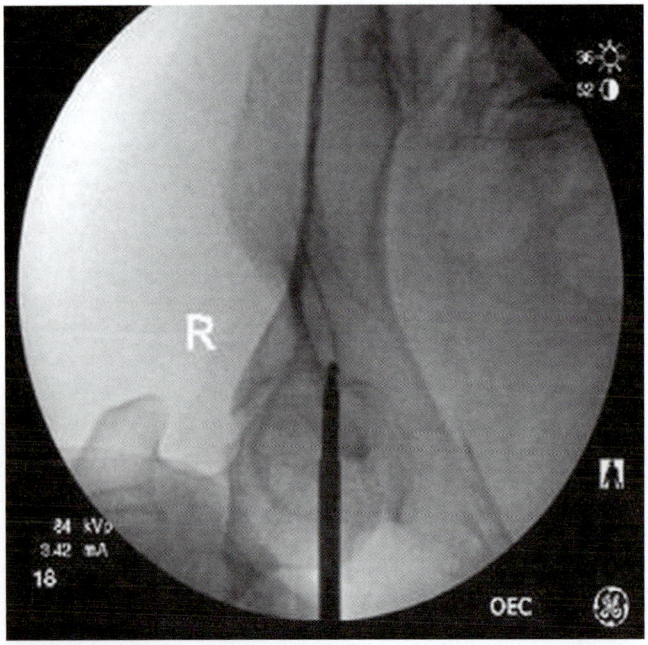

Figure 9.15 Intraoperative fluoroscopic view demonstrating down the wing view and entry of pin.

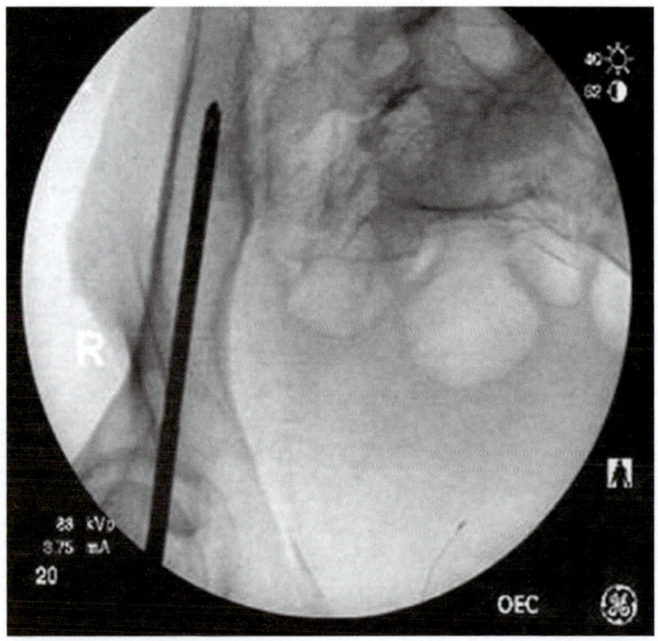

Figure 9.16 Intraoperative fluoroscopic view demonstrating pin down the wing.

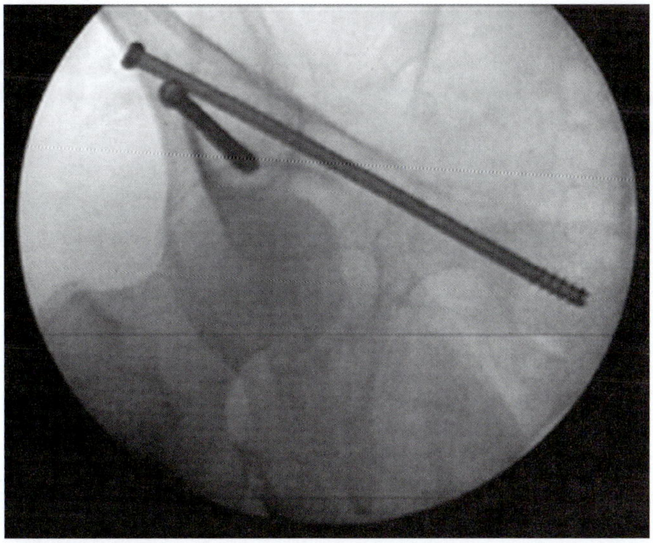

Figure 9.17 Intraoperative x-rays demonstrating placement of both an anterior column and LC II screw and how close these screws may be placed together.

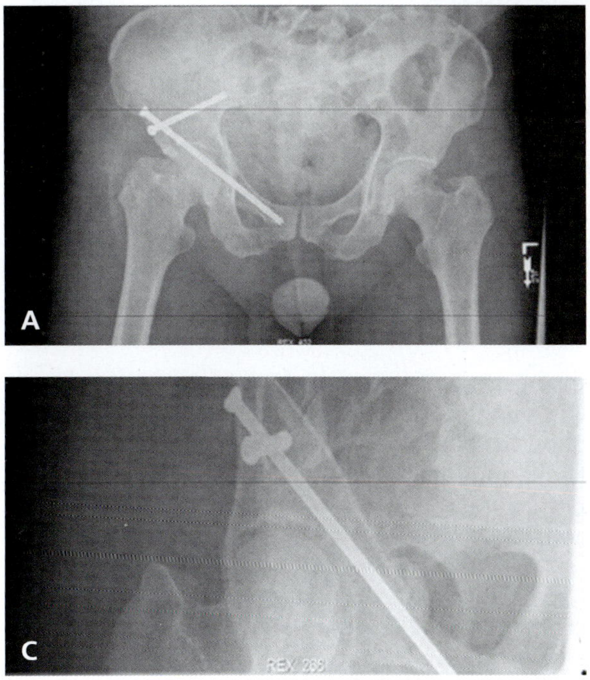

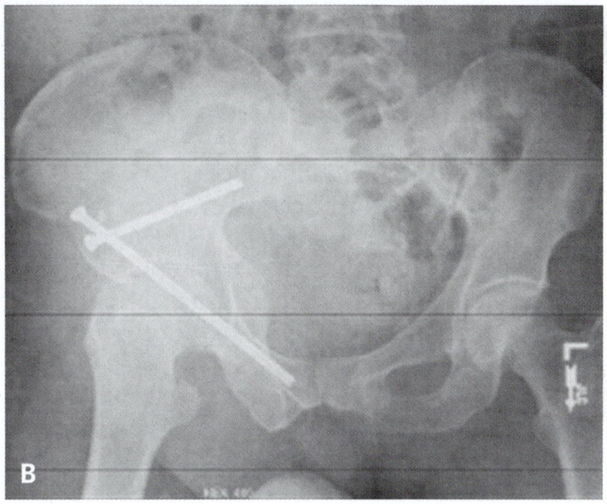

Figure 9.18 Postoperative x-rays demonstrating placement of both an anterior column and LC II screw.

columns equivalent, a fracture may benefit from both an anterior column and LC II screw (Figs. 9.17 and 9.18).

THE "MAGIC SCREW"

Starr et al.[24] have described the placement for the "magic screw." This screw may be used to hold the quadrilateral plate after reduction. The surgeon begins the guidewire on the oblique surface of the iliac wing proximal and posterior to the acetabulum. The guidewire exits the quadrilateral plate near the ischial spine (Fig. 9.19). The fluoroscopic views to obtain to place the magic screw include the AP, inlet, and iliac oblique views. The guidewire and/or screw cannot penetrate into the true pelvis.

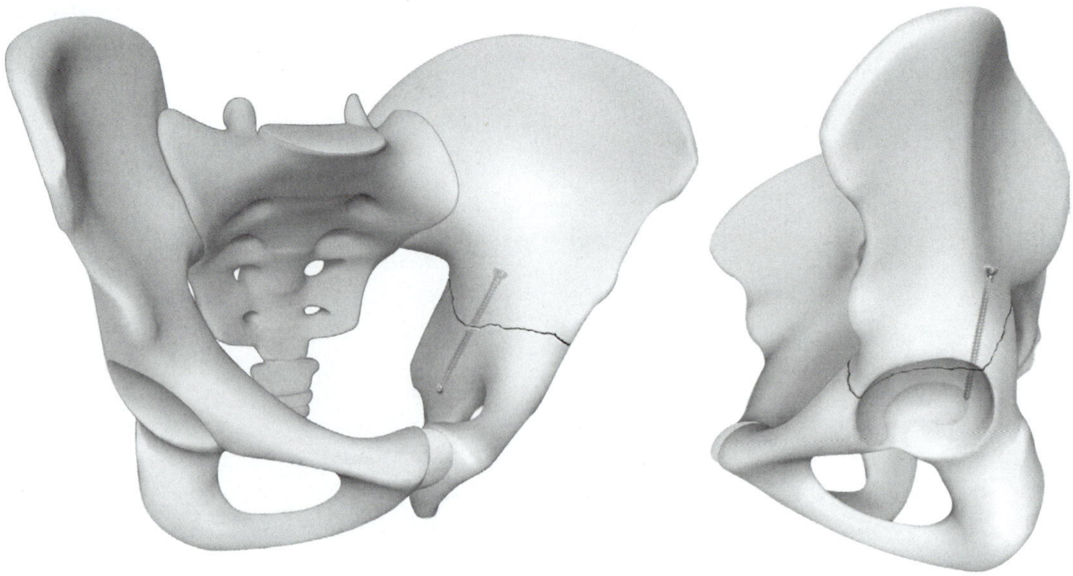

Figure 9.19 Placement of the magic screw.

NAVIGATION AND INTRAOPERATIVE CT

In some circumstances, we use navigated pelvic and acetabular fracture fixation methods. We use intraoperative CT analysis to visualize both the reduction as well as the internal fixation. We find that by using intraoperative CT we have been able to correct any inaccuracies in our reductions or internal fixation. Also, we believe that intraoperative CT may allow the surgeon better visualization of bony anatomy, especially in patients with osteoporosis or morbid obesity as fluoroscopy images in these patients are often difficult to visualize (Fig. 9.20).

We presented our early results using intraoperative CT in which we demonstrated in at least 7% of the cases the fluoroscopic images might not accurately define the reduction and implant position.[25] In our early series, we showed that through the use of intraoperative CT we were able to observe our errors in reduction and internal fixation, and then we were able to correct those errors after a review of the intraoperative CT. We have demonstrated what we believe to be an improvement in standard stress examinations of acetabular fractures by adding intraoperative CT during stress examination of posterior wall fractures (Fig. 9.21A–C).[26] We have also found that with improvements in intraoperative CT imaging, such as that found with the O-Arm (Medtronic, Minneapolis, MN), we are better able to define bony anatomy, field of view, and bony/internal fixation resolution (Fig. 9.22).[27] Intraoperative CTs may be useful in reviewing intraoperative fracture reductions and implants without the need for postoperative CTs, which may require a return to the operating room if the surgeon is not pleased with the postoperative CT results.

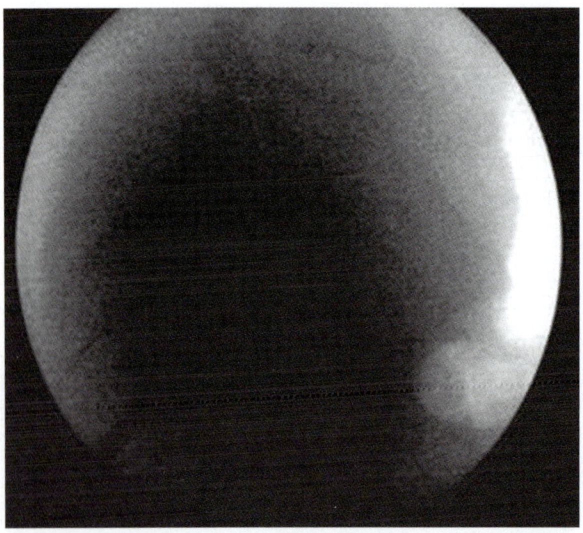

Figure 9.20 Preoperative fluoroscopic image of pelvis of patient with BMI greater than 50. Image displays inability for surgeon to visualize bony anatomy with fluoroscopy alone.

As surgeons increase their use of navigation to place acetabular screws, the accuracy of navigation-based fixation[28–30] has been analyzed. Hong et al.[29] examined the accuracy of two-dimensional (2D) fluoroscopy-based computer-assisted navigation, and they found that in 18 adult patients their average fracture gap went from 10 to 3 mm and that their wire tip deviated 2.5 mm at the tip of the wire. Rosenberger et al.[30] have also looked at noninvasive tracking methods with less favorable results.

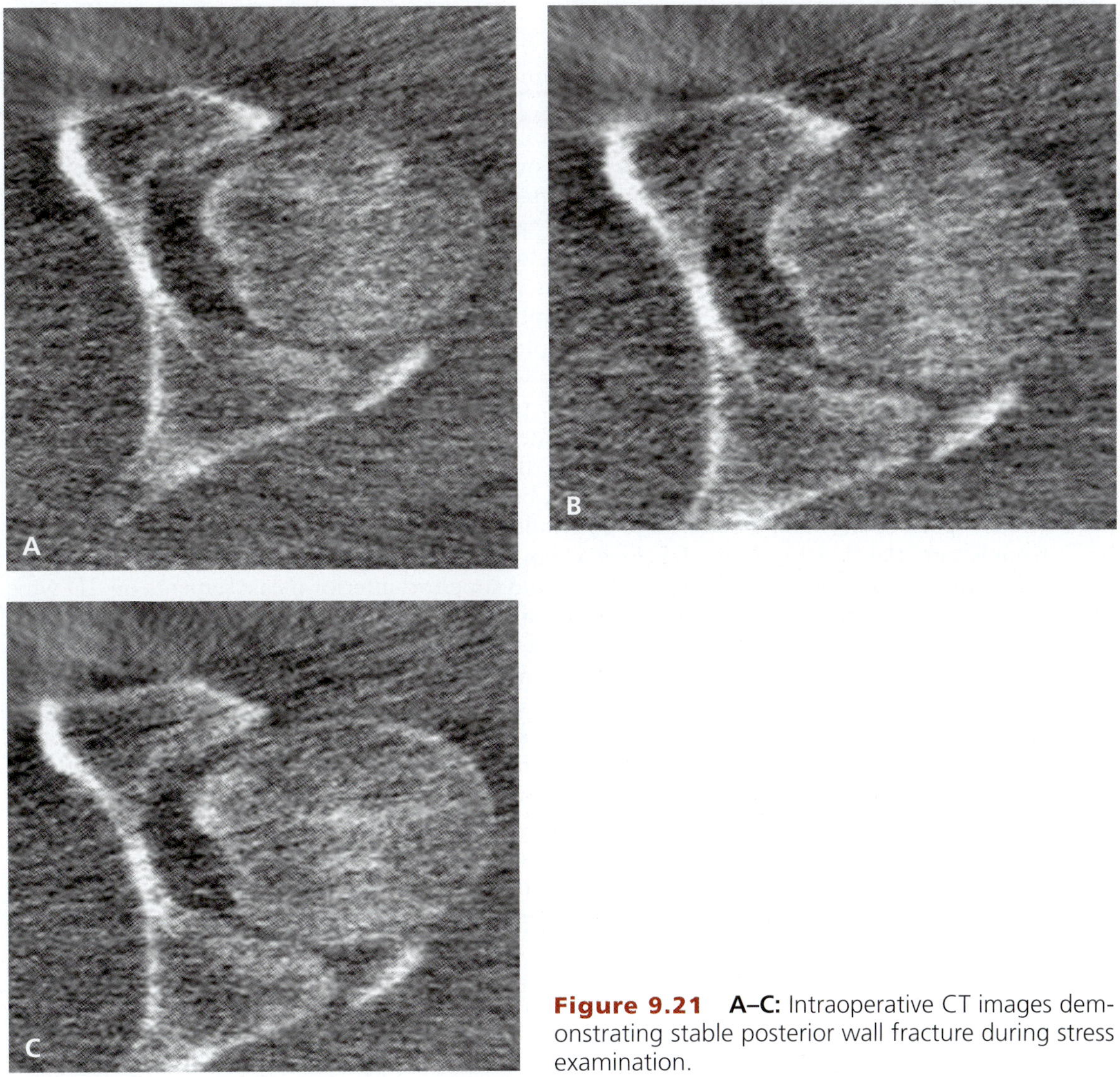

Figure 9.21 **A–C:** Intraoperative CT images demonstrating stable posterior wall fracture during stress examination.

Figure 9.22 Use of O-Arm (Medtronic, Minneapolis, MN) intraoperatively for intraoperative CT assessment of reduction and internal fixation. Photo demonstrates setup for intraoperative CT including the use of sterile fluoroscopy cover over patient.

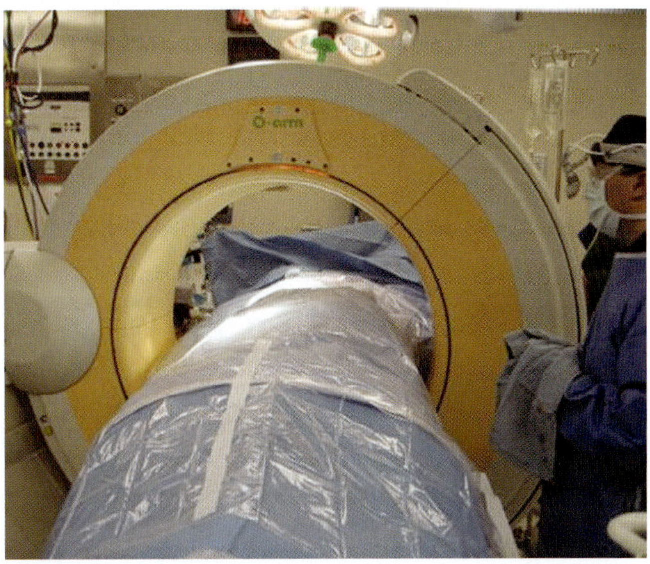

COMPLICATIONS

The risks and complications associated with minimally invasive acetabular fracture reduction and internal fixation techniques include the following: Infection, bleeding, neurovascular injury, malunion, nonunion, loss of reduction, loss of fixation, and/or anesthetic complications. The complication risks are dependent on several factors including patient physiology, fracture pattern, bony anatomy, surgeon experience, and/or intraoperative imaging. Before using the techniques used in this chapter, the surgeon must understand the diagnosis, patient anatomy and physiology, and standard open techniques.

In regard to bony anatomy, examinations of previously placed percutaneous screws on cadavers and postoperative CT scans prompted some to question the space available for screw insertion, especially in the anterior column.[31–33] Attias et al.[31] created virtual three-dimensional (3D) reconstruction models from CT scans of the intact hemipelvis from patients with acetabular fractures. They attempted to place virtual implants to determine the largest diameter screw that the anterior column, posterior column, and LC II corridor would safely accommodate. The posterior column and LC II corridor both had ample room to accommodate 11.4- and 12.1-mm screws, respectively, but the anterior column had a mean maximum virtual space of 6.4 mm. The authors concluded that they agree with the recommendations from Routt et al.[21] in 1995 that 3.5- or 4.5-mm screws should be used in the anterior column. Interestingly, the smallest anterior–posterior and superior–inferior measurements on 2D were 16.5 and 19.5 mm, respectively. Chen et al.[32] also evaluated the anterior column anatomy in a similar fashion but compared males to females. They found a 6.5-mm screw would fit in the anterior column in males, but warned against using 6.5-mm screws in females.

The strength of limited fixation acetabular constructs[34–36] has also been explored. Chang et al.[34] used a cadaveric model to compare traditional plating method versus percutaneously placed 6.5-mm screws in the anterior and posterior columns. The authors showed that although the plate and screw method had statistically greater yield and maximum strength, the stiffness was actually 39% greater with the column screws. In addition, Simonian et al.[35] used a T-type fracture model and stabilized them with an anterior plate with one screw traversing the posterior column or a posterior plate with one screw traversing the anterior column versus two plates and found no difference.

REHABILITATION PROTOCOL

The goals of minimally invasive acetabular surgery need to also consider the rehabilitation process. Although every fracture pattern and patient is different, we generally allow our patients to be weight-bearing as tolerated and perform range of motion of the hip, knee, and ankle as tolerated after their surgery. We believe that by placing any restrictions on weight-bearing status or range of motion that patients may impede rehabilitation. However, the surgeon must consider his/her confidence in the fracture reduction, internal fixation, and bone quality. If we are not confident in any of these three variables, then we limit the patients to touchdown weight-bearing 4.5 to 6.8 kg (10 to 15 lb) and/or limitation of hip active flexion beyond 90 degrees. If we use either or both of these restrictions, we will only use them for 6 weeks. We also offer our patients the option of aquatherapy in which they are allowed to fully weight-bear in a controlled pool environment with the pool water up to their chest level. We find this rehabilitation option allows patients to gain confidence in their walking gait when they transition to full weight-bearing on land.

OUTCOME

Kazemi and Archdeacon[37] treated 28 patients with anterior column or anterior column posterior hemitransverse fractures with closed reduction and percutaneous supra-acetabular screw fixation. All of their patients were allowed and encouraged to immediately bear weight on postoperative day 1, and at final follow-up they reported no patients with a loss of reduction; in addition, no infections, thromboembolic disease, or any heterotopic ossification occurred. Mouhsine et al.[38] reported on an elderly population of 21 patients with minimally displaced acetabular fractures treated with closed reduction and percutaneous fixation with weight-bearing at 4 weeks. At 3.5 years, 18 patients followed up with no evidence of degenerative changes, loss of fixation, or hardware failures.

Starr et al.[11] reported their preliminary results of 24 patients with acetabular fractures treated with closed or limited open reduction and percutaneous fixation. They divided their patients into a group of elderly patients with pre-existing signs of degenerative changes in which an anatomic reduction was not felt to be a necessity. Their second group consisted of young patients with simple fracture types. Their preoperative displacement averaged 10 mm in the elderly and 7 mm in the young group, and postoperatively measured 3 mm and 1 mm, respectively. No loss of reduction was seen in the young group and two minor losses in the elderly group. Crowl and Kahler[9] reported on 23 patients who were treated in a similar fashion and no patients experienced a loss of reduction.

We believe that in the appropriate circumstances minimally invasive surgical techniques offer patients an option for reduction and internal fixation of acetabular fractures. Surgeons that utilize minimally invasive techniques in acetabular fractures must be experienced in open approaches. Overall, when surgeons utilize minimally invasive acetabular fracture techniques, the same goals of surgery must include optimal reduction and stable internal fixation.

REFERENCES

1. Judet R, Judet J, Letournel E. Fractures of the acetabulum: Classification and surgical approaches for open reduction. Preliminary report. *J Bone Joint Surg Am.* 1964;46:1615–1646.
2. Matta JM. Fractures of the acetabulum: Accuracy of reduction and clinical results in patients managed operatively within three weeks after the injury. *J Bone Joint Surg Am.* 1996;78(11): 1632–1645.
3. Moed BR, Carr SE, Gruson KI, et al. Computed tomographic assessment of fractures of the posterior wall of the acetabulum after operative treatment. *J Bone Joint Surg Am.* 2003;85-A(3): 512–522.
4. Matta JM. Operative treatment of acetabular fractures through the ilioinguinal approach. A 10-year perspective. *Clin Ortho Relat Res.* 1994;(305):10–19.
5. Letournel EM, Judet R, Elson R. *Fractures of the Acetabulum.* 2nd ed. Berlin, New York: Springer-Verlag; 1993.
6. Tile M. *Fractures of the Pelvis and Acetabulum.* 2nd ed. Baltimore, MD: Williams & Wilkins; 1995.
7. Matta JM, Anderson LM, Epstein HC, et al. Fractures of the acetabulum. A retrospective analysis. *Clin Orthop Relat Res.* 1986;(205):230–240.
8. Matta JM, Mehne DK, Roffi R. Fractures of the acetabulum. Early results of a prospective study. *Clin Orthop Relat Res.* 1986;(205):241–250.
9. Crowl AC, Kahler DM. Closed reduction and percutaneous fixation of anterior column acetabular fractures. *Comput Aided Surg.* 2002;7(3):169–178.
10. Gay SB, Sistrom C, Wang GJ, et al. Percutaneous screw fixation of acetabular fractures with CT guidance: Preliminary results of a new technique. *AJR Am J Roentgenol.* 1992;158(4):819–822.
11. Starr AJ, Jones AL, Reinert CM, et al. Preliminary results and complications following limited open reduction and percutaneous screw fixation of displaced fractures of the acetabulum. *Injury.* 2001;32(Suppl 1):SA45–SA50.
12. Starr AJ, Reinert CM, Jones AL. Percutaneous fixation of the columns of the acetabulum: A new technique. *J Orthop Trauma.* 1998;12(1):51–58.
13. Olson SA, Matta JM. The computerized tomography subchondral arc: A new method of assessing acetabular articular continuity after fracture (a preliminary report). *J Orthop Trauma.* 1993; 7(5):402–413.
14. Parker PJ, Copeland C. Percutaneous fluoroscopic screw fixation of acetabular fractures. *Injury.* 1997;28(9–10):597–600.
15. Tornetta P 3rd. Non-operative management of acetabular fractures. The use of dynamic stress views. *J Bone Joint Surg Br.* 1999;81(1):67–70.
16. Porter SE, Russell GV, Dews RC, et al. Complications of acetabular fracture surgery in morbidly obese patients. *J Orthop Trauma.* 2008;22(9):589–594.
17. Heeg M, Oostvogel HJ, Klasen HJ. Conservative treatment of acetabular fractures: The role of the weight-bearing dome and anatomic reduction in the ultimate results. *J Trauma.* 1987;27(5): 555–559.
18. Keith JE Jr., Brashear HR Jr., Guilford WB. Stability of posterior fracture-dislocations of the hip. Quantitative assessment using computed tomography. *J Bone Joint Surg Am.* 1988;70(5):711–714.

19. Vailas JC, Horowitz S, Wiesel SW. Posterior acetabular fracture dislocation: Fragment size, joint capsule, and stability. *J Trauma.* 1989;29:3.
20. Helfet DL, Borrelli J Jr., DiPasquale T, et al. Stabilization of acetabular fractures in elderly patients. *J Bone Joint Surg Am.* 1992;74(5):753–765.
21. Routt ML Jr., Simonian PT, Grujic L. The retrograde medullary superior pubic ramus screw for the treatment of anterior pelvic ring disruptions: A new technique. *J Orthop Trauma.* 1995;9(1):35–44.
22. Starr AJ, Walter JC, Harris RW, et al. Percutaneous screw fixation of fractures of the iliac wing and fracture-dislocations of the sacro-iliac joint (OTA Types 61-B2.2 and 61-B2.3, or Young-Burgess "lateral compression type II" pelvic fractures). *J Orthop Trauma.* 2002;16(2):116–123.
23. Sen M, Harvey EJ, Steinitz D, et al. Anatomical risks of using supra-acetabular screws in percutaneous internal fixation of the acetabulum and pelvis. *Am J Orthop (Belle Mead NJ).* 2005;34(2):94–96.
24. Starr AJ, Borer D, Reinert CM. Technical aspects of limited open reduction and percutaneous screw fixation of fractures of the acetabulum. *Oper Tech Orthop.* 2001;11(3):9.
25. Ortega GR, Rhorer AS, Miller B, et al. Use of intraoperative 3-dimensional CT imaging in the treatment of pelvic fractures. Abstract presented at: Orthopaedic Trauma Association Annual Meeting; 2008; Denver, CO.
26. Ortega GR, Cunningham B. Intraoperative 3D CT imaging in the assessment of posterior wall acetabular fracture stability during stress examination under anesthesia. Abstract presented at: AONA Challenges in Fracture Care Meeting; 2010; Phoenix, AZ.
27. Ortega GR, Cunningham B. A comparative study using a new 3D intraoperative CT image intensifier, the O-Arm®, verus the Iso-C 3D CT image intensifier. Abstract presented at: AONA Challenges in Fracture Care Meeting; 2010; Phoenix, AZ.
28. Mosheiff R, Khoury A, Weil Y, et al. First generation computerized fluoroscopic navigation in percutaneous pelvic surgery. *J Orthop Trauma.* 2004;18(2):106–111.
29. Hong G, Cong-Feng L, Cheng-Fang H, et al. Percutaneous screw fixation of acetabular fractures with 2D fluoroscopy-based computerized navigation. *Arch Orthop Trauma Surg.* 2010;130(9):1177–1183.
30. Rosenberger RE, Dolati B, Larndorfer R, et al. Accuracy of minimally invasive navigated acetabular and iliosacral fracture stabilization using a targeting and noninvasive registration device. *Arch Orthop Trauma Surg.* 2010;130(2):223–230.
31. Attias N, Lindsey RW, Starr AJ, et al. The use of a virtual three-dimensional model to evaluate the intraosseous space available for percutaneous screw fixation of acetabular fractures. *J Bone Joint Surg Br.* 2005;87(11):1520–1523.
32. Chen KN, Wang G, Cao LG, et al. Differences of percutaneous retrograde screw fixation of anterior column acetabular fractures between male and female: A study of 164 virtual three-dimensional models. *Injury.* 2009;40(10):1067–1072.
33. Shahulhameed A, Roberts CS, Pomeroy CL, et al. Mapping the columns of the acetabulum—implications for percutaneous fixation. *Injury.* 2010;41(4):339–342.
34. Chang JK, Gill SS, Zura RD, et al. Comparative strength of three methods of fixation of transverse acetabular fractures. *Clin Orthop Relat Res.* 2001;(392):433–441.
35. Simonian PT, Routt ML Jr., Harrington RM, et al. The acetabular T-type fracture. A biomechanical evaluation of internal fixation. *Clin Orthop Relat Res.* 1995;(314):234–240.
36. Giordano V, do Amaral NP, Pallottino A, et al. Operative treatment of transverse acetabular fractures: Is it really necessary to fix both columns? *Int J Med Sci.* 2009;6(4):192–199.
37. Kazemi N, Archdeacon MT. Immediate full weightbearing after percutaneous fixation of anterior column acetabulum fractures. *J Orthop Trauma.* 2012;26(2):73–79.
38. Mouhsine E, Garofalo R, Borens O, et al. Percutaneous retrograde screwing for stabilisation of acetabular fractures. *Injury.* 2005;36(11):1330–1336.

CHAPTER 10

Minimally Invasive Hip Fracture

Yoram A. Weil and Rami Mosheiff

BACKGROUND

Hip fracture has become a modern epidemic. The incidence of hip fractures is increasing throughout the world, as is the cost of treatment.[1] Despite the existing surgical treatment, the mortality from hip fracture is still high, and reported to be about 15% to 20% in the first year post fracture. In older patients with severe comorbidities the mortality is tripled due to the fracture.[2]

Optimally, minimally invasive procedures are performed on these often frail patients. The goals of such surgery should include minimal blood loss, efficient and reliable procedures, and adequate stability allowing immediate postoperative mobilization.

As numerous types of implants and techniques are available, this chapter will discuss three types of modern, minimally invasive techniques, all well supported in the orthopaedic literature. This includes navigated-assisted percutaneous screw fixation for femoral neck fractures, percutaneous compression plating for stable intertrochanteric fractures, and intramedullary nailing for unstable pertrochanteric fractures. Arthroplasty for displaced femoral neck fractures is beyond the scope of this chapter.

NAVIGATED PERCUTANEOUS SCREW FIXATION FOR FEMORAL NECK FRACTURES

Nondisplaced fractures and displaced fractures in young patients are best treated with closed or open reduction and internal fixation, most commonly with cannulated cancellous screws.[3] The rationale for using this fixation technique is to enable healing by controlled fracture impaction across parallel placed screws, allowing early weight-bearing and mobilization.

Although placement of screws is often trivialized, most surgeons tend to underestimate the technical requirements for accuracy of screw placement in terms of drill attempts, fluoroscopic time, and desired implant placement. Computerized navigation allows better accuracy for screw placement in terms of parallelism and screw spread within the femoral neck.[4] Evidence shows that this leads to less mechanical complications.[5]

Fluoroscopic navigation is a modality that enhances the capacity of the intraoperative, conventional 2D fluoroscopy by displaying multiple orthogonal views simultaneously (such as anteroposterior and lateral) without actually performing live fluoroscopy.[6,7] The advantages of this system are that trajectories of implants can be planned prior to their insertion, thus minimizing drilling attempts, reducing radiation, and decreasing operative time after setting up the system. A typical fluoroscopic navigation system comprises a computer, a tracking optical system, trackable surgical tools, and c-arm.

Optical trackers are attached to the patient's bony anatomy (such as the iliac crest) and to the surgical tools and drill guides. Tracked fluoroscopic images are captured using either a calibration target on the c-arm or a mobile targeting device that should be displayed to the optical tracking device ("camera") (Fig. 10.1). As the camera tracks the anatomical trackers and the c-arm tracker, the computer builds a coordinate system (x, y, z) on which the virtual image of the tracked instruments and their trajectories can be overlaid and displayed on all previously taken fluoroscopic images.

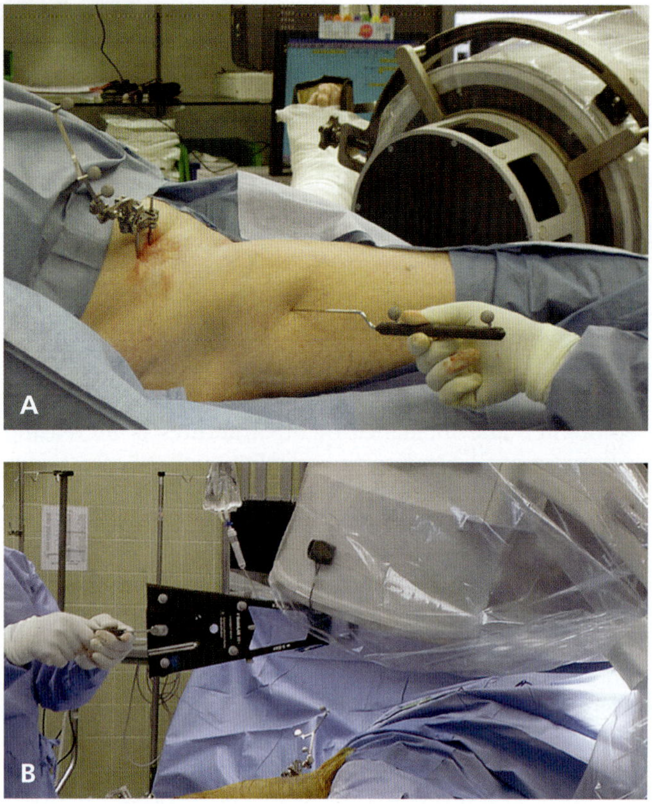

Figure 10.1 Setup for fluoroscopic navigation using optical tracking system. **A:** A tracker is mounted on the iliac crest and an optical calibration target is mounted on the c-arm fluoroscope. Alternatively, a mobile, handheld targeting device (X-spot) can be used instead **(B)** allowing more flexibility in image registration.

INDICATIONS

Nondisplaced femoral neck fractures or displaced femoral neck fractures in young (<60 years) patients—after closed or open reduction.

PATIENT POSITIONING, PREPPING, AND DRAPING

The patient is positioned supine on a fracture table. The contralateral leg is placed in a well leg support or abducted, and the operative limb is draped free or a shower curtain is used based on surgeon preference. The ipsilateral iliac crest should be prepped as well for the placement of optical trackers.

FRACTURE REDUCTION

For nondisplaced fractures, gentle positioning without the use of excessive force is recommended. For displaced fractures several closed maneuvers are described. The Leadbetter maneuver consists of flexing the hip to 90 degrees, applying traction and internally rotating and then extending the hip with slight abduction. Traction, internal rotation, and extension can be performed using the fracture table. If satisfactory reduction cannot be achieved, especially on the lateral view (e.g., posterior sag of the femoral head is the usual deformity), open reduction should be then performed either through a separate Smith-Petersen approach[8] or through an anterolateral extension of the Watson-Jones approach.[9] The description of these approaches can be found elsewhere and is beyond the scope of this chapter. After satisfactory reduction, fixation can be inserted.

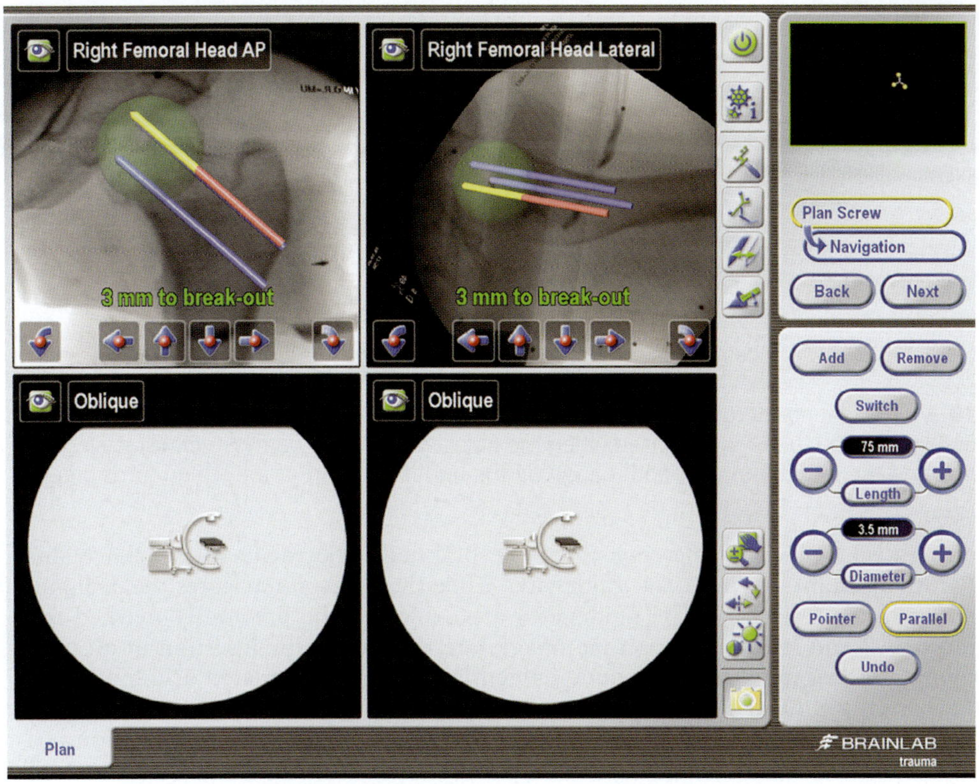

Figure 10.2 Screenshot of the navigation system at the time of intraoperative planning of screws' trajectories. The "active" screw is designated in red (superior posterior one). A special feature in newer software version is "break-in" or "break-out" spheres allowing estimation of screw length before penetrating the joint. The sphere representing the borders of the femoral head is marked in green.

FRACTURE FIXATION

The principle of fracture fixation is the creation of a stable construct consisting of three parallel cancellous screws in an inverted triangle formation—a proximal base consisting of an anterior and a posterior screw with an inferior screw supporting the femoral calcar and situated in the center of the femoral neck on the lateral view. It should be noted that the most distal starting point for the most distal screw should not be below the level of the lesser trochanter due to the risk of a subtrochanteric stress fracture, previously reported with these low starting points.[10] Maximal parallelism and spread, especially in the lateral view should be achieved, in order to create as much stable construct as possible to avoid varus collapse and implant failure.[5] The trajectory of the three screws can be planned on the computer screen prior to their actual insertion (Fig. 10.2). Then, sequential guidewire insertion, matching the plan, can be done using the navigation system.

The computerized navigation system allows virtual trajectory monitoring in all views while inserting the guidewires. One major drawback of this system is that long guidewires can bend during insertion, and since the computer cannot track the actual guidewire but only the trajectory of the drill guide, a few precautionary measures should be taken. First, a long navigated drill guide should be selected to create as straight a trajectory as possible. Second, tactile feedback during insertion is essential, and drill bit-tipped guidewires can improve tactile sensation. If any doubt exists, a verification fluoroscopy should be taken. Third, since the goal is to limit fluoroscopy to avoid radiation exposure, a simple measure of precalibrating guidewires' length is performed—the guidewire is inserted through the drill guide, and the length of 75 to 80 mm of trajectory (the most common screw size for this procedure) is marked at the proximal part of the guidewire. This mark is copied to the rest of the guidewires.

The next step is actual navigation. The drill guide is placed over the patient's skin until the trajectory of the inferior screw is appropriate while looking at the computer screen. A 3- to 4-cm incision is made proximal to this point and continued 0.5 cm distal to it. The skin, subcutaneous tissue, fascia, and vastus lateralis muscle are sharply dissected. At this point,

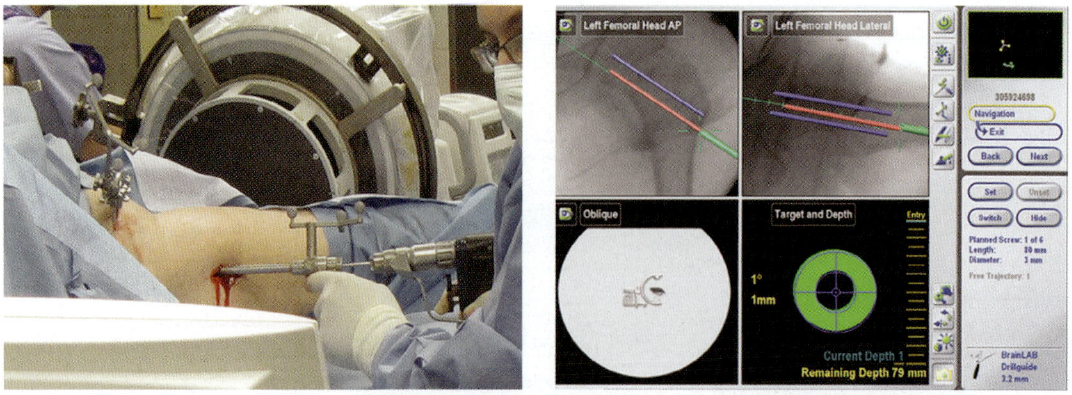

Figure 10.3 Navigating the guidewire to its desired position—the tracked drill guide is placed on the right entry point and the k-wire is drilled when the trajectory of the lowermost screw (active screw, in red) is met and the target and the depth gauge on the right hand part of the screen turns green.

navigation can take place by meeting all of the planned trajectories in a serial fashion (Fig. 10.3). An assistant can place the guidewires while the surgeon navigates the drill guide to meet the planned trajectory. The guidewires are drilled to the previously marked area. Verification of AP and lateral fluoroscopic images are done after the insertion of all guidewires. Opening of the lateral cortex is done sequentially with a cannulated drill bit, and 6.5 or 7.3 mm partially threaded screws are inserted. As recent evidence shows that excessive femoral neck shortening can occur and can affect function,[11,12] we prefer to insert long partial thread (32 to 40 mm) screws that cross the fracture, or one short thread screw to create intraoperative compression, and then to use two long-threaded or fully threaded screws to avoid further sliding (Fig. 10.4).

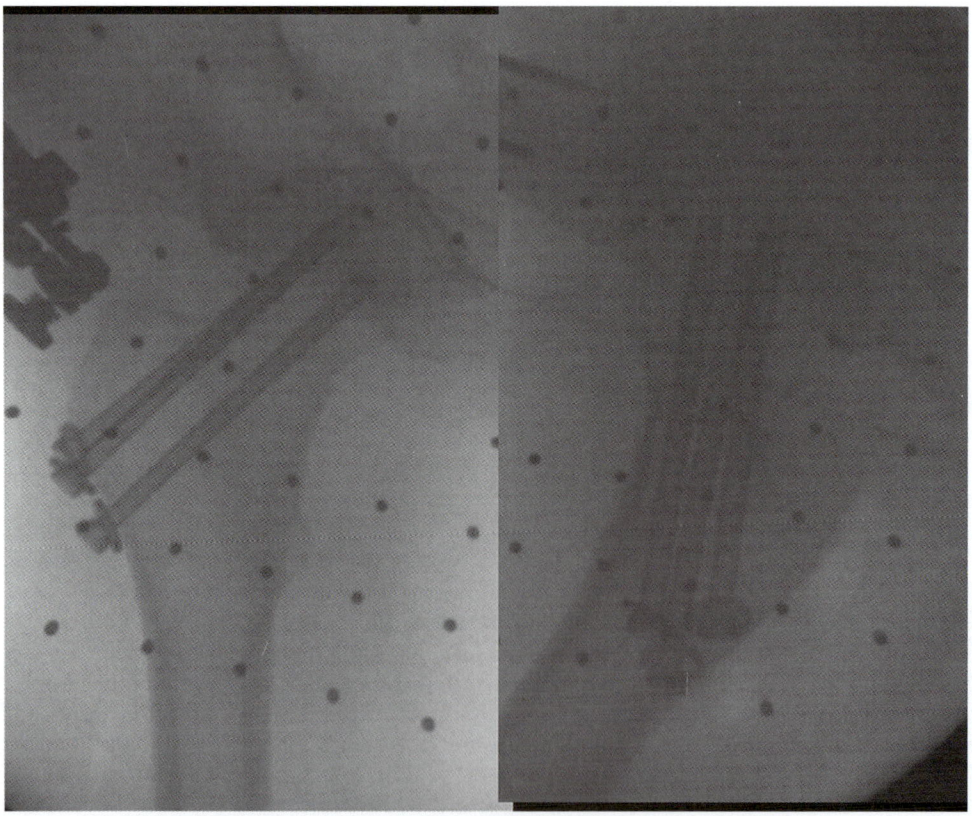

Figure 10.4 An intraoperative fluoroscopic image demonstrated the actual position of screws in both AP and lateral views.

POSTOPERATIVE CARE

The wound is closed in layers: Fascia, subcutaneous tissue, and skin. In elderly patients, weight-bearing as tolerated is encouraged, with DVT prophylaxis for several weeks. In younger patients with unstable fractures, toe touch weight-bearing is commenced and progressed to weight-bearing as tolerated at 6 weeks postoperatively.

OUTCOME AND COMPLICATIONS

The incidence of complications in nondisplaced or valgus-impacted fractures is low. Screw protrusion into the femoral head can occur and screw implant removal is warranted in these cases. While infection is not common, it can be a devastating complication in elderly patients since arthroplasty after infected, failed fixation is not a viable option. Osteonecrosis and varus collapse are more common after displaced fractures and should be monitored. In cases of nonunion with a viable femoral head, a Pauwels type intertrochanteric osteotomy should be considered in young patients, while arthroplasty should be reserved for older, lower-demand patients.

STABLE INTERTROCHANTERIC FRACTURES WITH PERCUTANEOUS SLIDING HIP SCREW DEVICE

Despite the popularity and success of nailing systems for intertrochanteric hip fractures, the sliding hip screw (SHS) is still considered the gold standard with less mechanical and technical complications. However, the integrity of the lateral wall, as proven by Gotfried,[13] and later by Langford et al.,[14] is sometimes compromised in certain stable fractures, therefore rendering them unstable. The Per Cutaneous Compression Plate (PCCP) device offers several advantages over a standard SHS by the use of two (antirotational) neck screws that are smaller diameter (7.6 mm as compared to the 11.2 mm of the SHS) that are drilled in a sequential, atraumatic fashion. In addition, the plate extends more proximal compared to a standard SHS, protecting somewhat against excessive lateralization of the proximal fragment. Published evidence supports the mechanical advantages as well as the decrease in pain as compared with the SHS.[15] In addition, the procedure is truly "percutaneous" and can be performed in a minimal access fashion.

INDICATIONS

Stable (AO/OTA 31A1) and certain unstable (31A2) trochanteric fractures. Contraindications include unstable (31A3) fractures and those with fracture lines extending 2 cm below the lesser trochanter.

PATIENT POSITIONING

Patients are positioned supine on a fracture table. Since the procedure is entirely percutaneous, posterior fragment sag must be reduced prior to surgery. A posterior reduction device can be placed under the fracture site and elevated until the fracture is reduced on the lateral view, similar to the application of a crutch (Fig. 10.5). Reduction of the remainder of the deformity is done by closed means with the fracture table, most commonly involving traction, adduction, internal rotation, and extension of the limb. Additional techniques such as percutaneous ball spike pushers or hooks to manipulate the fragments through small incisions can be invaluable.

PREPPING AND DRAPING

Similar to femoral neck fractures as described previously.

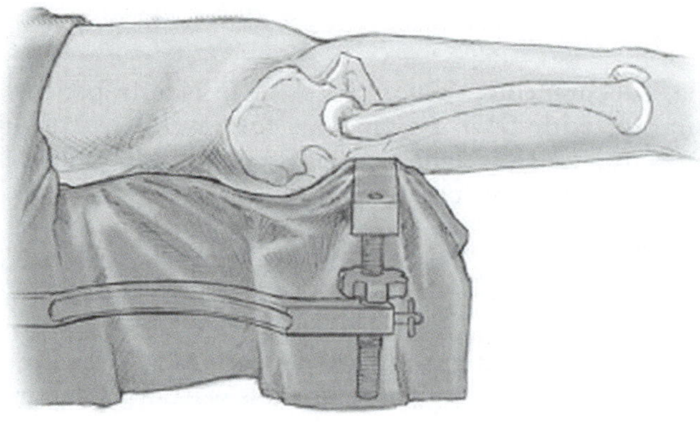

Figure 10.5 The limb is placed on the traction table. The reduction tool is placed under the thigh in order to prevent posterior sag of the fracture. It can be raised or lowered according to fracture deformity in the axial (lateral) view. (From: Peyser A, Weil Y, Liebergall M, et al. Percutaneous compression plating for intertrochanteric fractures. Surgical technique, tips for surgery, and results. *Oper Orthop Traumatol.* 2005;17(2):158–177, with permission.)

APPROACH

A spinal needle is used to verify the position of the proximal incision. It should be aligned at the center of the femur on the lateral view and at the upper border of the lesser trochanter. A 2.5-cm incision is made from this point, extending distally, cutting the skin, subcutaneous layer, and fascia. The muscle is gently dissected from the bone using Metzenbaum scissors. The plate is assembled on the provided gig and inserted into the wound using subperiosteal dissection with the plate's sharp end. Verification of the plate's position is done using AP and lateral fluoroscopic views. A two c-arm setup is a useful adjunct to this procedure. The next step is clamping the plate to the bone. A second 2.5-cm incision is made at the position of the second hole from the top of the gig (Fig. 10.6A). The skin, subcutaneous tissues, and fascia are incised. The scissors are gently used to percutaneously create room for the distal jaw of the clamp. This is done by spreading the muscle fibers at the anterior edge of the bone. The clamp is inserted next, first at a 45-degree angle and then straightened. The distal jaw is inserted under fluoroscopic control into the hole made earlier by the scissors medial to the bone. Both jaws are now turned 90-degree clockwise and the clamp is provisionally tightened, allowing some freedom in positioning, and fixed to the clamp adaptor, previously inserted into the second hole from the top of the gig (Fig. 10.7). Verification of AP and lateral fluoroscopy views are done to ensure proper plate positioning: Inferior to the greater trochanter flare on the AP view and center on the femur on the lateral view.

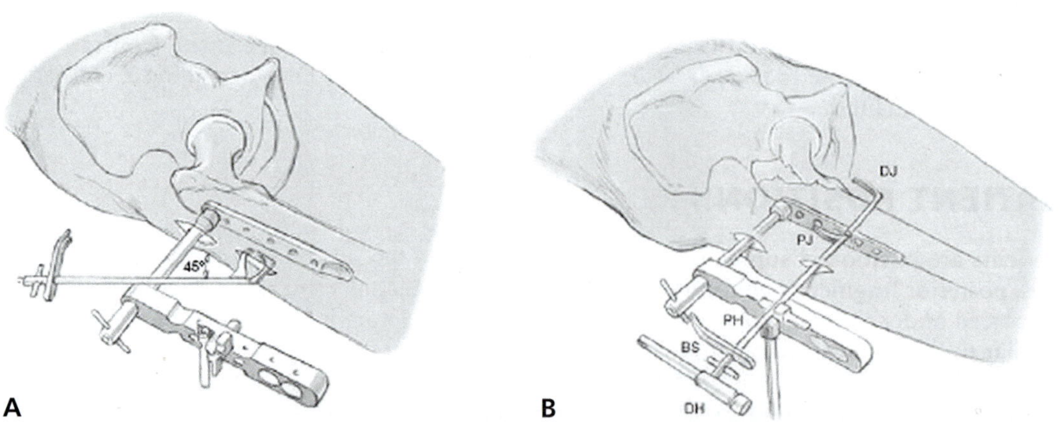

Figure 10.6 The distal incision is made around the second hole in the gig **(A)**. After mounting the bone clamp adaptor on the gig, the bone clamp is inserted in a 45-degree angle into the dissected plane anterior to the femoral bone. **B:** The distal jaw (designated DJ) and the proximal jaw (PJ) are controlled by the handles. The clamp is then rotated 90-degree clockwise. DH;distal handle, PH; proximal handle. (From: Peyser A, Weil Y, Liebergall M, et al. Percutaneous compression plating for intertrochanteric fractures. Surgical technique, tips for surgery, and results. *Oper Orthop Traumatol.* 2005;17(2):158–177, with permission.)

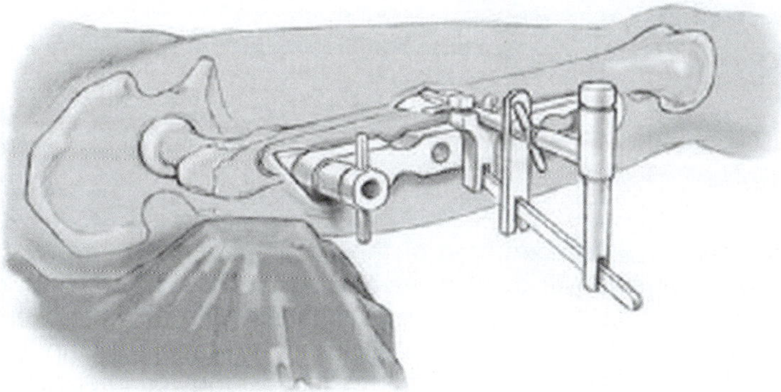

Figure 10.7 The gig is now assembled after the tightening of the bone clamp. Verification of fluoroscopic views should be done on the AP and lateral views to verify the desired plate position. (From: Peyser A, Weil Y, Liebergall M, et al. Percutaneous compression plating for intertrochanteric fractures. Surgical technique, tips for surgery, and results. *Oper Orthop Traumatol.* 2005;17(2):158–177, with permission.)

The first guidewire is inserted next. A sharp trocar coupled with the main sleeve is inserted through the lowermost hole of the gig. The first drill sleeve is screwed into the main sleeve, and the main guidewire is inserted using a power drill. It should be adjacent to the calcar on the AP view and centered in the femoral head on the lateral view (Fig. 10.8). The following adjustments can be made.

a. If the wire is excessively superior or inferior, the clamp is loosened and the plate is repositioned distally or proximally.
b. If the wire is too anterior or posterior, the plate should be either repositioned on the lateral view or rotated down or up respectively.

When the desired position of the main guide is reached, the trochanteric pin is inserted in the appropriate hole in the gig to secure the plate. At this point, the clamp is further tightened. Length is measured by alignment of the measuring block. The main guide is then removed. Sequential drilling using the step drills is done next under fluoroscopic control.

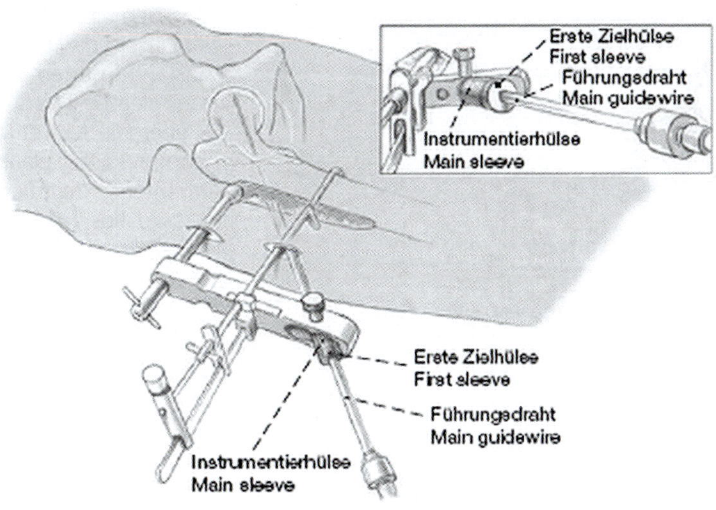

Figure 10.8 The position of the main guide should be adjacent to the calcar in the AP view and in the center of the femoral head at the lateral view. This illustration demonstrates the assembly of the gig, main sleeve, and main guide. (From: Peyser A, Weil Y, Liebergall M, et al. Percutaneous compression plating for intertrochanteric fractures. Surgical technique, tips for surgery, and results. *Oper Orthop Traumatol.* 2005;17(2):158–177, with permission.)

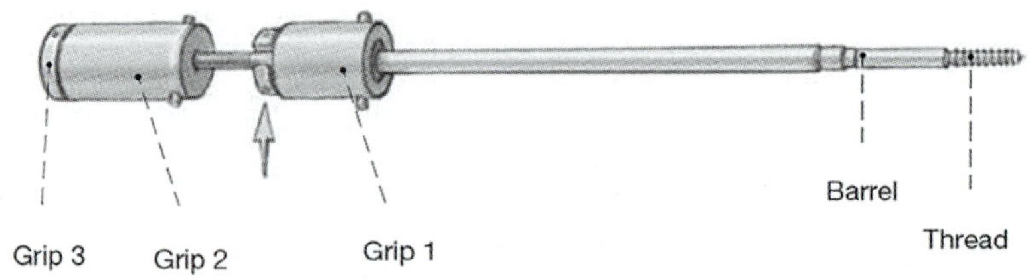

Figure 10.9 The screwdriver is composed of three grips and a nut (*arrow*). Grip 3 is used to attach the screw to the screwdriver by pressure and clockwise rotation. Grip 1 screws the barrel of the screw until it locks into the plate and the nut is then turn backward (anticlockwise) to allow the insertion of the telescopic part done through rotation of Grip 2. (From: Peyser A, Weil Y, Liebergall M, et al. Percutaneous compression plating for intertrochanteric fractures. Surgical technique, tips for surgery, and results. *Oper Orthop Traumatol.* 2005;17(2):158–177, with permission.)

The neck screws are telescoping screws composed of a barrel (proximal part) and a distal part. The neck screw is mounted on the screwdriver turning the top part of the driver, using slight compression and rotation (Fig. 10.9). The distal grip of the screwdriver inserts into the proximal (barrel) part and locks it to the plate, while the proximal grip of the screwdriver will insert into the distal (telescoping) part of the screw and advance it into the femoral head. A nut separates the two grips. The barrel is first inserted by rotating the distal grip until the barrel is locked to the plate. Then, the telescoping part is screwed into the subchondral bone on both AP and lateral views. The screw is dismounted by releasing the most proximal grip and the threads are tapped with the impactor.

The shaft screws are then inserted into holes 1 and 3 using the 3.2-mm drill through the appropriate drill sleeve and trocar (Fig. 10.10) through the distal incision. Length is measured using the depth gauge provided in the set. The shaft screwdriver is used on a power drill to advance the self-tapping screws. The bone clamp is removed by loosening the bone clamp adaptor, rotating both jaws at 45 degrees and removing it. Screw 2 is then drilled and placed in a similar fashion. The last step in the procedure is removal of the trochanteric pin and insertion of the superior neck screw (Fig. 10.11). This is done in a similar fashion to the insertion of the distal neck screw. The gig is dismounted and the wounds are irrigated. The fascia, subcutaneous fascia, and skin are closed. A drain is optional.

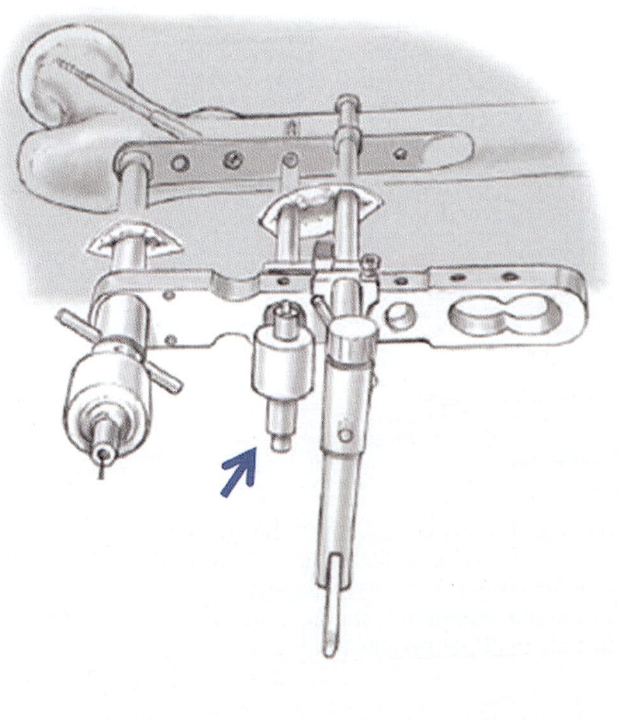

Figure 10.10 The shaft screws are inserted with the aid of the trocar (*arrow*) inserted with the dedicated drill sleeve. (From: Peyser A, Weil Y, Liebergall M, et al. Percutaneous compression plating for intertrochanteric fractures. Surgical technique, tips for surgery, and results. *Oper Orthop Traumatol.* 2005;17(2): 158–177, with permission.)

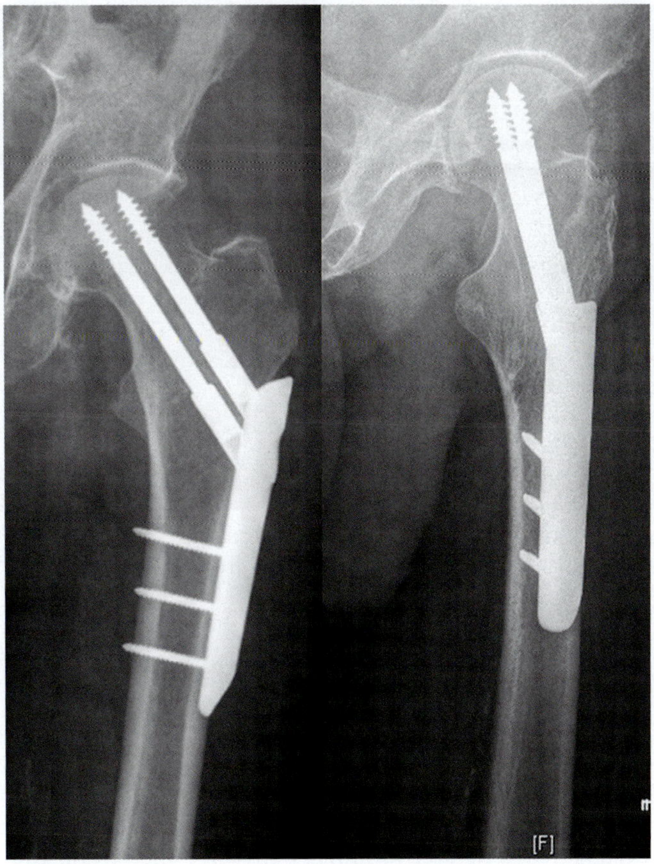

Figure 10.11 Final (AP and lat) views of the completed PCCP construct.

POSTOPERATIVE CARE

Patients are encouraged to weight-bear as tolerated. Low-molecular-weight heparin (enoxaparin, 40 mg qd) DVT prophylaxis is prescribed for 4 weeks.

PITFALLS AND COMPLICATIONS

Care must be taken to avoid an inadequate reduction. A good reduction with 135 degrees of neck–shaft angle is desired, although recreation of the patient's anatomy is optimal. In cases of excessive varus, the plate will sit rather distal but this can result in the superior screw penetrating the proximal neck. If this occurs, traction from the table can increase valgus alignment and the screws are repositioned. In excessive valgus reduction, the plate will sit rather high, sometimes sliding due to the trochanteric ridge. In that case, the trochanteric pin should be inserted before tightening the clamp to avoid this distal migration.

In cases where a closed reduction cannot be achieved, semi open maneuvers can be added. This includes such things as pulling the calcar using a bone hook (Fig. 10.12) or pushing a proximal spike using a ball-tipped spike pusher through a stab anterior incision.

It is important to keep the system stable, since it is not cannulated, until the insertion of the first screw. All drilling, especially the inferior neck screw placement, should be monitored using fluoroscopy.

OUTCOME

Peyser et al.[15] described the outcome of the PCCP in a prospective randomized study. Two patients out of fifty had mechanical failure (2.5%), and there was significantly less collapse and loss of reduction as compared to the SHS. Overall, medical complications are similar in all hip fracture groups.

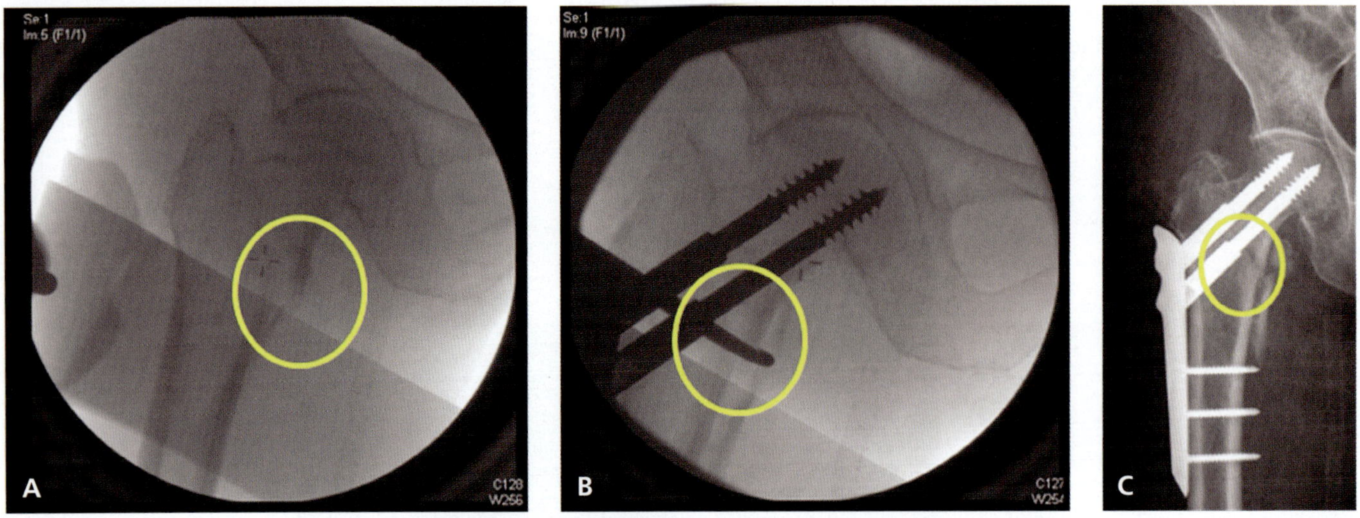

Figure 10.12 **A:** A case of an unstable A2 fracture with gapping at the calcar. **B:** Percutaneous bone hook is used to pull the proximal fragment medially resisting the forces of the screw the further open up the gap. **C:** Despite the comminution of the posteromedial fragment the calcar is well opposed.

UNSTABLE TROCHANTERIC FRACTURES—FIXATION WITH A CEPHALOMEDULLARY NAIL

Cephalomedullary nails have become increasingly popular in recent years due to better designs, ease of use, minimally invasive insertion, and compatibility with all fracture patterns. One theoretical advantage includes a shorter lever arm between the fixed-angle device and the bone. In addition, medialization and telescoping of the sliding device are limited due to the decreased distance of the nail from the medial cortex, thus less shortening occurs, especially in unstable fractures. Also, some biomechanical evidence demonstrates superiority over extramedullary implants.[16]

Newer implants offer antirotation mechanisms of various types, including a set screw to lock a single lag screw, two points of fixation in the head/neck, or a helical blade, which is the authors' preferred implant. Older designs of intramedullary nails resulted in complications such as fractures below the tip of the nail due to bulky design and short distance between the distal locking bold and the nail tip.[17] These have been largely eliminated with the improvement of nails over the years. However, clinical evidence for clear-cut superiority of these implants over extramedullary devices is still lacking in the literature[17,18] and their cost remains higher.

INDICATIONS

Indications for cephalomedullary nails include unstable trochanteric fractures (31A2 and A3 AO/OTA classifications) and subtrochanteric fractures.

PREOPERATIVE PLANNING

The use of a manual or a digital template can be helpful in determining the nail's length and angle, as well as the insertion point, since trochanteric shapes vary. A 125- or 130-degree nail can be chosen according to the contralateral neck–shaft angle. Nail diameters vary with most manufacturers offering a range of sizes. Whether to use a short or long nail remains controversial for most intertrochanteric and high reverse oblique fractures, but most agree that a long nail is required for subtrochanteric fractures, for pathologic fractures, and for combined femoral neck and shaft fractures when using one implant.

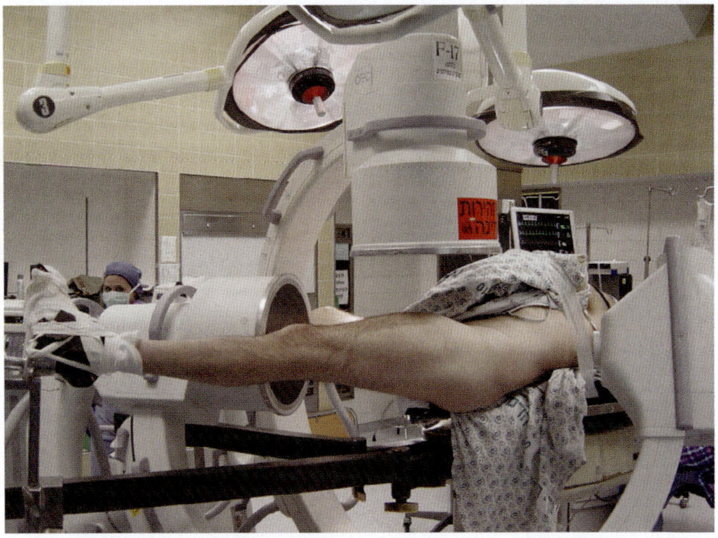

Figure 10.13 Positioning with two c-arm setup of a patient for cephalomedullary nailing. The body should be abducted from the extremity to allow easy nail insertion.

PATIENT POSITIONING

Patients are positioned supine on a fracture table. The affected extremity should be adducted (10 to 15 degrees) in order to facilitate insertion. Another option is abduction of the patient's torso toward the contralateral side using a side support and tape (Fig. 10.13). Extreme caution should be applied while adducting the extremity to avoid the patient falling off the table. A closed reduction is affected using traction, rotation, an external support for posterior sag as needed. The two c-arm fluoroscopic setup is a useful adjunct in assessing reduction and implant placement in both anteroposterior and lateral views simultaneously.

The affected extremity should be prepped in a standard sterile fashion. The authors prefer to drape using an adhesive vertical isolation drape ("shower curtain") supported by two posts on either side of the patient. If an additional c-arm is used for concomitant fluoroscopy, a sterile drape is applied over it.

APPROACH AND TECHNIQUE

The starting point varies according to the nail's design. The authors' preferred implant utilizes a proximal 6-degree valgus bend. Therefore, the insertion should be at the tip or slightly medial to the tip of the greater trochanter depending on the patient's anatomy. The tip of the greater trochanter and the trajectory of the proximal femur on both AP and lateral views can be identified using fluoroscopy and drawn on the patients' skin prior to incision. This can minimize soft tissue dissection and may facilitate the location of the entry point (Fig. 10.14). A 3- to 4-cm incision is created from the tip of the trochanter proximally in-line with the center of the trochanter on the lateral view.

A threaded guidewire is inserted into the greater trochanter and the medullary canal under fluoroscopic control on both AP and lateral views (Fig. 10.15). A cannulated starter reamer is then introduced over the guidewire after a soft tissue protection sleeve is inserted to minimize injury to the hip abductors. It should be stressed that this reamer is utilized through its entire length to ensure easy passage of the nail, otherwise nail incarceration may occur (Fig. 10.16). The nail should be introduced by hand or with gentle mallet strikes. Insertion depth is determined by the AP fluoroscopic view. A virtual line corresponding with the center of the femoral head should be the landmark. A lateral view is mandatory to ensure that the nail is seated within the medullary canal. An insufficient radius of curvature of the nail in a bowed femur can result in anterior perforation of the cortex or a fracture of the femoral shaft. In cases where short nails are not used, a long nail with the appropriate anatomical bend is preferable.

Insertion of the implant into the head and neck is next. A 2- to 3-cm incision is made after marking the skin with the targeting device. The skin, subcutaneous tissues, and fascia

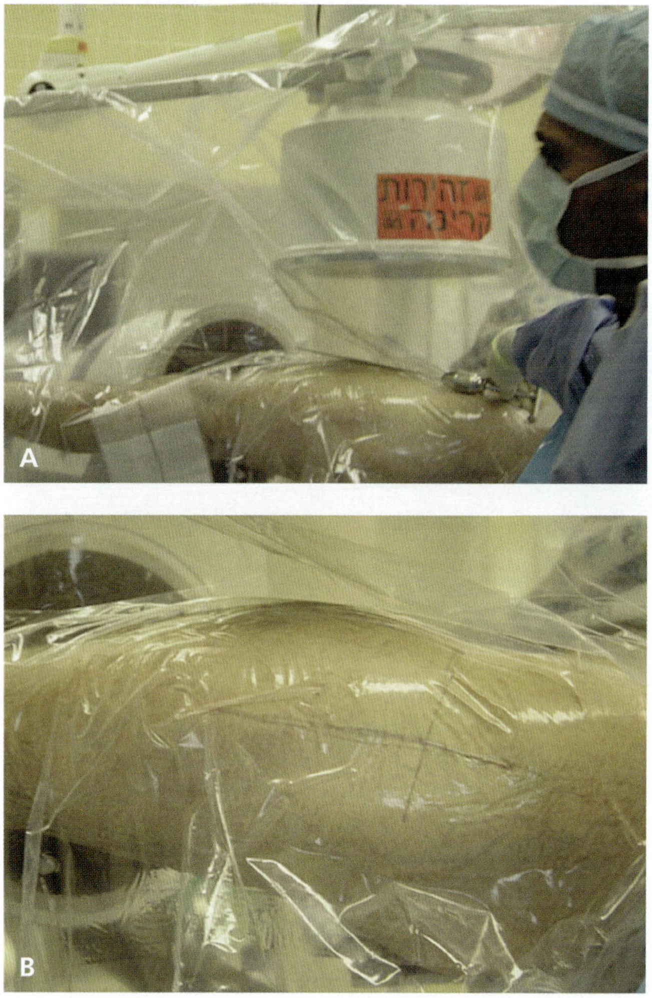

Figure 10.14 Use of fluoroscopy minimizes dissection by finding the trajectory and entry point—an AP and lateral views with the guidewire held on the patients' thigh **(A)** is used to mark the projected shaft of the femur (**B**—horizontal line on the lateral view) and the level of the greater trochanter tip (**B**—vertical line). The incision is made from the intersection of lines 3 to 4 cm proximally.

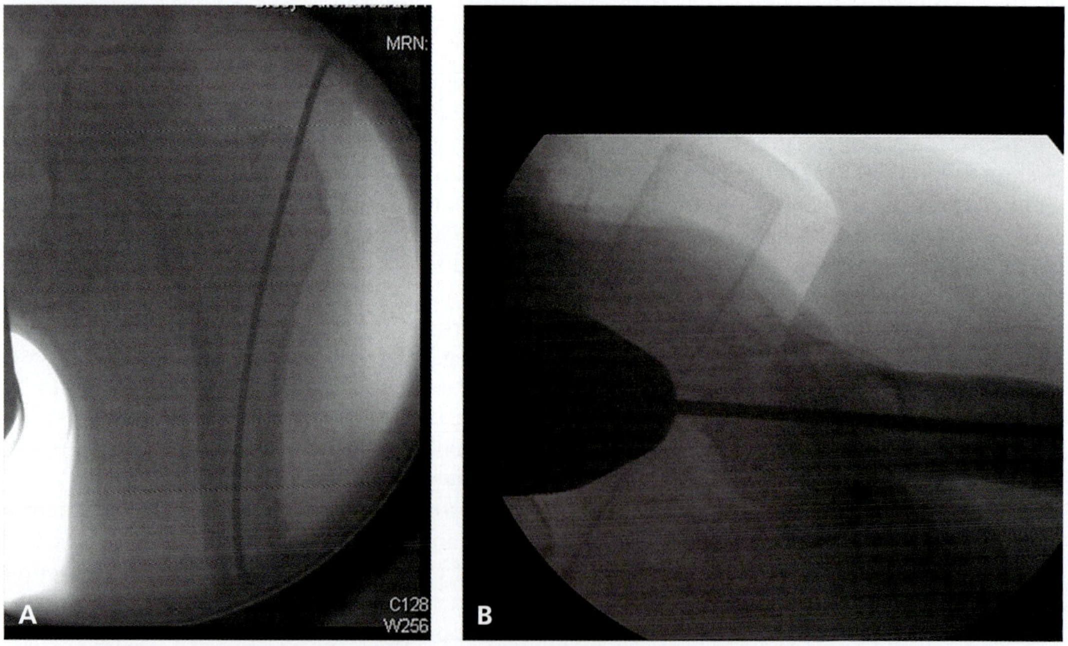

Figure 10.15 The entry point is slightly lateral or medial to the tip of the greater trochanter, depending on the patient's anatomy **(A)** and lined with the femoral shaft on the lateral view **(B)**.

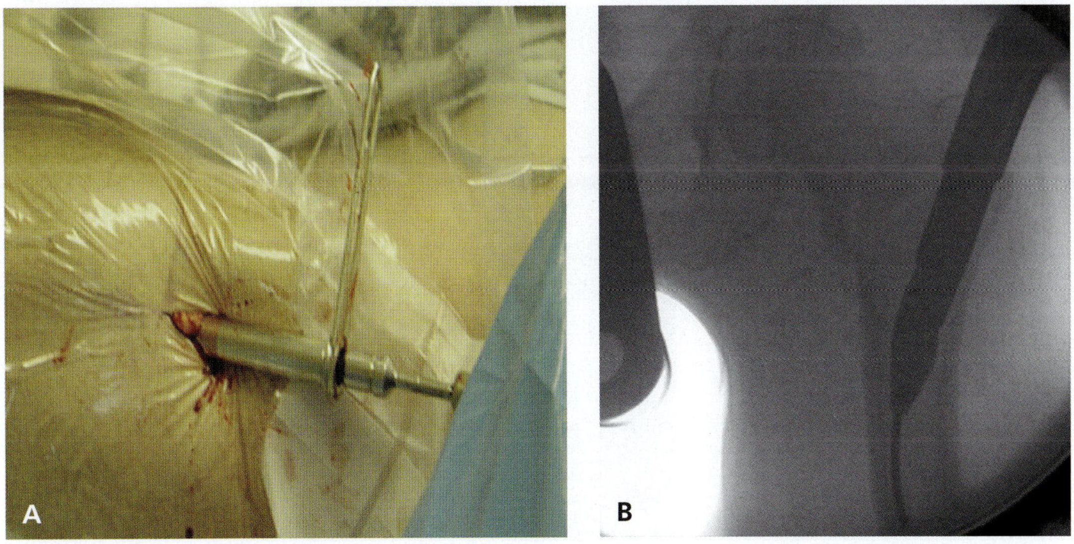

Figure 10.16 The 17-mm cannulated drill bit should be inserted with the protection sleeve to avoid damage to the abductor muscles **(A)** and should be inserted to its entire depth under fluoroscopic control to avoid nail jamming **(B)**.

are sharply dissected. The insertion sleeve is inserted until the aiming guide is on the lateral femoral cortex (Fig. 10.17). This step is pertinent since lack of bone contact can result in inaccurate guidewire placement. A guidewire is then drilled into the femoral head under fluoroscopy. It should be in the center or slightly inferior in the head on the AP view and in the center of the femoral head on the lateral view (Fig. 10.18). If the guidewire is too superior in position, the wire should be removed and the nail should be driven further into the bone. If the guidewire is too anterior or posterior on the lateral fluoroscopic view, the aiming guide should be rotated to correct guidewire placement. The wire should reach the subchondral bone. The ideal implant length is unknown but most surgeons attempt to be as deep as possible in the femoral head without penetrating the femoral head. Measurement is done and the lateral cortex is drilled. Depending on the patient's bone quality and the device being used, further drilling into the femoral neck must be decided. Typically in young, nonosteopenic patients, the guidewire should be overdrilled. The implant is inserted into the femoral neck and position is verified on both AP and lateral fluoroscopic views (Fig. 10.20). If compression along the fracture is required, then a compression device is utilized.

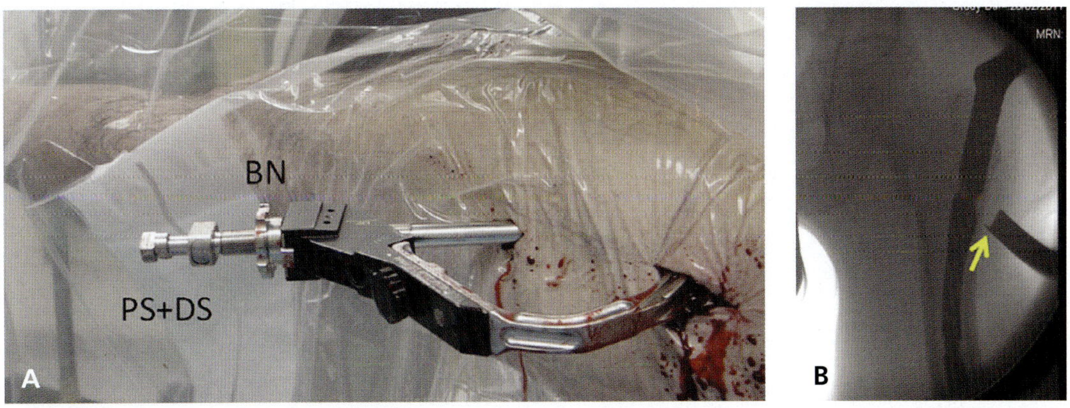

Figure 10.17 **A:** The second incision is made and the protection sleeve (PS), drill sleeve (DS), and trocar are inserted into the wound through the carbon aiming guide. The buttress nut (BN) should be rotated clockwise until the protection sleeve's sharp end is touching the bone (*arrow*). **B:** It should be felt as well as seen in fluoroscopy.

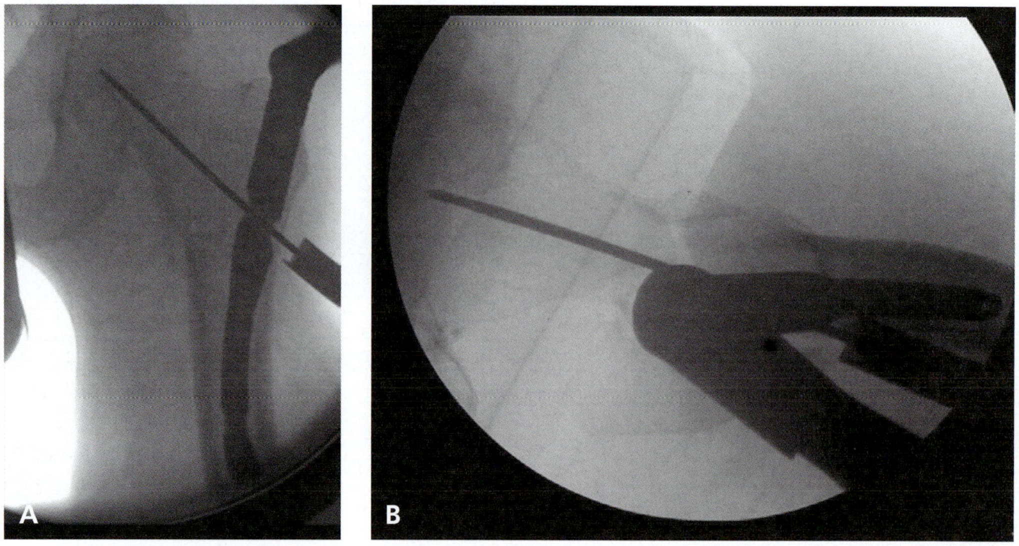

Figure 10.18 The guidewire for the helical blade should be in the center of the femoral neck or slightly inferior to it on the AP view **(A)** and in the center of the femoral neck and head on the lateral view **(B)**.

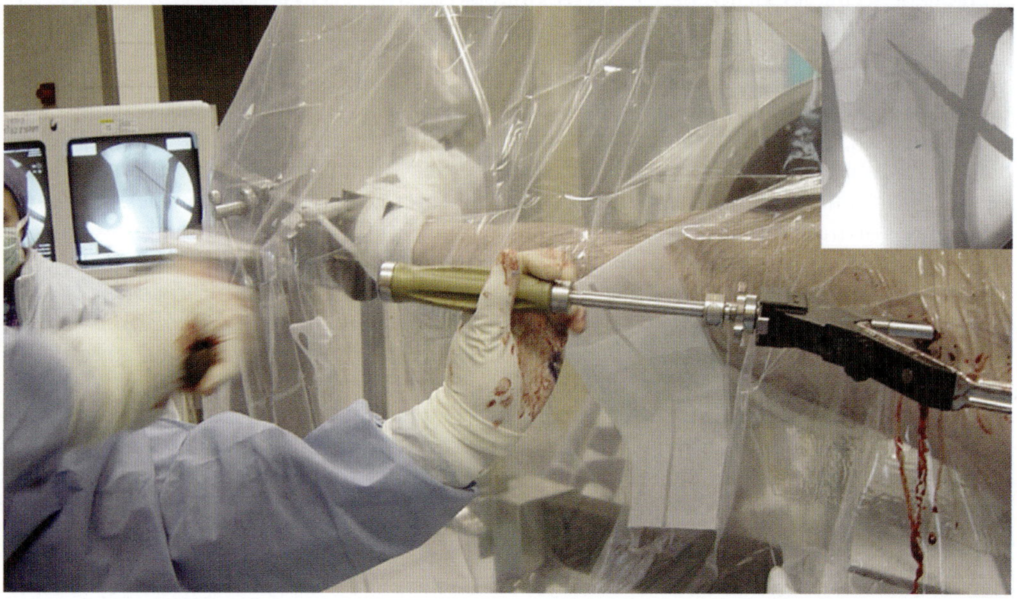

Figure 10.19 The blade should be inserted by slight hammer blows and followed by fluoroscopic control.

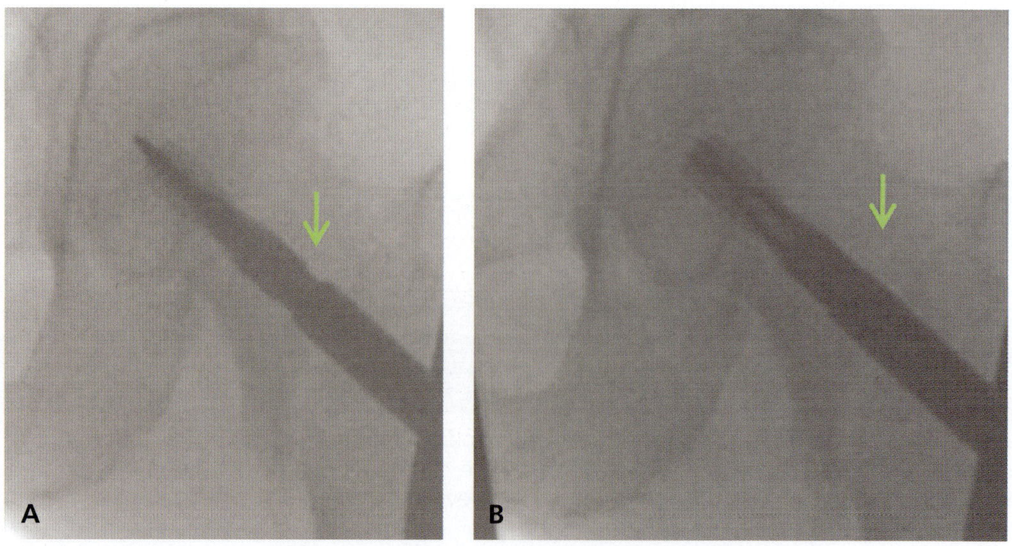

Figure 10.20 The locking of the helical blade can be evidently seen on the fluoroscopy by closing of the gap (**A** and **B**, *arrows*). At that point the insertion handle is automatically dismounted from the blade.

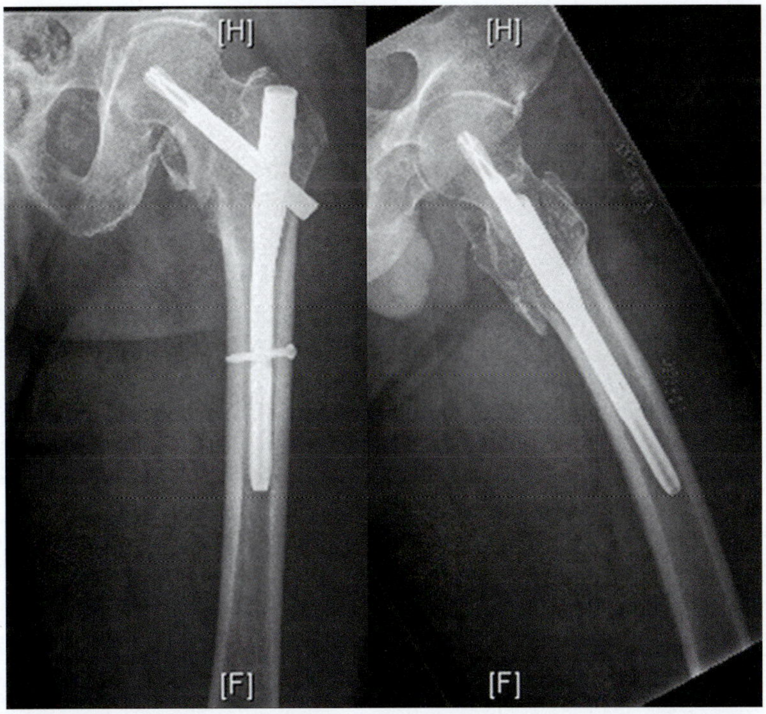

Figure 10.21 AP and lateral radiographs after the completion of procedure.

A distal, usually static locking screw is inserted either with the gig (short nails) or using the "perfect circle" technique (long nails). After verification using fluoroscopic AP and lateral views (Fig. 10.21), the insertion gig handle is dismounted and the wounds are closed in layers.

POSTOPERATIVE CARE

Aftercare for A2 fractures is weight-bearing as tolerated on the first postoperative day. In unstable reverse obliquity (A3) and subtrochanteric fracture, partial weight-bearing according to the surgeon's preference is prescribed for 6 weeks and progressed to full weight-bearing subsequently.

COMPLICATIONS AND PITFALLS

In certain subtrochanteric fractures, inadequate closed reduction often occurs. The deforming forces typically cause the proximal fragment to rotate externally, abduct, and flex by the pull of the short rotators, abductors, and iliopsoas muscles, respectively. As in any fracture, the nail should not be inserted prior to fracture reduction. There are two options to achieve reduction. A small incision is made at the fracture site, directly laterally, where the insertion of the blade will take place. A Verbrugge clamp is then inserted and a reduction is affected and confirmed under fluoroscopic guidance (Fig. 10.22). Nail insertion then proceeds as above. Another option is a small anterolateral incision over the flexed fragment. A ball spike pusher can be used to push the flexed fragment to realign the fracture on the lateral view.

OUTCOME

As prospective randomized trials comparing modern, third generation nail designs to standard SHSs are still lacking, only evidence from more limited literature is available. However, performance of helical-blade type implants is comparable to nail-screw type constructs with less than 2% cut-out in recently published studies.[19,20]

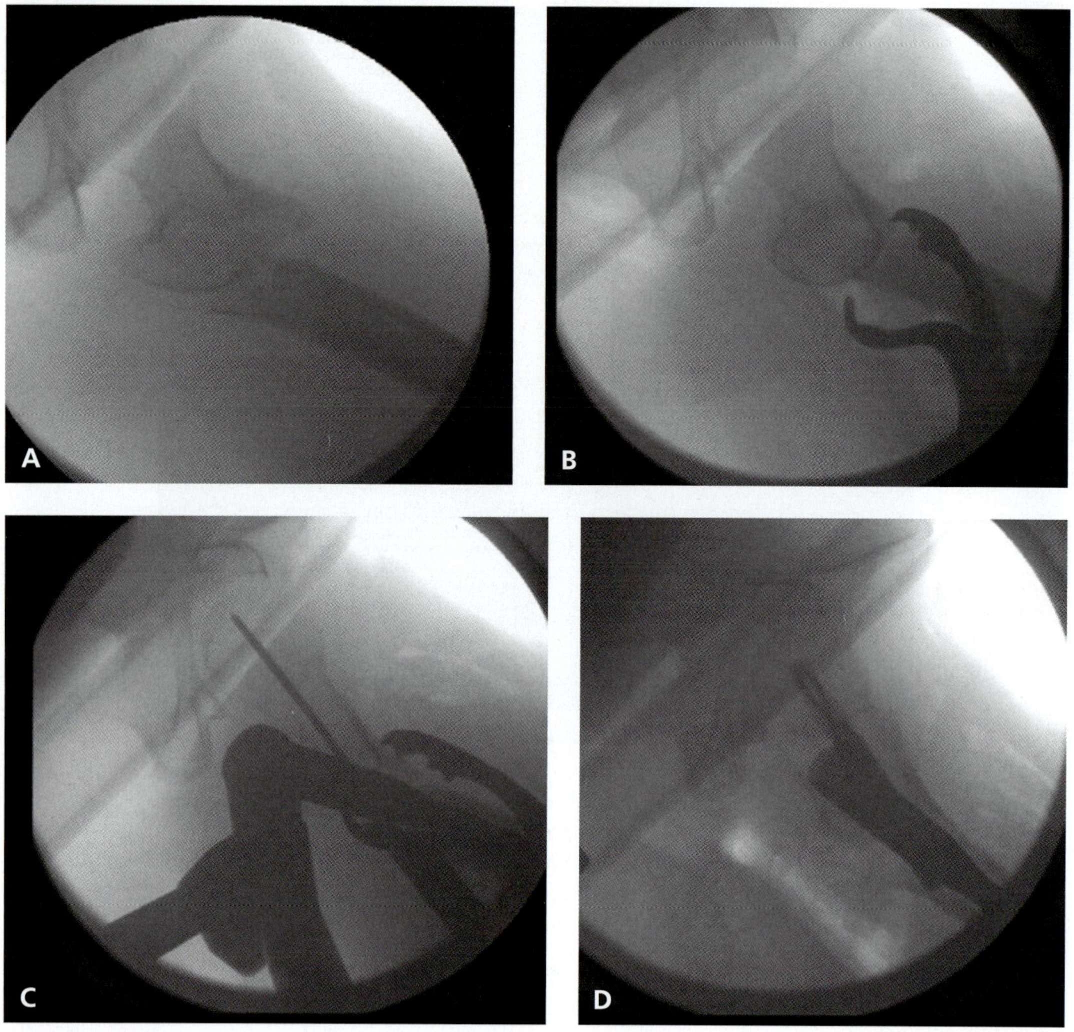

Figure 10.22 In cases where flexion deformity of the proximal fragment occur **(A)**, a small incision centered in the fracture site is done and a Verbrugge clamp is used percutaneously to clamp the fracture **(B)**. It is pertinent to maintain the clamp throughout the procedure **(C)** until the blade and distal locking are placed **(D)**.

REFERENCES

1. Gullberg B, Johnell O, Kanis JA. World-wide projections for hip fracture. *Osteoporos Int*. 1997;7:407–413.
2. Pillai A, Eranki V, Shenoy R, et al. Age related incidence and early outcomes of hip fractures: A prospective cohort study of 1177 patients. *J Orthop Surg Res*. 2011;6:5.
3. Parker MJ. The management of intracapsular fractures of the proximal femur. *J Bone Joint Surg Br*. 2000;82:937–941.
4. Liebergall M, Ben-David D, Weil Y, et al. Computerized navigation for the internal fixation of femoral neck fractures. *J Bone Joint Surg Am*. 2006;88:1748–1754.
5. Gurusamy K, Parker MJ, Rowlands TK. The complications of displaced intracapsular fractures of the hip: The effect of screw positioning and angulation on fracture healing. *J Bone Joint Surg Br*. 2005;87:632–634.
6. Weil Y, Mosheiff L, Joskowicz L, et al. Principles of computer-aided surgery in trauma surgery. In: Stiehl JB, Konermann WH, Haaker RG, DiGioia AM III, eds. *Navigation and MIS in Orthopedic Surgery*. Heidelberg: Springer; 2007:476–485.
7. Weil YA, Gardner MJ, Helfet DL, et al. Computer navigation allows for accurate reduction of femoral fractures. *Clin Orthop Relat Res*. 2007;460:185–191.
8. Boraiah S, Paul O, Hammoud S, et al. Predictable healing of femoral neck fractures treated with intraoperative compression and length-stable implants. *J Trauma*. 2010;69(1):142–147.

9. Ly TV, Swiontkowski MF. Treatment of femoral neck fractures in young adults. *Instr Course Lect.* 2009;58:69–81.
10. Kloen P, Rubel IF, Lyden JP, et al. Subtrochanteric fracture after cannulated screw fixation of femoral neck fractures: A report of four cases. *J Orthop Trauma.* 2003;17:225–229.
11. Zlowodzki M, Ayieni O, Petrisor BA, et al. Femoral neck shortening after fracture fixation with multiple cancellous screws: Incidence and effect on function. *J Trauma.* 2008;64:163–169.
12. Zlowodzki M, Jonsson A, Paulke R, et al. Shortening after femoral neck fracture fixation: Is there a solution? *Clin Orthop Relat Res.* 2007;461:213–218.
13. Gotfried Y. The lateral trochanteric wall: A key element in the reconstruction of unstable pertrochanteric hip fractures. *Clin Orthop Relat Res.* 2004;425:82–86.
14. Langford J, Pillai G, Ugliailoro AD, et al. Perioperative lateral trochanteric wall fractures: Sliding hip screw versus percutaneous compression plate for intertrochanteric hip fractures. *J Orthop Trauma.* 2011;25:191–195.
15. Peyser A, Weil YA, Brocke L, et al. A prospective, randomised study comparing the percutaneous compression plate and the compression hip screw for the treatment of intertrochanteric fractures of the hip. *J Bone Joint Surg Br.* 2007;89:1210–1217.
16. Roderer G, Moll S, Gebhard F, et al. Side plate fixation vs. intramedullary nailing in an unstable medial femoral neck fracture model: A comparative biomechanical study. *Clin Biomech (Bristol, Avon).* 2011;26:141–146.
17. Parker MJ, Handoll HH. Gamma and other cephalocondylic intramedullary nails versus extramedullary implants for extracapsular hip fractures in adults. *Cochrane Database Syst Rev.* 2005;(4):CD000093.
18. Verettas DA, Ifantidis P, Chatzipapas CN, et al. Systematic effects of surgical treatment of hip fractures: Gliding screw-plating vs intramedullary nailing. *Injury.* 2010;41:279–284.
19. Yaozeng X, Dechun G, Huilin Y, et al. Comparative study of trochanteric fracture treated with the proximal femoral nail anti-rotation and the third generation of gamma nail. *Injury.* 2010;41:1234–1238.
20. Stern R, Lubbeke A, Suva D, et al. Prospective randomised study comparing screw versus helical blade in the treatment of low-energy trochanteric fractures. *Int Orthop.* 2011;35(12):1855–1861.

CHAPTER 11

Femoral Shaft

Theerachai Apivatthakakul and Chang-Wug Oh

INDICATIONS

The standard treatment of femoral shaft fractures is closed intramedullary nailing.[1] However, in some situations an intramedullary nail may be contraindicated or technically not feasible. These may include polytrauma patients, associated femoral shaft and neck fractures, pelvic and acetabular fractures, spinal fractures, patients with pulmonary compromise, pediatric femoral shaft fractures, a deformed or stenotic femoral canal, and periprosthetic femoral fractures. In these situations, plate fixation has many advantages and is often the only feasible option.[2–6] Conventional open plating requires extensive exposure, stripping of muscle and periosteum around the bone fragments, and injury to the blood supply, all of which can lead to delayed union, nonunion, infection, or implant failure.[7] With the evolution of the plate fixation in the past decade,[8] minimally invasive plate osteosynthesis (MIPO) has gained popularity with acceptable clinical outcomes.[9–13]

PATIENT POSITIONING

The patient is positioned supine on a radiolucent operating table. A padded bolster is placed under the distal thigh and knee to maintain it in 30 degrees of knee flexion. A small bump should be placed under the ipsilateral hip to offset external rotation of the limb such that the patella faces directly anteriorly. However, the presence of a hip bump must be remembered and removed at the end of the procedure when determining limb rotation. A standard fracture table with traction is not recommended because manipulation of the fracture is difficult. Instead, a fully radiolucent flat top table is used.

Preparation of the lower limb is performed depending on the configuration of the fractures. In simple transverse, oblique, spiral, or wedge fractures, determination of the length can be done by using the apposition of the fragments. In these cases, the injured lower extremity is prepared with the uninjured lower extremity elevated in a hemilithotomy position in order to obtain an AP and lateral x-ray of the fractured femoral shaft. In comminuted or segmental comminuted fractures in which the length cannot be determined by fragment apposition, both the lower extremities may be sterilized and prepared in the field to directly compare the length and rotation. With this method, the lateral x-ray view is obtained by lifting the uninjured limb upward to avoid obstruction of the x-ray. The image intensifier is positioned on the contralateral side of the patient. The c-arm is tilted so that the fluoroscopy beam is able to obtain orthogonal images along the entire length of the femur.

SURGICAL APPROACHES

A direct lateral approach is the standard approach for MIPO of the femur, as it provides access to the entire femur with no main neurovascular structures at risk. Before making incisions, the fracture must be provisionally reduced to restore the alignment as close to anatomic as possible. Mark the location of the fractures on the skin, and determine the plate length by the desired plate-span ratio and plate–screw density.[14] In general, we prefer to err on the side of using longer plates with fewer screws to maximize stability while minimizing the biologic insult. Make incisions proximally and distally corresponding to the proximal and distal ends of the plate (Fig. 11.1). Dissect deep through the iliotibial band, and split the vastus lateralis longitudinally. The lateral femoral cortex is exposed with two Hohmann retractors.

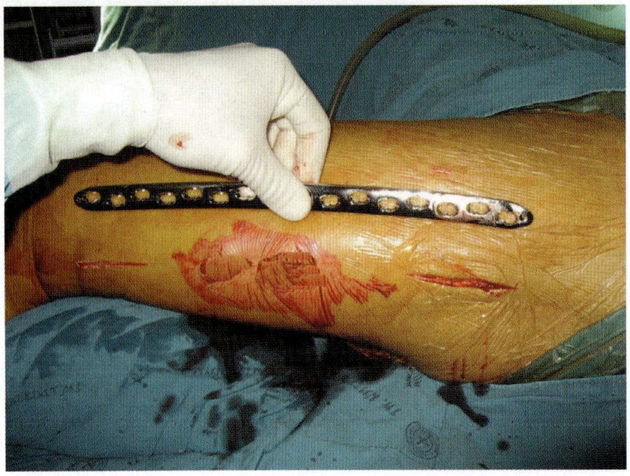

Figure 11.1 The incisions are made several centimeters in length, based on the planned plate length and position.

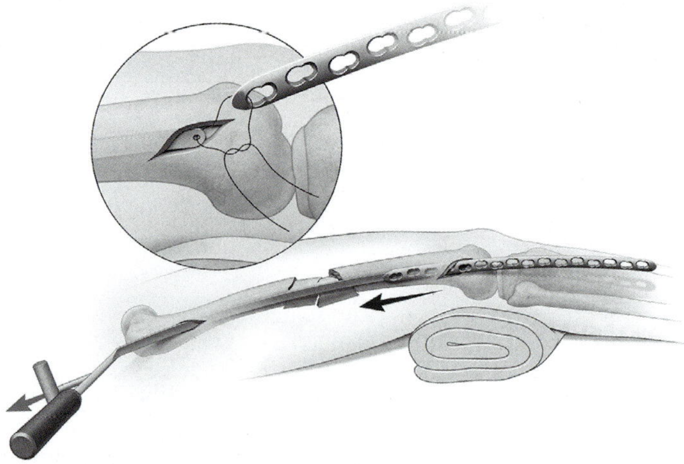

Figure 11.2 Tie a suture to the tip of the tunneling instrument and the plate hole and pull the plate back into the tunnel.

Preparation of the submuscular tunnel under the vastus lateralis can be done either proximal to distal or distal to proximal. A tunneling instrument can be a helpful tool to prepare the tunnel over the lateral cortex, as it is easier to advance and change direction than with the beveled end of a plate. This tunnel should be created in a submuscular but extraperiosteal plane. Once the tunneler is passed through the far incision, use a suture to connect the tunneler to the plate and pull it back into the tunnel to preserve the track (Fig. 11.2).

In osteoporotic fractures with previous proximal plate fixation, open fractures, or when a lateral external fixator is in place, an anterior approach can be considered to avoid implant removal or pin tract contamination. This involves splitting the rectus and vastus intermedius, and should be avoided when possible.

REDUCTION TECHNIQUES

There are two general methods for reduction of the femoral shaft fractures when using a minimally invasive technique. First, the fracture is reduced and the desired reduction is maintained with devices such as cerclage wires, collinear reduction forceps, an external fixator, Schanz pin joysticks, an intramedullary splint, or a femoral distractor. Collinear reduction forceps or cerclage wires are useful in reduction and maintain reduction of simple long oblique or spiral fractures. In fracture patterns with a single butterfly fragment, two wire loops around the proximal and distal end of the butterfly is a very effective provisional reduction tool. External fixators or Schanz pin joysticks are typically the first choice for simple transverse, short oblique or comminuted fractures in which cerclage wiring or a collinear clamp cannot be used.

The second general reduction strategy involves introducing the plate first adjacent to an unreduced fracture, and reducing the fracture indirectly “under” the plate, using traction, bumps, percutaneous reduction tools, or screws through the plate. This method is recommended in wedge or comminuted fractures, since anatomical reduction is not needed or possible. After fixation of the plate to one fragment, reduction is done to achieve correct length, angulation, and rotation. Then, using a cortical screw through a plate hole or a collinear clamp, the other fragment is realigned and reduced to the plate. In simple transverse or short oblique fractures, this technique is more difficult because the fracture must be anatomically reduced before using reduction screw.

Reduction with Mini-Open Cerclage Wiring

Cerclage wiring for reduction of long oblique or spiral fractures has been well described. The mechanism of reduction is that the wire applies circumferential force around the bone to bring the fragments to their anatomic position and maintains the reduction while the plate

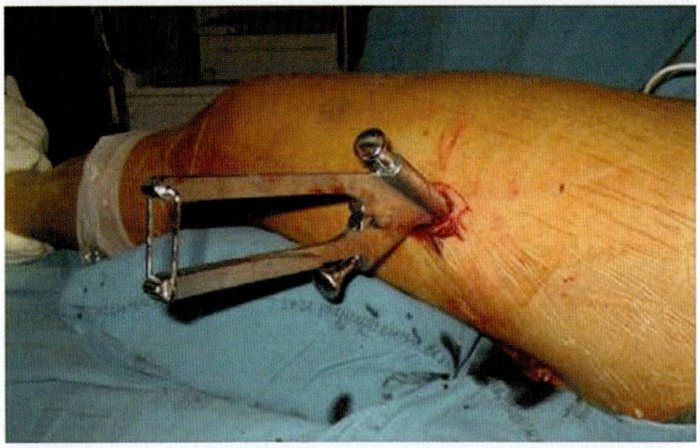

Figure 11.3 The arms of the modular wire passer are passed around the femur through a small incision. The arms are connected to mate the tubes at the fracture site.

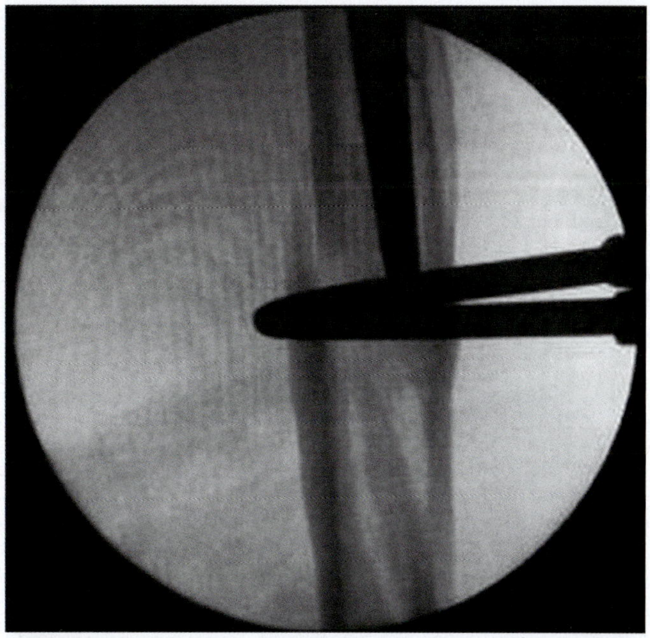

Figure 11.4 The mated position of the wire passer is verified fluoroscopically.

and screw are applied. Historically, the disadvantage of cerclage wiring in the femur is that a large exposure is often needed, which can involve stripping of the muscle and periosteum and disruption of the blood supply. Traditional wire passers for cerclage techniques were designed for open wiring through large incisions. Newer modular cerclage wire passers have been designed specifically for minimally invasive techniques.[15,16] These devices have a larger curve and angle of the handle away from the skin, making them amenable to use through much more limited exposures. Two detachable arms can be independently inserted anteriorly and posteriorly around the femur at the fracture site through a 2-cm incision, minimizing insult to the local biology.

To perform this technique, first make an incision approximately 2 cm long in the region of the fracture site. Longitudinally split the fascia lata and vastus lateralis to access the fracture site. Use a long clamp to penetrate the intermuscular septum and the linea aspera.

Preparation of the wire path using a tunneling device is necessary to facilitate insertion of the cerclage passer through the fascia lata and the muscle envelope. Place one trocar in each tube of the cerclage passer to prevent the soft tissue from entering the cannulated tubes of the passer. Insert one-half of the cerclage passer into the prepared tunnel and pass it around the femur posteriorly. It is critical to contact bone while passing the device to avoid injury to the sciatic nerve. Next, insert the other half of the forceps. Connect the flat parts of the forceps and close the handles, allowing the tips to mate around the femur (Fig. 11.3). The correct closed position can be verified by the image intensifier (Fig. 11.4). Remove the trocar from each side of the forceps, and pass the wire through the tube until it passes through the opposite side. Unlock the forceps and disconnect the two halves of the forceps (Figs. 11.5 and 11.6). For long spiral fractures, a second wire can be helpful to achieve a more concentric reduction and distribute the forces during wire tightening (Fig. 11.7).

Indirect reduction of the fracture can now be performed by manual traction and internal and external rotation of the leg to close the fracture gap. The wire loops are sequentially tightened to allow circumferential fracture reduction (Fig. 11.8).

Collinear Reduction Forceps

This clamp consists of an aiming arm that functions like a bone hook and the collinear closing mechanism. These allow percutaneous direct clamp reduction of long oblique or spiral

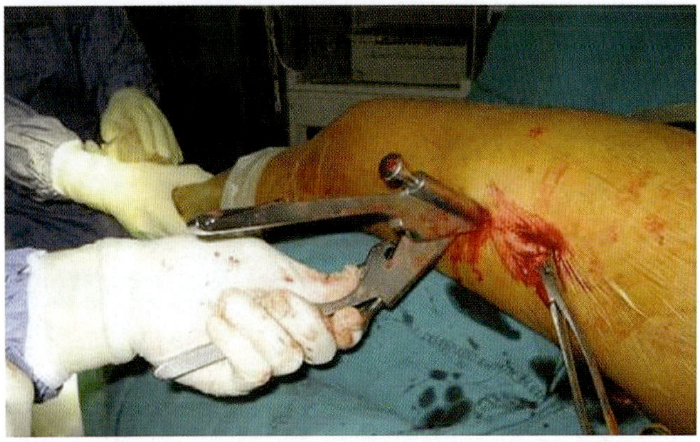

Figure 11.5 After the wire is passed, the handles are disconnected.

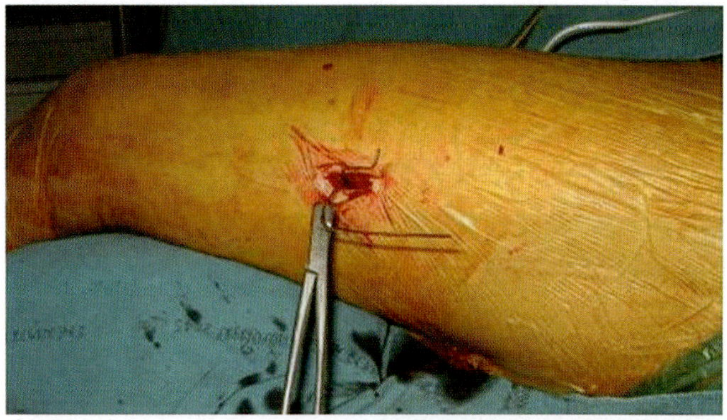

Figure 11.6 The wire ends can then be tightened.

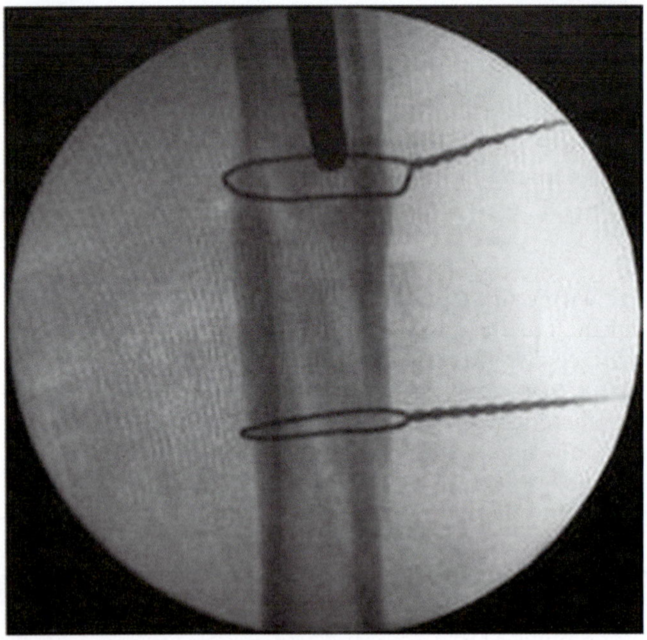

Figure 11.7 A second wire can be used for long spiral fractures to facilitate reduction.

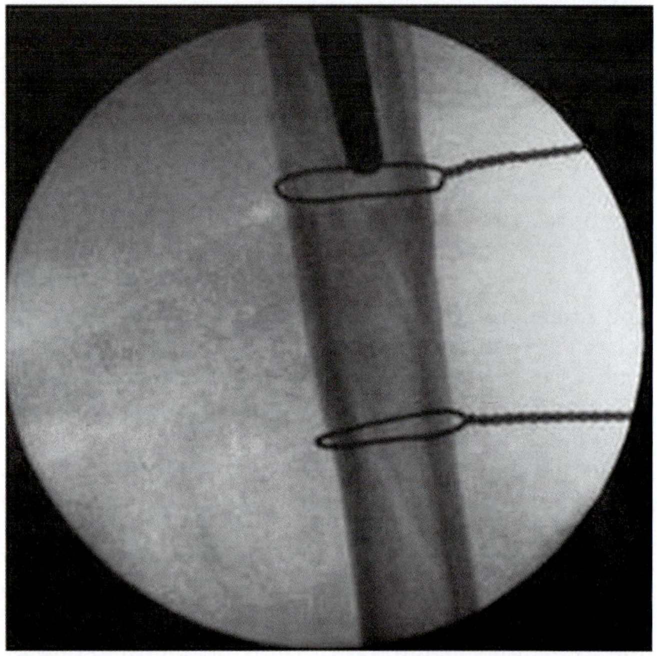

Figure 11.8 The wires are sequentially tightened while traction and rotation on the limb is applied.

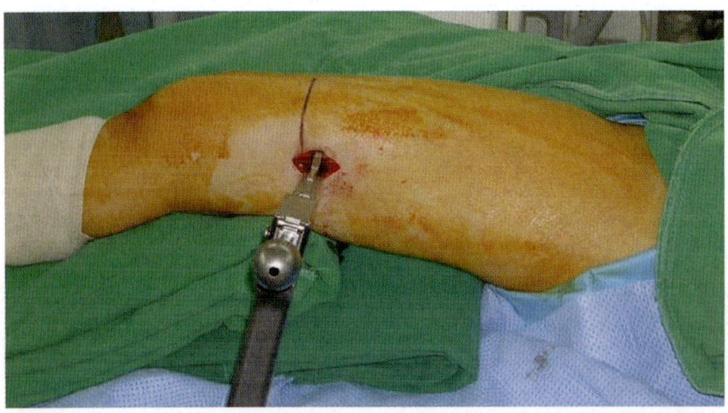

Figure 11.9 A collinear clamp is a powerful reduction tool for spiral or sagittal plane oblique fractures, and can be used through small incisions.

fractures through a small incision (Fig. 11.9). Longitudinal traction and rotation, while simultaneously deploying the clamp, can achieve anatomical reduction (Fig. 11.10). After the reduction is obtained, the fracture is provisionally stabilized by a percutaneous lag screw or K-wire, and the clamp is removed for plate passage (Fig. 11.11). This instrument can also be used as a bone-plate reduction clamp to draw the bone to the plate. In fracture patterns with a widely displaced butterfly fragment, the collinear clamp can be used to reduce each side of the butterfly fragment and maintain the reduction for percutaneous screw fixation.

Manipulator

"Manipulators" consist of threaded guide pin and cannulated handles which can be attached to the pins with a

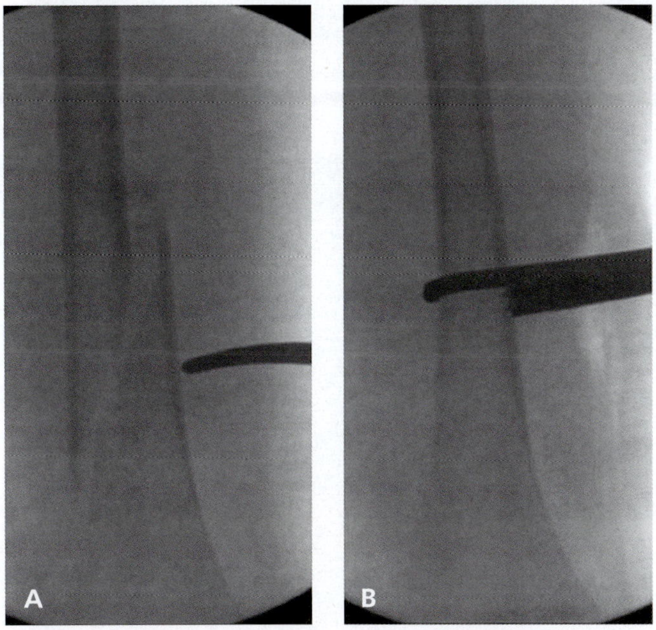

Figure 11.10 A collinear clamp is positioned across a spiral fracture **(A)**. With limb manipulation during clamp deployment, the fracture is anatomically reduced **(B)**.

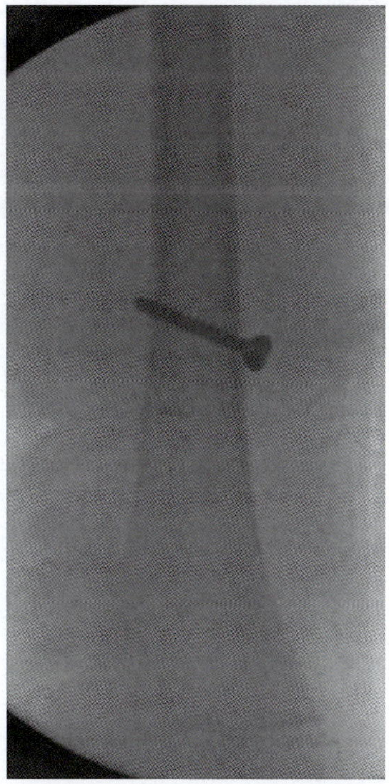

Figure 11.11 A lag screw can then be placed and the clamp removed.

wing nut. The tips of the handles have teeth that can be used to gain traction on the cortex and assist in controlling the fracture fragment in multiple planes. After fracture reduction is achieved, the handles can be connected with clamps and a rod, similar to an external fixation system, to maintain the provisional reduction.

This technique first involves making 1-cm incisions anteriorly in each fracture fragment and placing a trocar onto the femoral shaft (Fig. 11.12). Threaded pins are then inserted bicortically (Fig. 11.13). The cannulated handle is

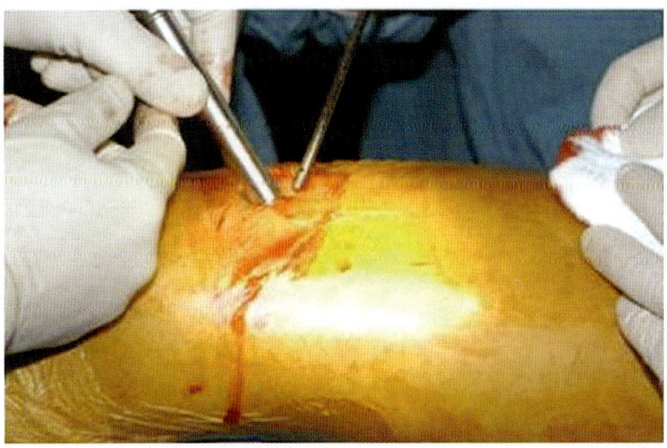

Figure 11.12 Threaded guide pins for manipulators are best placed anteriorly to avoid obstruction with plate passage. A trocar is first inserted anteriorly through a small incision.

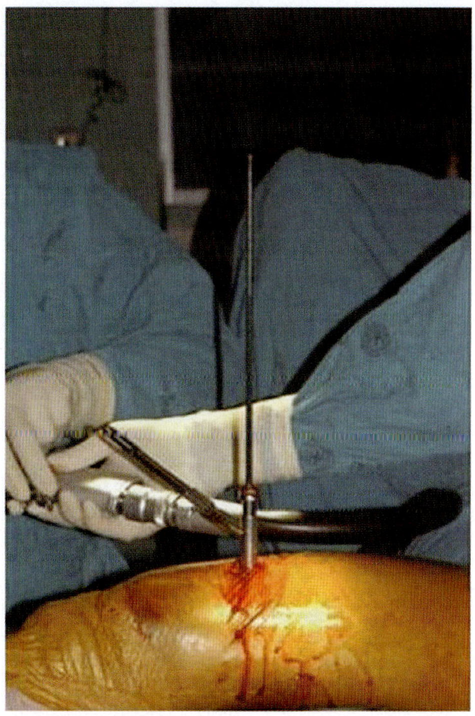

Figure 11.13 The trocar is removed from the sleeve and a threaded guide pin is inserted.

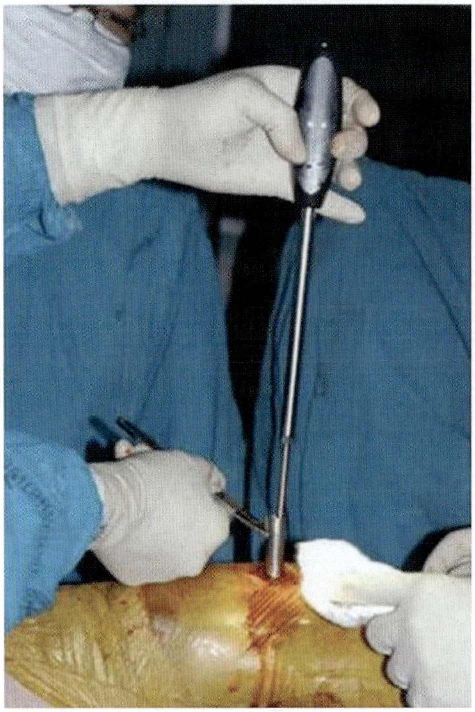

Figure 11.14 A cannulated handle is placed over the threaded guide pin.

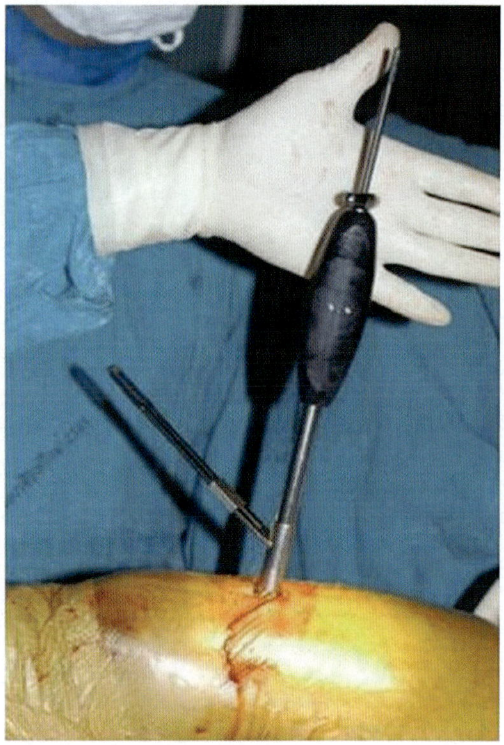

Figure 11.15 Tightening the wing nut over the handle stabilizes the handle, and drives the teeth on the tip of the handle into the periosteum, providing excellent control for joystick reduction maneuvers.

then inserted over the pin and advanced to bone (Fig. 11.14). A wing nut is then threaded over the protruding portion of the pin and tightened to stabilize the handle (Fig. 11.15). When the pins and handles are attached to each fragment, these are used as joysticks to reduce the fracture under fluoroscopic visualization (Fig. 11.16). A carbon fiber rod is then connected between both manipulator handles, and when a final reduction is achieved, the clamps are locked (Fig. 11.17). A percutaneous laterally based plate is then inserted for fracture stabilization.

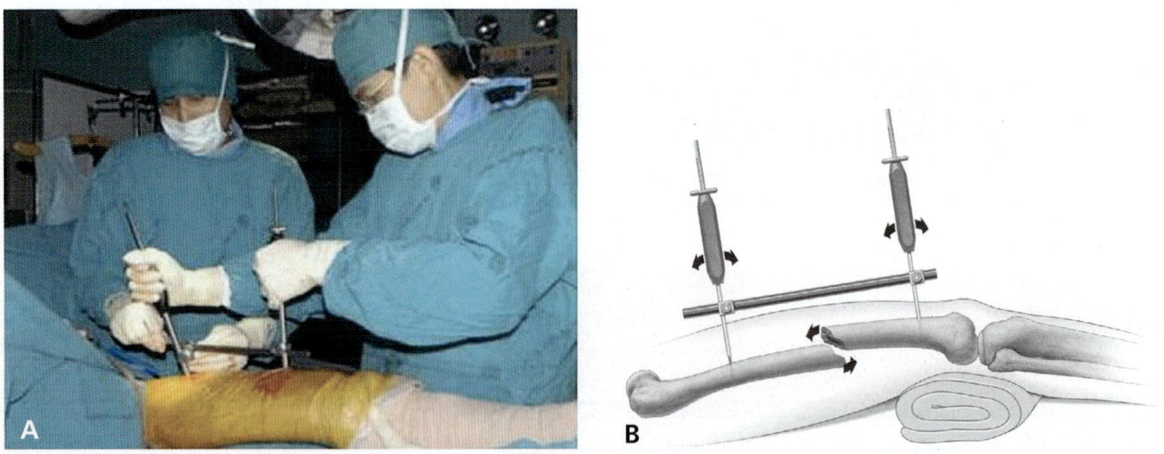

Figure 11.16 With the handles tightened, the fracture fragments can be manipulated to achieve reduction. **A:** Clinical photograph. **B:** Schematic of joystick fracture reduction.

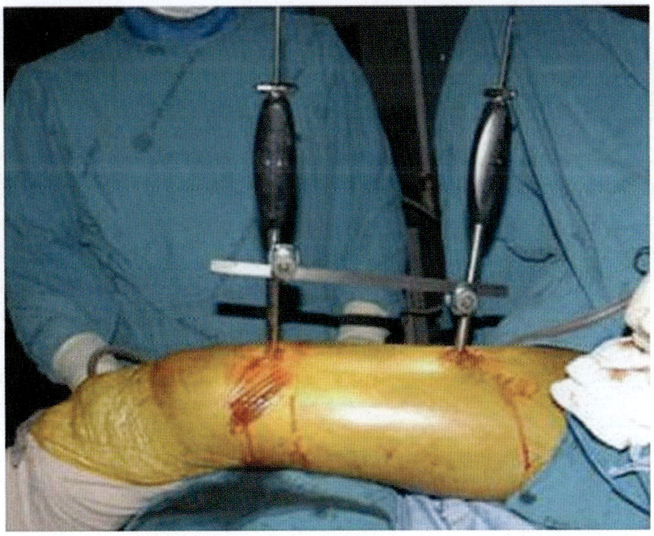

Figure 11.17 Provisional stabilization of the reduction is achieved by connecting a carbon fiber external fixation bar to the handles with external fixation clamps.

Plate as a Reduction Tool

Femur-specific plates which contain an anterior bow can be used as templates to restore the patient's anatomy. After inserting the plate submuscularly beneath the vastus lateralis, the plate is aligned in the center of the bone on both proximal and distal fragments. Temporary fixation is applied initially with a screw or threaded pin through the end plate hole in one fragment, most commonly the proximal fragment. Reduction is then performed by manual traction until appropriate length and rotation are achieved. The plate is then stabilized to the other (distal) fragment with another screw or pin at the other end of the plate. Next, ensure that the bone ends at the fracture site are also aligned and centered under the plate. The bone is then reduced to the plate to complete the reduction using cortical screws or a collinear clamp (Fig. 11.18).

Percutaneous Bone-Plate Clamp

Clamps can be used through small incisions at the fracture site, first to grossly realign the fracture as well as to centralize the bone beneath the plate (Fig. 11.19). Proximal and distal incisions are made and the reduction is optimized with indirect techniques, such as traction and angulation of the limb, as well as strategically placed towel bumps. Paralytic anesthesia greatly facilitates this process. The plate is then inserted submuscularly along the lateral aspect of the femur. The clamps are then used to center the plate at the fracture site (Fig. 11.20),

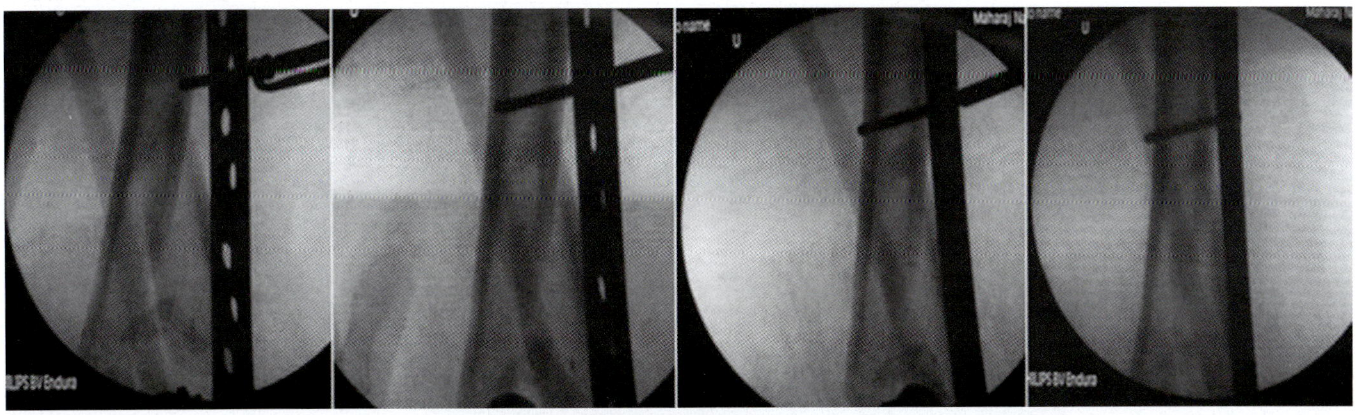

Figure 11.18 A mainstay of percutaneous femoral shaft plating is using the plate as a reduction tool. Tightening a cortical screw will pull the fracture fragment to the plate and improve the reduction.

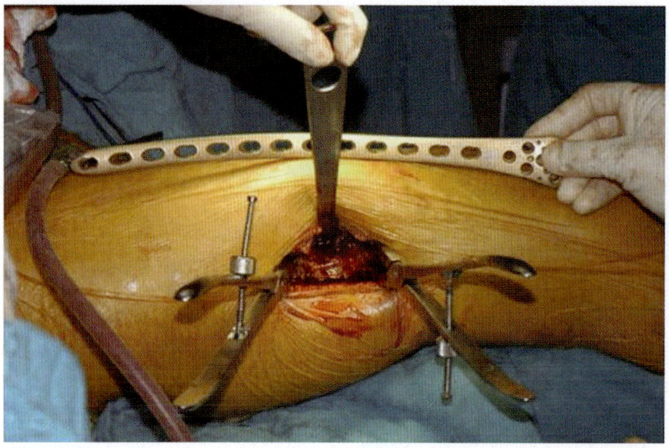

Figure 11.19 In difficult situations when indirect reduction maneuvers have failed, clamps can be inserted directly on to the bone through a small incision.

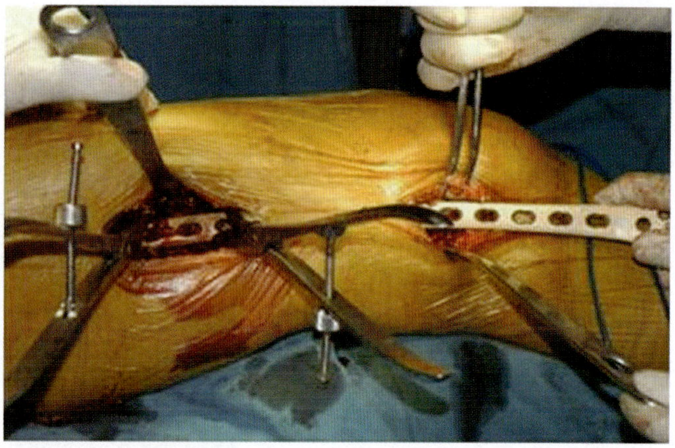

Figure 11.20 Later in the reduction sequence, the clamps can be used to center the plate on both the proximal and distal fragments.

and the plate is fixed to one fragment provisionally with a cortical screw. The reduction is once again verified fluoroscopically and fine-tuned, and the plate is fixed to the other fragment. The remainder of the screws is placed to complete the construct.

FIXATION

The plate length in diaphyseal fracture is determined by plate-span ratio (plate length/fracture length). The goal should be a ratio of greater than 3 in comminuted fractures and greater than 8 in simple fractures.[14] Longer plates provide increased stability to the fixation.[17] The number of screws is determined by plate–screw density (number of screws/number of plate holes) which is usually approximately 0.5. Locking screws are indicated in patients with osteoporotic bone or very short-end segments. In young patients with good bone quality, nonlocking screws provide adequate fixation.[18]

Plate Fixation after Temporary Reduction

After provisional reduction and stabilization, the plate must be inserted and sequentially stabilized to improve or not alter the reduction, depending on the situation. Curved, broad, large fragment plates generally fit well along the lateral cortex. If the fixation needs to extend proximally to the vastus ridge or distally to the supracondylar flare, some additional contouring may be required.

Two Hohmann retractors can be placed through small incisions at the proximal and distal ends of the diaphysis (Fig. 11.21). Newer devices allow the Hohmann's to be maintained in a stable and retracted position to free the surgeon's hands to manipulate the plate or insert

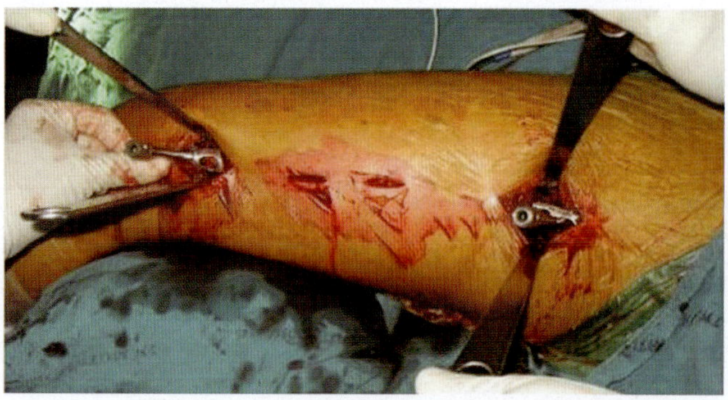

Figure 11.21 Hohmann retractors anteriorly and posteriorly to the femoral shaft allow visualization and precise positioning of the plate.

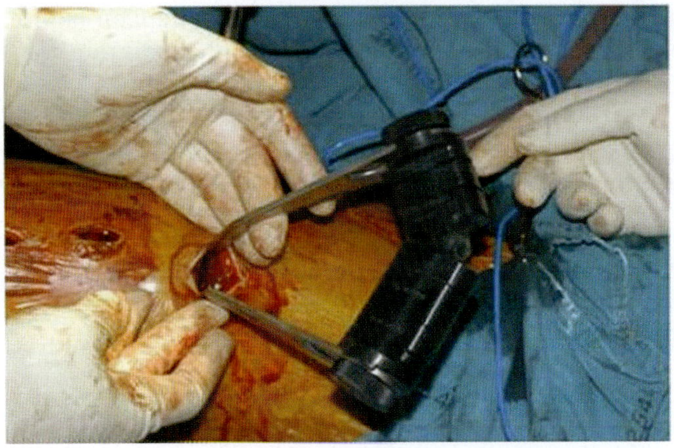

Figure 11.22 Attachments are available that convert Hohmann retractors into self-retaining retractors.

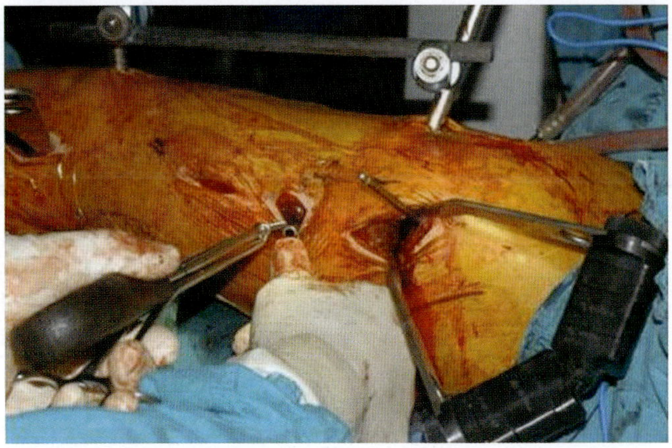

Figure 11.23 With the plate in position and the fracture reduced, wires should be placed at the ends of the plate for provisional fixation.

the fixation (Fig. 11.22). Temporary fixation of the plate at each end hole can be inserted through these windows. This can be done by using the 2-mm K-wire through a threaded drill guide (Fig. 11.23). The first and the last hole of the plate are then fixed with a cortical screw, to draw the bone to the plate if the reduction needs to be adjusted, or with a locking screw if the reduction is accurate. The rest of the screws are spread evenly among each fragment, typically using three screws in each fragment.

Once the end holes are filled, the next step is typically placing screws adjacent to the fracture site. This can be done percutaneously or through a small open incision, depending on the reduction method that has been used. The fracture fragments must be centered under the plate at this stage. Percutaneous screw fixation with conventional screws can be done by using drill sleeves that seat within the screw holes, and this can be confirmed fluoroscopically. Insertion of percutaneous locking screws can be difficult. After making a 1-cm incision, the fascia and muscle are split and dissection continues deep until the plate is identified. One trick is to use a 2-mm Steinmann pin or drill bit to palpate the center of the locking hole, and slide the threaded locking guide over the pin, perpendicular to the plate, to find the locking hole.

COMPLICATIONS

Most of the complications are caused by technical error and are preventable.[19] Malalignment is the most common intraoperative complication, especially sagittal plane angulation and malrotation. Coronal plane angulation is not as common, because the diaphysis shaft is generally straight in the coronal plane and the plate can be used to reduce fracture in this plane. Malalignment is prevented by vigilant intraoperative fluoroscopic assessment of alignment.[20] Sagittal plane malreduction is prevented by obtaining an adequate lateral view to make sure that the plate lies on the center of the bone. If long straight plates are used on the femur, the plate typically needs to reside posterior to the center of the shaft at the fracture site to account for the femoral bow. In subacute situations with soft tissue contraction or malunion with deformity, mini-open reduction at the fracture site is recommended to manipulate the fracture directly in order to reduce the surgical time and radiation exposure to the surgeon.

A hip rotation test can be used to detect malrotation by flexing the hip and the knee 90 degrees and assessing internal and external rotation of the hip compared to the uninjured limb. The lesser trochanter shape sign can also be used to detect malrotation by using the fluoroscopic appearance of the lesser trochanter on a perfect AP view of the hip compared to the contralateral side. Shortening can be grossly detected by using a radioopaque ruler or cautery cord intraoperatively, measuring from the anterior superior iliac spine to the distal femoral articular surface.

Postoperative complications include infection, delayed- or nonunion, and implant failure. A carefully performed minimally invasive technique likely decreased the infection rate compared to traditional open plating. Delayed- or nonunion is infrequent because of the preservation of the blood supply and hematoma at the fracture site. However, it can occur specifically in case with large defects or widely displaced comminution. Percutaneous reduction of the grossly displaced or large butterfly fragments is recommended to minimize this risk. Implant failure is usually followed by delayed- or nonunion. The use of a longer plate with at least three well-spread screws provides relative stability and typically stimulates abundant callus formation. In elderly patients with osteoporosis, the use of a long plate that spans from the proximal femur to the supracondylar area avoids stress risers and decreases the chance of fracture above or below the plate.[17,21]

REHABILITATION PROTOCOL

The patient is allowed to exercise the hip and knee as soon as the pain is subsided, usually around 2 to 3 days postoperatively. External immobilization is not required. Partial weight-bearing is allowed in the first week to load the bone slightly and prevent the disused osteoporosis. The bridge plate principle requires some fracture motion in order to stimulate callus formation. The patient obtains clinical examination and radiographs at 6 weeks, 12 weeks, 20 weeks, 6 months, and 12 months until complete healing. Progressive weight-bearing is allowed when the callus is seen usually after 8 to 12 weeks. Full weight-bearing is recommended after the callus bridges the fracture more than three cortices and the patient has no pain during weight-bearing. If radiographs do not show callus progression in a timely fashion, especially in open fracture or bone defects, bone grafting is recommended at an early stage which reduces the risk of implant failure.

OUTCOME

Minimally invasive plate fixation of the femoral shaft is intended to respect the biology of bone healing. When it is done in the correct steps, healing rates are extremely high. Unfortunately to date, little high-quality published evidence is available.[5,6,22]

REFERENCES

1. Winquist RA, Hansen ST Jr, Clawson DK. Closed intramedullary nailing of femoral fractures. A report of five hundred and twenty cases. *J Bone Joint Surg Am.* 1984;66(4):529–539.
2. Apivatthakakul T, Chiewcharntanakit S. Minimally invasive plate osteosynthesis (MIPO) in the treatment of the femoral shaft fracture where intramedullary nailing is not indicated. *Int Orthop.* 2009;33(4):1119–1126.
3. Babst S, Bavonratanavech S, Pesantez R. Femur, shaft. In: *Minimally Invasive Plate Osteosynthesis (MIPO).* 2nd ed. Stuttgart, Germany: Georg Thieme Verlag; 2012:375–410.
4. Kanlic EM, Anglen JO, Smith DG, et al. Advantages of submuscular bridge plating for complex pediatric femur fractures. *Clin Orthop Relat Res.* 2004; 426:244–251.
5. Ricci WM, Borrelli J Jr. Operative management of periprosthetic femur fractures in the elderly using biological fracture reduction and fixation techniques. *Injury.* 2007;38(Suppl 3):S53–58.
6. Sink EL, Hedequist D, Morgan SJ, et al. Results and technique of unstable pediatric femoral fractures treated with submuscular bridge plating. *J Pediatr Orthop.* 2006;26(2):177–181.
7. Thompson F, O'Beirne J, Gallagher J, et al. Fractures of the femoral shaft treated by plating. *Injury.* 1985;16(8):535–538.
8. Mast J, Jakob R, Ganz R. *Planning and Reduction Technique in Fracture Surgery.* 1st ed. Berlin, Heidelberg, New York: Springer-Verlag; 1989.
9. Farouk O, Krettek C, Miclau T, et al. Minimally invasive plate osteosynthesis: does percutaneous plating disrupt femoral blood supply less than the traditional technique? *J Orthop Trauma.* 1999;13(6):401–406.
10. Heitemeyer U, Kemper F, Hierholzer G, et al. Severely comminuted femoral shaft fractures: treatment by bridging-plate osteosynthesis. *Arch Orthop Trauma Surg.* 1987;106(5):327–330.
11. Perren SM. The concept of biological plating using the limited contact-dynamic compression plate (LC-DCP). Scientific background, design and application. *Injury.* 1991;22(Suppl 1):1–41.

12. Park KC, Oh CW, Byun YS, et al. Intramedullary nailing versus submuscular plating in adolescent femoral fracture. *Injury*. 2012;43(6):870–875.
13. Perren SM. Evolution of the internal fixation of long bone fractures. The scientific basis of biological internal fixation: choosing a new balance between stability and biology. *J Bone Joint Surg Br.* 2002;84(8):1093–1110.
14. Gautier E, Sommer C. Guidelines for the clinical application of the LCP. *Injury.* 2003;34(Suppl 2): B63–B76.
15. Apivatthakakul T, Phornphutkul C, Bunmaprasert T, et al. Percutaneous cerclage wiring and minimally invasive plate osteosynthesis (MIPO): A percutaneous reduction technique in the treatment of Vancouver type B1 periprosthetic femoral shaft fractures. *Arch Orthop Trauma Surg.* 2012;132(6):813–822.
16. Apivatthakakul T, Phornphutkul C. Percutaneous cerclage wiring for reduction of periprosthetic and difficult femoral fractures. A technical note. *Injury*. 2012;43(6):966–971.
17. Stoffel K, Dieter U, Stachowiak G, et al. Biomechanical testing of the LCP–how can stability in locked internal fixators be controlled? *Injury.* 2003;34(Suppl 2):B11–B19.
18. Stoffel K, Stachowiak G, Forster T, et al. Oblique screws at the plate ends increase the fixation strength in synthetic bone test medium. *J Orthop Trauma*. 2004;18(9):611–616.
19. Apivatthakakul T. Complications and solutions. In: *Minimally Invasive Plate Osteosynthesis (MIPO)*. 2nd ed. Stuttgart, Germany: Georg Thieme Verlag; 2012:121–140.
20. Krettek C, Miclau T, Grun O, et al. Intraoperative control of axes, rotation and length in femoral and tibial fractures. Technical note. *Injury.* 1998;29(Suppl 3):C29–C39.
21. Egol KA, Kubiak EN, Fulkerson E, et al. Biomechanics of locked plates and screws. *J Orthop Trauma*. 2004;18(8):488–493.
22. Krettek C, Muller M, Miclau T. Evolution of minimally invasive plate osteosynthesis (MIPO) in the femur. *Injury*. 2001;32(Suppl 3):SC14–SC23.

CHAPTER 12

Minimally Invasive Fixation of Fractures of the Distal Femur

Hobie Summers

INDICATIONS

Minimally invasive techniques for the fixation of distal femur fractures have evolved over time as a result of a better understanding of these fractures as well as improvements in the implants available for fixation. Distal femur fractures represent an interesting diversity of complexity and decision making with regards to surgical approach, reduction techniques, and fixation strategies. In general, simple fracture patterns are well treated with direct, open, anatomic reduction and compression. Minimally invasive techniques may be attractive, yet counterproductive for simple fracture patterns in the metadiaphyseal region, or in simple B-type articular fractures. Multifragmentary fractures of the metadiaphyseal region, on the other hand, have a higher nonunion rate with direct, anatomic reduction techniques and are more amenable to indirect reduction with bridge plating techniques. The development of locked plating has further expanded our ability to treat some fractures of the distal femur with minimally invasive techniques. The best indications for minimally invasive techniques for fixation of distal femur fractures include the following.

Multifragmentary metadiaphyseal supracondylar fractures
Periprosthetic fractures around total knee and hip arthroplasties
Pediatric distal femur fractures

Contraindications for minimally invasive techniques include the following.

Simple fracture patterns in the supracondylar region that are more amenable to direct visualization, anatomic reduction, and compression.

B-type articular fractures

So how do intra-articular fractures fit into minimally invasive techniques? Intra-articular fractures must be treated with an open approach to provide an anatomic reduction and compressive fixation of the articular surface. This may then be followed by percutaneous application of a plate to realign the articular block to the shaft. Locked plates are frequently used for minimally invasive fixation of the distal femur, although traditional implants may be used in this fashion as well.

PATIENT POSITIONING

The patient should be positioned on a radiolucent table to allow for appropriate intraoperative imaging. The image intensifier should come into the field from the opposite side of the table so that it may be used during the procedure. Tourniquets are rarely used as they typically get in the way and blood loss should be minimal with careful dissection. A "sloppy" lateral position will work well for the majority of cases. A one-blanket bump is placed under the operative hip and shoulder to internally rotate the limb. This makes imaging on the AP significantly easier by not constantly fighting the tendency toward external rotation. It also raises the hip to assist with imaging on the lateral x-ray by getting the operative femur above the normal side. Sterile bolsters may be used (10, 12, or 14 towels wrapped together) to elevate the distal segment. This allows for improved lateral imaging as well as providing assistance with overcoming the pull of the gastroc on the distal fragment. The upper extremity may be placed across the chest and secured with sufficient padding.

SURGICAL APPROACHES

The surgical approach for minimally invasive fixation of the distal femur will depend upon the amount of work that needs to be done to achieve an anatomic reduction of the joint. The direct lateral approach is sufficient for extra-articular fractures, and those with a simple intercondylar split. This approach avoids incising the quadriceps tendon and spares the vastus lateralis. The incision is made from Gerdy's tubercle, which is palpable over the lateral proximal tibia, and directly over the mid-lateral portion of the distal femur. After incising the subcutaneous tissue, the tensor fascia is incised in-line with the skin incision. The vastus lateralis is then easily elevated from the posterior intermuscular septum, and all periosteum and muscle attachment to the femur are left attached. The capsular attachment of the suprapatellar pouch should be left attached to the articular fragment to maintain its blood supply. The capsule may be incised in-line with the skin incision to enter the joint and visualize the lateral aspect of the distal femur. If there is no intercondylar fracture line, the capsule may be elevated to just visualize the vermilion border of the articular lateral condyle. If an intercondylar split is present and visualization of the distal articular surface is necessary, the tensor fascia is split slightly anterior to Gerdy's tubercle, as is the capsule. The capsule is incised along the lateral border of the patellar tendon so the articular surface may be better visualized. If necessary, the skin incision may curve closer to the tibial tuberosity, rather than Gerdy's tubercle. This allows easier dissection close to the patellar tendon and retraction of the patella medially to visualize the joint surface.

In C3 fracture patterns, articular reconstruction requires a lateral parapatellar approach. When significant comminution or coronal plane fractures are present, the lateral parapatellar approach will make the reconstruction significantly easier, and still allow for subcutaneous application of a plate for fixation to the proximal segment. The lateral parapatellar approach may be performed through a midline or a (lateral) paramedian incision. After incising the skin, the deep portion of the approach hugs the lateral aspect of the patella and incising the lateral portion of the quad tendon and muscle is performed in a full thickness manner for later repair. This allows the surgeon to enter the joint more anteriorly and medially, making intercondylar and medial access easier. The capsule is dissected from the lateral condyle, once inside the joint, for plate application in its appropriate position. Again, the soft tissue attachment to the condylar fragments should not be dissected from the bone. This blood supply to the condyle should be preserved.

Occasionally, a small medial approach may be necessary to deal with coronal plane fractures on the medial side of the joint, or in rare cases where the medial condyle is comminuted. A medial parapatellar arthrotomy can be carefully performed in conjunction with the standard, direct lateral incision in these rare cases. Being cautious to leave a sufficient skin bridge between the medial and lateral incisions is paramount to avoid wound problems. Keeping the incisions only as long as they absolutely need to be is likewise helpful.

It should be noted that in cases of simple fracture patterns, B-type articular or simple supracondylar, a direct lateral approach can be performed nicely without devascularizing the bone. The same skin incision for a direct lateral approach to the distal femur may be extended along the lateral femoral shaft. The vastus lateralis is elevated from the posterior intermuscular septum while perforating vessels are carefully cauterized. A Cobb elevator is used to gently release the vastus from the septum as well as from the periosteum from the lateral aspect of the shaft. The periosteum and anterior musculature is not detached. This maintains the vascularity to the femur while providing a "working window" to visualize the lateral aspect of the fracture line. Reduction forceps may be passed without further soft tissue stripping to afford an anatomic reduction for simple fracture patterns.

REDUCTION TECHNIQUES

For simple extra-articular fracture patterns, the dissection just described may be used for anatomic reduction and compressive fixation. While this may not be minimally invasive in terms of skin incision, it is soft tissue sparing by not stripping the bone of its vascularity. Having a nice "working window" with soft tissues minimally dissected from the septum and periosteum, anatomic reduction of simple fracture patterns can be performed in a biologically friendly manner. Large pointed reduction forceps may be placed around muscle to maintain the bone's vascularity and anatomic reduction can be performed. This is typically followed by lag screw fixation and/or compression plating. Independent lag screws may be placed followed by neutralization plating, or compression plating using an articulated tension device may be performed, followed by lag screw application through the plate when appropriate (Fig. 12.1 with x-rays).

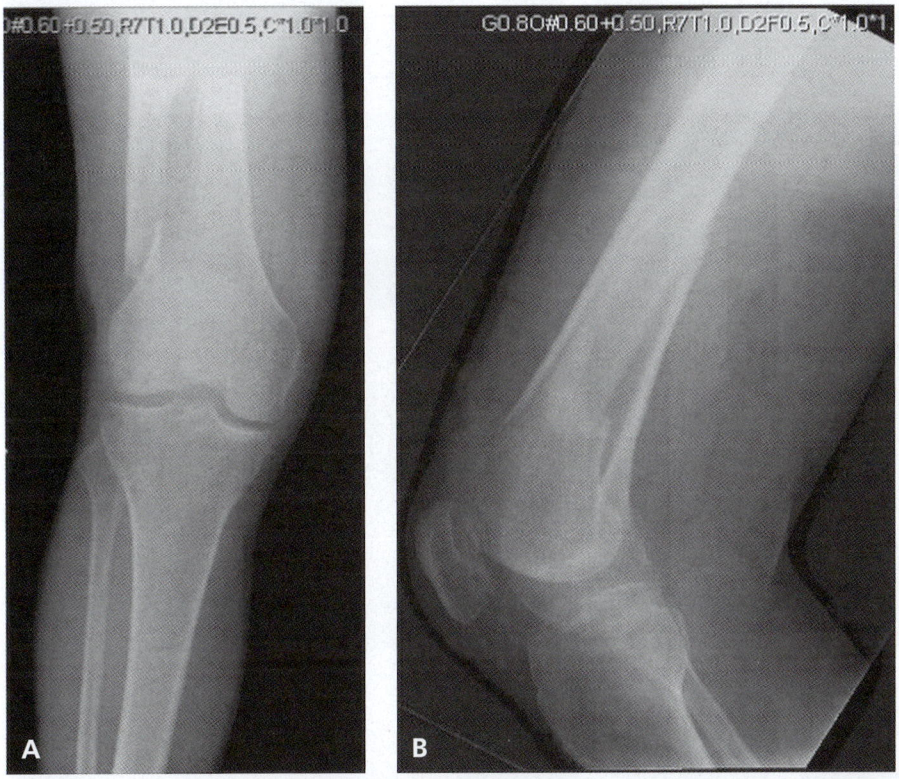

Figure 12.1 A and B: AP and lateral radiographs of a 43-C1 injury. Note the simple articular and simple metadiaphyseal components. **C through G:** Fluoroscopic images showing the intraoperative steps for anatomic reduction and absolute stability for this simple fracture pattern. **C:** Demonstrates articular reduction and fixation followed by appropriate plate positioning to the distal fragment. **D and E:** Demonstrate clamp application on AP and lateral images with the plate well positioned. **F:** Shows the use on the articulated tension device. **G:** Illustrates lag screw application after compression with the plate has been completed. **H:** Limited open exposure for a simple fracture pattern with respect for the soft tissues was performed to achieve an anatomic reduction and compressive fixation. **I and J:** The completed anatomic reconstruction through a limited exposure. *(continued)*

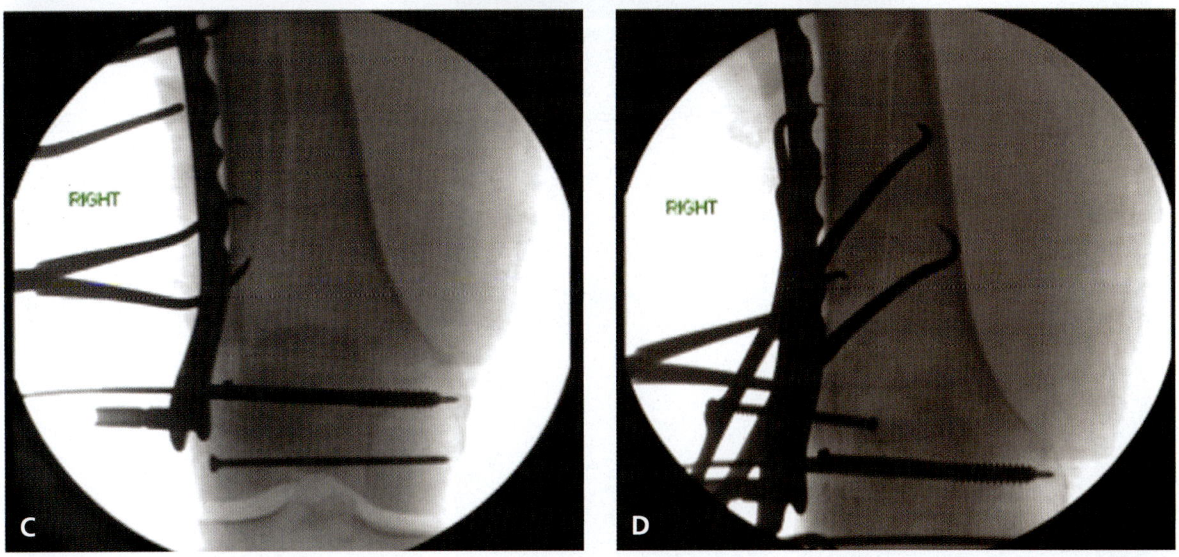

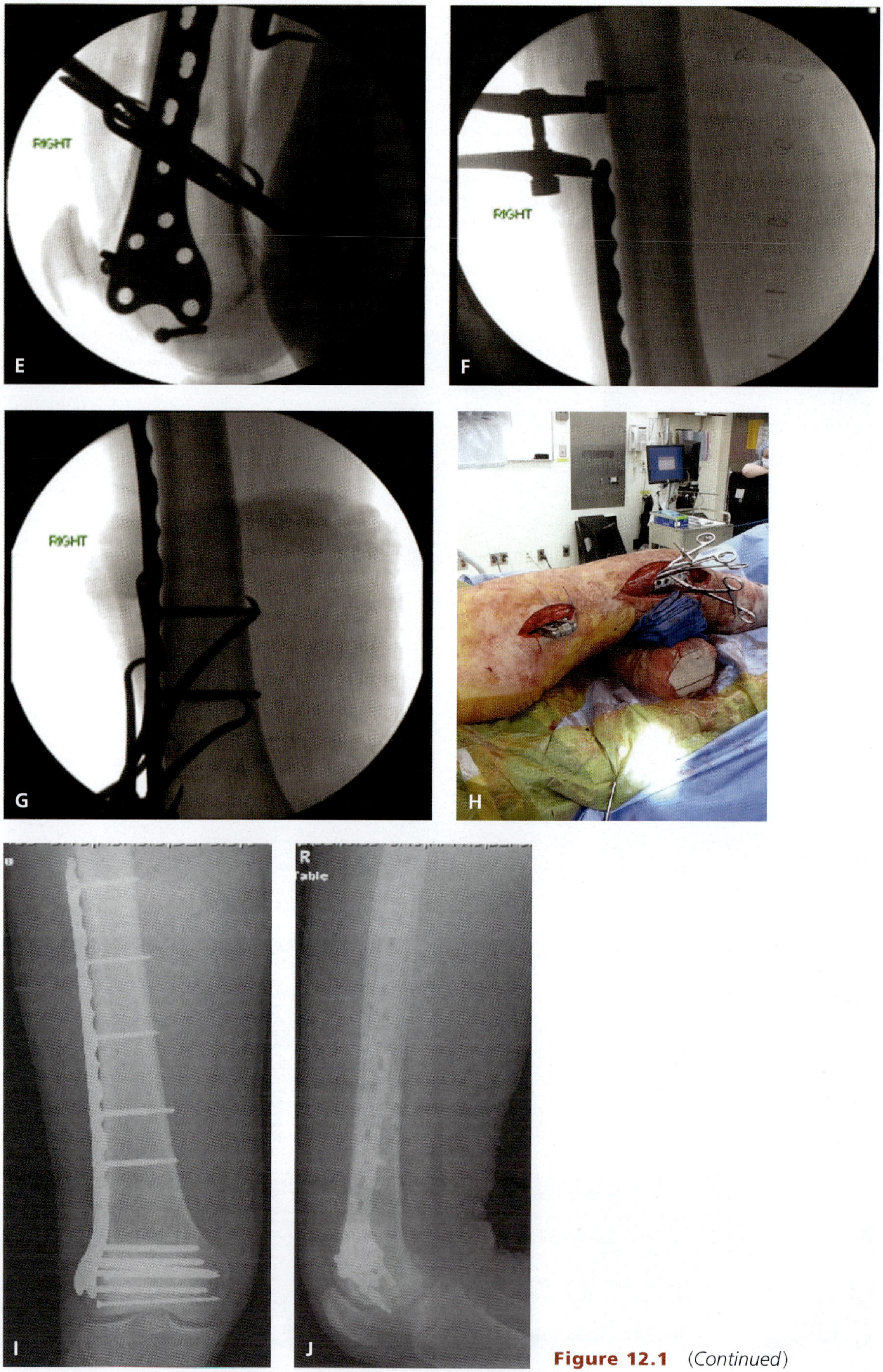

Figure 12.1 *(Continued)*

For comminuted extra-articular fractures, bridge plating may be performed in a minimally invasive fashion. The key to reduction is restoring length, alignment, and rotation. Multiple reduction aids are available and knowledge in their appropriate use is the key. Some simple patterns may reduce with simple manual traction over soft, sterile towel bumps. It is not uncommon to have medial comminution with a simple fracture line laterally. Once brought out to length, the lateral cortex may reduce quite nicely to maintain length. This "lateral read" may be visible or palpable through the lateral approach at its most proximal extent. When obtaining length proves difficult, first make sure the patient is adequately paralyzed by anesthesia to reduce muscle tone necessary for reduction. A femoral distractor or external fixator may be used to help achieve length as well. Schantz pins are placed from anterior to posterior in the femoral shaft and proximal tibia to keep them out of the way for plate application. After restoring length, carefully evaluate the lateral fluoroscopic imaging, as the pull of the gastroc on the distal fragment tends to cause an extension deformity. A bolster placed under the apex of the metaphyseal spike of the distal fragment may be very useful in controlling this deformity. When the distal fragment will not reduce with closed/positioning means, a carefully inserted Schantz pin in the distal fragment will provide excellent control to reduce this fragment. The Schantz pin may be placed through a small stab incision from anterior to posterior, and should be placed outside the articular surface (just proximal to it) in the metaphyseal portion of the distal fragment. Flexion/extension control is excellent with this single pin and the fragment may be reduced. Once the articular segment is appropriately aligned with the more proximal shaft, definitive fixation may be completed. A laterally based locked plate is most commonly used for fractures with metadiaphyseal comminution. When using locked implants, the reduction of the fracture should be performed prior to plate application. The plate is inserted in a submuscular fashion, deep to the vastus lateralis, and extraperiosteally along the femoral shaft. The position of the plate is carefully evaluated on AP and lateral fluoroscopic images, keeping in mind the recommended position for the implant selected. Once the implant is correctly positioned, k-wires may be used to provisionally keep the plate in position until it has been fixed to the bone. Fixation typically begins with the distal fragment and many implant manufacturers have designed a central screw that should be positioned parallel to the articular surface on the AP image. It is critical to understand the implant you are using so that deformity is not induced by incorrect application of the implant. Only after the implant is perfectly positioned and attached to the distal fragment can one move on to proximal fixation.

It should be noted that many fracture patterns, even comminuted patterns, have a simple fracture line laterally that may be amenable to compression. When there is an opportunity to compress the lateral cortex, this should be taken advantage of. Tensioning the plate and compressing the fracture will improve the overall stability of the construct. When using a long plate, a separate incision at the proximal end of the plate may be made; the vastus lateralis elevated from the posterior intermuscular septum, and a push–pull screw may be inserted outside the plate for application of the articulated tensioning device.

Understanding the shape of the distal femur is critical to being able to effectively and accurately apply fixation for these fractures (Fig. 12.2). If looking up at the distal femur from below (looking directly at the articular surface) it is trapezoidal in shape being narrower anteriorly and wider posteriorly. The angle of inclination on the lateral side is 10 degrees and on the medial side 25 degrees. Therefore, a lateral plate should sit in 10 degrees of internal rotation relative to neutral rotation of the femur, thereby sitting flush on the lateral femoral condyle. Screws inserted for Hoffa (coronal plane) fractures should be angled appropriately as well. Screws from anterior to posterior on the medial side should start slightly lateral and angle 25 degrees to remain central in the condyle and cross the fracture in a perpendicular fashion for most patterns (Fig. 12.2). The same holds true for the lateral Hoffa fractures except the screws start slightly medial and angle 10 degrees laterally. When placing screws for sagittal plane fractures, one should remember that the more anteriorly placed screws should be shorter than the more posteriorly placed screws due to the trapezoidal shape of the distal segment. Therefore, on the AP image, the anterior screws will appear to be too short, when in fact they are not. Making these screws too long can be very irritating to the medial soft tissues.

For simple intercondylar fractures, a standard lateral approach will typically allow for adequate visualization and reduction of the articular fracture. Allowing the fracture to

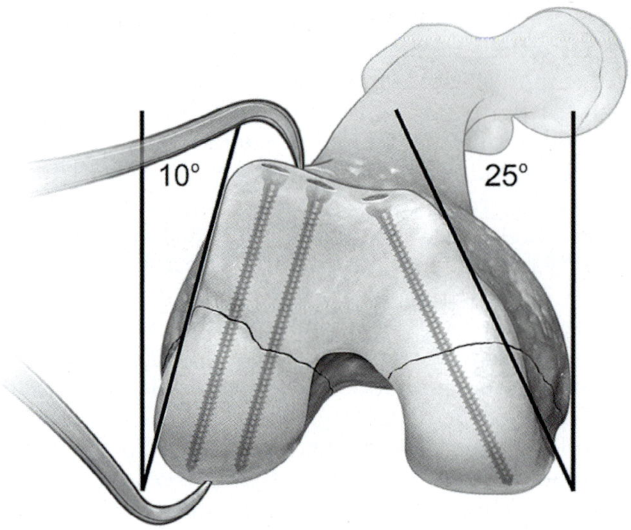

Figure 12.2 Note the 10-degree inclination laterally and 25-degree inclination medially. This anatomy is important for appropriate plate placement and lag screw orientation when Hoffa plane fractures are present. (From: Gardner MJ, Henley MB. Distal femur fractures. In: Gardner MJ, Henley MB, eds. *Harborview Illustrated Tips and Tricks in Fracture Surgery.* Philadelphia, PA: Lippincott Williams & Wilkins; 2011:221–240.)

shorten by telescoping the shaft fragment around the articular block will allow easier access to visualize the joint. Large periarticular clamps and large pointed reduction forceps are typically sufficient for reduction. When rotation of the fragments proves difficult, 2-mm k-wires can be inserted into the condyles to assist with rotation. Alternatively, a Schantz pin may be inserted through a small incision into the medial femoral condyle to provide better control of the fragment. Be careful to clamp the fracture symmetrically. It is very easy to place the clamp too anteriorly and gap the fracture posteriorly (Fig. 12.3). A central periarticular clamp or two large pointed forceps may be needed to evenly compress the intercondylar split.

Complex articular patterns require patience. After a lateral parapatellar approach, identifying and cleaning clot from the articular fragments is performed. When Hoffa fragments are present, resist the temptation to reduce the intercondylar split first. Instead, take advantage of the intercondylar fracture line and work through it to help visualize, reduce, and clamp the

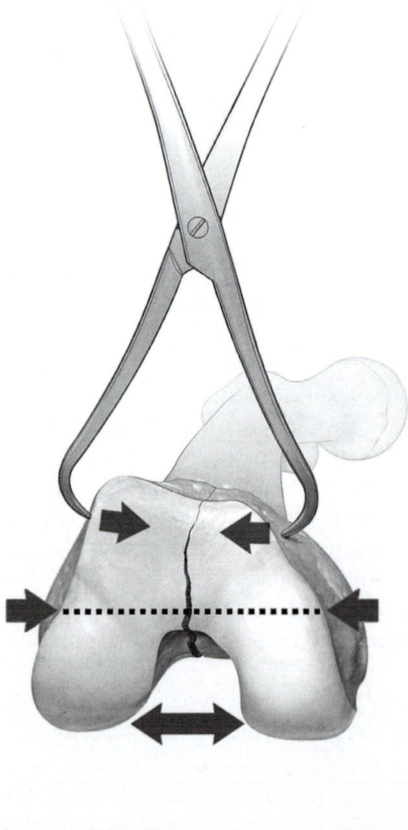

Figure 12.3 If the intercondylar clamp is placed too anteriorly, the posterior condyles risk becoming distracted (*bottom double arrow*). The ideal clamp placement for balanced fracture compression is relatively posterior on the condyles (*middle arrows and dashed line*) at the level of Blumensaat line. (From: Gardner MJ, Henley MB. Distal femur fractures. In: Gardner MJ, Henley MB, eds. *Harborview Illustrated Tips and Tricks in Fracture Surgery.* Philadelphia, PA: Lippincott Williams & Wilkins; 2011:221–240.)

Hoffa fragment. These can be provisionally fixed with k-wires or definitively fixed with lag screws. Be sure to angle the screws appropriately for the medial and lateral sides according to the angle of inclination, and use your tactile senses as well as fluoroscopy to avoid placing a screw that is too long and protrudes into the joint. After the Hoffa plane fractures have been addressed, reduce the intercondylar fracture line. When the central portion, or "notch" fragment, is a separate piece, it may be beneficial to reduce this to one of the two condyles, provisionally secure this, and then reduce to two large fragments together. It is common to have multiple k-wires for joysticks, a Schantz pin, a few clamps, and multiple provisional k-wires for temporary fixation used at the same time. Once again, patience is the key and sometimes you have to revise your reduction strategy and sequence as you go. Once the articular block is reduced, it should be definitively fixed with screws before reducing the block to the more proximal fragments. Keep in mind the position of the plate to be used for fixation, and try to keep the articular screws outside the zone of the plate screws. This can be difficult, but one can frequently place a template of the distal portion of the implant to be used on the lateral aspect of the femur to ensure the screws for articular fixation are out of the way. The intercondylar screws may be countersunk so they rest under the plate if necessary.

FIXATION

For the articular fracture fragments, 3.5-mm and 2.7-mm screws are typically used in lag fashion for fixation. Using larger screws is difficult as they interfere with the path of screws for the plate. These screws can be used with washers as the lateral metaphyseal and anterior bone where the head engages may be rather soft and the washers will assist with providing sufficient compression.

Plate fixation for simple patterns may use nonlocking implants, in compression mode, very effectively. Most implants for the distal femur are technically locked plates, but they can be used in combination mode with both locking and nonlocking screws. It may be wise to use locking screws in the distal fragment to provide secure fixation in this metaphyseal bone, while nonlocking screws may be used in the more proximal diaphyseal bone. This will maintain some flexibility in the construct to provide the correct strain environment for callous formation. Locking screws may be used to protect nonlocking screws in the shaft for osteoporotic patients. Paying careful attention to bone quality is important. Avoiding a construct that is too short and too stiff, by using multiple-locked screws in the proximal fragment, is important to avoid nonunion and hardware failure. Whether performing an anatomic reduction with compression or a bridge plate construct, with or without compression of the lateral side, maintaining some flexibility is desirable. Long implants with sufficiently spaced screws will perform this task much better than shorter implants with screws bunched up close to the fracture site.

COMPLICATIONS

One of the most common complications with minimally invasive fixation of fractures of the distal femur is related to malreduction and has been reported as high as 26%.[1] Careful attention must be paid to length, alignment, and rotation. Establishing appropriate length may be very difficult in osteoporotic fractures as they can be significantly impacted. Femoral components in periprosthetic fractures can make visualization of the reduction as well as plate and screw position very difficult. In these cases, obtain an accurate reduction and provisionally stabilize these fractures before plate application. Varus–valgus alignment can be difficult in the significantly comminuted fracture patterns. Using the plate as a reduction tool can be very helpful if used correctly. Like a 95-degree blade plate, many implants manufactured today have a central screw that is 95 degrees to the plate and can be used to drive the reduction of the comminuted segment when the plate is applied distally first, and then brought to the proximal fragment. This requires knowledge of the implant chosen for the case and should be understood before taking on these fractures. In addition, a bovie cord may be used to check alignment. Fluoroscopic images with the cord over the center of the hip and ankle should also pass through the center of the knee. Make sure the limb is straight with the patella pointing straight up when checking alignment with this method. If the cord falls medial, the resultant deformity is varus, and when it falls laterally, the deformity is valgus. Check the position of the central screw to see if it has been placed correctly and revise as necessary. In addition, the plate should be placed at a 10-degree angle on the distal fragment as illustrated previously. When this is not done correctly, the typical malreduction is both rotational and translational. Sagittal plane malreductions may be caused by posterior plate placement, as one should notice that the center of the articular block does not line up with the center of the femoral shaft. The femoral shaft is anterior to the center of the distal articular block; hence the plate should sit rather anterior on this fragment to avoid these malreductions.

Nonunion rates for fractures of the distal femur have decreased dramatically with the advent of fixed-angled devices and improvements in our understanding of indirect reduction techniques.[2] Several early series of locked plating have reported union rates of 90% or better.[3–5]

It has been discovered that union rates may not be as high as originally reported. A comprehensive review of the literature has demonstrated nonunion, delayed union, implant failures, and the need for secondary procedures after locked plating to be substantial.[6] In this review the reported nonunion rate ranged from 0% to 19% and delayed union ranged from 0% to 15%. Implant failure ranged from 0% to 20%. Patients requiring secondary procedures related to healing, including revision of implant or secondary bone grafting, ranged from 0% to 32%. The overall rate of healing difficulties, including nonunion, delayed union, implant revision, or secondary bone grafting, ranged from 0% to 32%. Of note, 50% of all implant failures occurred after 6 months. While 83% of all implant failures occurred in the first 12 months, 17% occur after a year. It is important to recognize that the advent of locked plating has improved the time to failure and there may be fractures that are partially healed and simply do not declare themselves nonunions for many months. Due diligence and long-term follow-up is important to ensure patients are truly treated to union.

Infection rates should be expected to be approximately 2% or less for closed injury and higher for open fractures. Early recognition and treatment should be employed for postoperative infections and antibiotic beads may be helpful in open fracture cases, particularly when a staged bone grafting procedure is anticipated.

REHABILITATION

For the majority of intra-articular distal femur fractures, the patient is kept non–weight-bearing for 10 to 12 weeks. Unrestricted range of motion exercises can be started immediately after surgery as can straight leg raises to work on quad strength. In elderly patients the articular fracture pattern is often simple or periprosthetic, and I typically allow them to perform 13.6 kg (30 lb) touch-down weight-bearing with a walker in order to mobilize them early. It is very difficult for them to maintain a non–weight-bearing status, and allowing partial weight-bearing will make it easier for them to get out of bed and perform self-cares. Once callous is seen on plain radiographs, weight-bearing may be advanced. Gait and strength training may be the focus after the patient is weight-bearing as tolerated.

OUTCOMES

There are relatively few long-term follow-up studies looking at functional results in patients with distal femur fractures. Rademakers et al. published their results of 65 operatively treated, intra-articular distal femur fractures treated by open reduction and internal fixation with plates and screws.{Rademakers:2004ws} At 1 year follow-up, the average knee range of motion was 111 degrees and 58% were pain free. Thirty-one percent had mild pain and 7% had moderate pain with weight-bearing. Seventy-five percent were able to walk for 30 minutes or longer. Over half of the patients involved in sporting activities returned to those activities in 1 year. Thirty-two patients returned for long-term follow-up at a mean of 14 years (5 to 25). Eighty-one percent of these patients had no pain while weight-bearing and approximately 9.5% had moderate pain and mild pain. Using the HSS knee score and the Neer score, good-to-excellent results were seen in 75% to 84%, respectively. There was no correlation between B and C type fractures, or age at injury, with regards to knee scores or secondary osteoarthritis. Overall, the grade of secondary osteoarthritis correlated with lower knee scores, although most patients with moderate-to-severe osteoarthritis continued to have scores in the good-to-excellent results ranges. It should be noted that only two patients had a varus or valgus malalignment of 5 to 10 degrees, indicating the importance of accurate reduction.

SUMMARY

Fractures of the distal femur are complex injuries requiring an intimate understanding of the anatomy and geometry to the distal femoral complex. Minimally invasive techniques may be employed for the treatment of these fractures when the patterns are appropriate. Anatomic reconstruction of the articular segment and correction of length, alignment, and rotation of that segment to the more proximal shaft are the primary goals. Bridge plating techniques through limited incisions may be used in the comminuted metadiaphyseal patterns, but open, direct reduction techniques can be performed in a biologically friendly manner when the fracture pattern is appropriate. Good-to-excellent results may be expected in the majority of these fractures when treated with appropriate techniques and attention to detail.

REFERENCES

1. Schutz M, Muller M, Regazzoni P, et al. Use of the less invasive stabilization system (LISS) in patients with distal femoral (AO33) fractures: A prospective multicenter study. *Arch Orthop Trauma Surg.* 2005;125(2):102–108.
2. Bolhofner BR, Carmen B, Clifford P. The results of open reduction and internal fixation of distal femur fractures using a biologic (indirect) reduction technique. *J Orthop Trauma.* 1996;10(6):372–377.
3. Ostrum RF, Geel C. Indirect reduction and internal fixation of supracondylar femur fractures without bone graft. *J Orthop Trauma.* 1995;9(4):278–284.
4. Weight M, Collinge C. Early results of the less invasive stabilization system for mechanically unstable fractures of the distal femur (AO/OTA types A2, A3, C2, and C3). *J Orthop Trauma.* 2004;18(8):503–508.
5. Kregor PJ, Stannard JA, Zlowodzki M, et al. Treatment of distal femur fractures using the less invasive stabilization system: Surgical experience and early clinical results in 103 fractures. *J Orthop Trauma.* 2004;18(8):509–520.
6. Henderson CE, Kuhl LL, Fitzpatrick DC, et al. Locking plates for distal femur fractures: Is there a problem with fracture healing? *J Orthop Trauma.* 2012;25(Suppl 1):S8–S14.

CHAPTER 13

Minimally Invasive Plating of the Distal Tibia

Daniel J. Stinner, Michael J. Beltran, and Cory A. Collinge

INDICATIONS

Minimally invasive percutaneous plate osteosynthesis (MIPPO) is a technique indicated for fractures of the distal tibial metaphysis, including those with simple involvement of the articular tibial plafond. This includes both low- and high-energy extra-articular metaphyseal fractures, and select high-energy axial loading plafond injuries (i.e., pilon fractures) without articular comminution (OTA type A and C1/2 fractures) (Figs. 13.1 and 13.2). While metadiaphyseal and metaphyseal distal tibia fractures may also be well treated with modern intramedullary nails—despite articular extension and short distal segments, recent literature has indicated a higher incidence of angular malalignment after nailing compared to plating, and anterior knee pain remains a common long-term outcome.[1–3] Strategies for minimally invasive surgery around the distal tibia are not new. External fixation has been used around the distal tibia with good results, where biology is preserved and stability provided by external fixation allows for early healing in most cases. The difference between internal and external fixation is in the risk/benefit profile, as well as the mechanics and the resulting healing process. For example, while scant metal is implanted at the fracture site with external fixation, pin problems exist, the fixator crosses the ankle making stiffness a concern, it requires removal, and high rates of malunion have been reported.

MIPPO of the distal tibia may be utilized when the surgeon desires either absolute or relative fracture stability based on the fracture pattern being treated. Noncomminuted oblique or spiral fractures with or without simple articular extension are well treated with absolute stability techniques and implants if they can be anatomically reduced. Adjuvant reduction tools (percutaneous clamps, joysticks, etc.) can often be used to help obtain an anatomic reduction, which is then stabilized with lag screws either through or outside of the plate. In the latter case, the percutaneous plate is applied in a neutralization mode. Highly comminuted fractures, conversely, are usually best managed with relative stability, and in these circumstances plates should be placed in a bridging mode. In these situations, the plate itself can be used as a reduction aid to restore mechanical alignment, in addition to other adjuvant reduction aids. In either circumstance, the goals of percutaneous fracture surgery are met—preservation of fracture biology and minimization of soft tissue complications.

Select situations pose particular challenges for distal tibia MIPPO, and under these conditions an alternative fixation strategy should be employed. Severe compromise of the distal leg soft tissue envelope, particularly medially, may increase the chances for infection and wound breakdown even when small incisions are used. Intramedullary nailing, open reduction through a different approach, or external fixation should be considered under these circumstances. Furthermore, type C3 pilon fractures with articular comminution are best managed, in most cases, with a fully open approach and anatomic reconstruction of the articular surface. This is especially true in the younger, more active population. Finally, simple fractures at the metaphysis or metadiaphyseal junction of the distal tibia, while amenable to MIPPO, may be well treated with intramedullary nailing. With intramedullary nailing, there may be theoretical benefit to apply a local bone graft in nailed distal tibias, as well as the ability to dynamically compress and load certain fracture patterns during weight bearing.

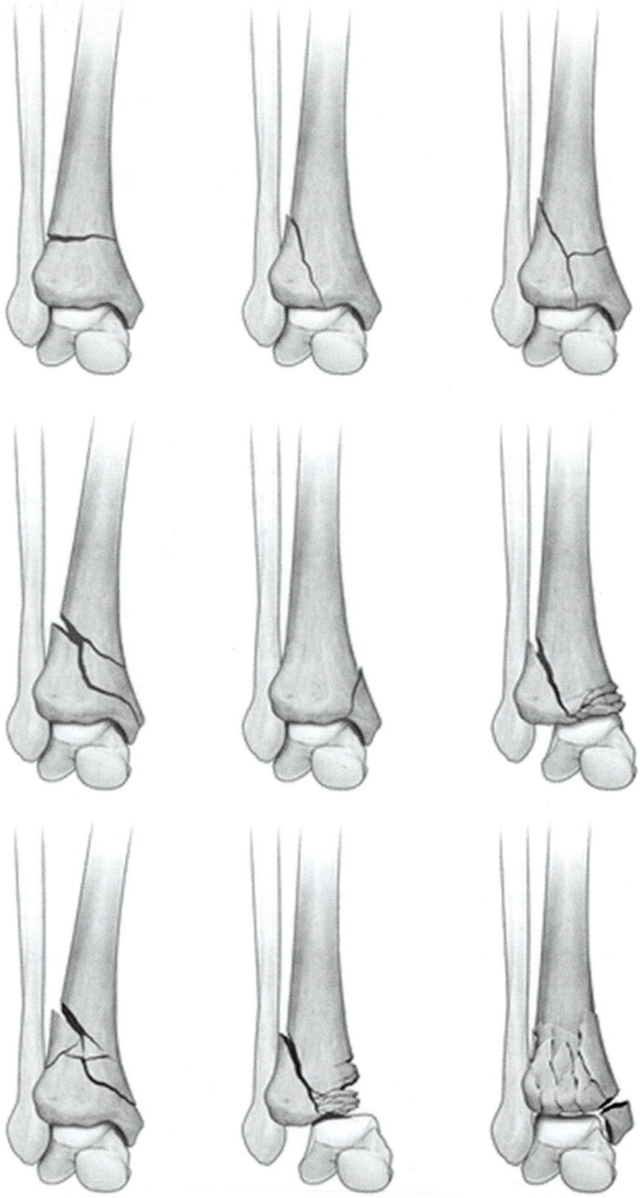

Figure 13.1 Orthopedic Trauma Association alphanumeric classification of distal tibia (43) fractures.

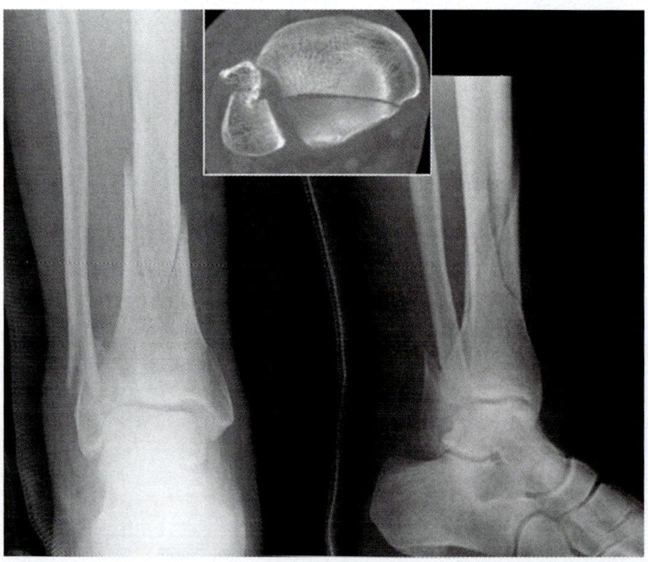

Figure 13.2 Illustrative case, a 43-year-old man with an OTA 43-C1 injury treated as demonstrated by associated figures.

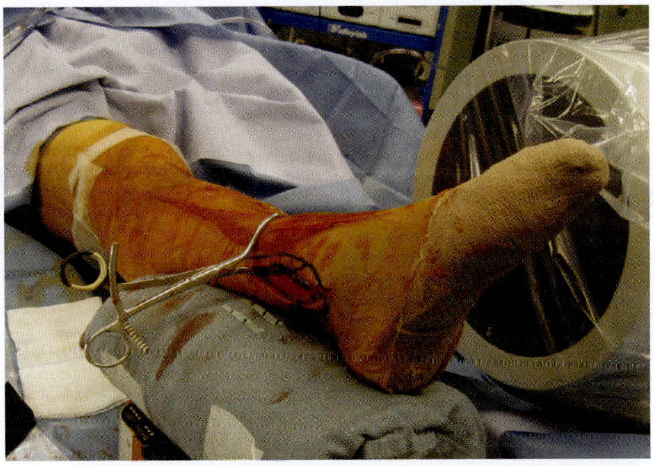

Figure 13.3 Positioning is supine and C-arm is brought in from the opposite side. Use of bumps and clamps are demonstrated.

PATIENT POSITIONING

The patient is positioned in the supine position on a radiolucent table (Fig. 13.3). A small bump is placed under the hip to place the entire lower extremity in a neutral position, which aids in obtaining orthogonal radiographs and does not compromise the surgical approaches necessary for the technique. If the fracture is already spanned with an external fixator and the pins are ideally placed to aid in indirect fracture reduction, the bar and clamp components are removed and the pins prepped into the field. After prepping, we prefer to isolate the pin sites with small sponges to reduce contamination of the sterile surgical wounds.

SURGICAL APPROACHES

Approaches for MIPPO of the distal tibia include the workhorse medial approach and, less commonly, the anterolateral approach. Nearly all metaphyseal fractures can be managed via the medial approach. While large, open medial incisions have previously been associated with high wound complication rates, the small incisions, preserve biology, and careful soft tissue handling used in MIPPO techniques have not led to adverse soft tissue problems in larger series of patients.[1,4,5]

The medial approach involves a 2- to 3-cm incision at the tip of the medial malleolus, taking care to preserve the saphenous vein and nerve with the superficial dissection (Figs. 13.4 and 13.5). Once the dissection reaches the periosteal level, a subcutaneous, extraperiosteal tunnel is developed proximally using an elevator or the plate itself, taking diligent care to stay along the anteromedial face of the tibia and not deviate anteriorly or posteriorly. A small 2- to 3-cm proximal window is often helpful to pass the plate centrally on the medial tibia and ensure its proper proximal position.

We prefer the use of modern, precontoured, locking small fragment plates medially because they can be used as indirect reduction aids themselves and allow for fixed-angle stability when managing short metaphyseal segments. In contrast, nonlocking plates can be used and have been associated with good results in a recent series.[1] If the surgeon is bending plates for the medial distal tibia, the local anatomy must be appreciated or else deformity may be imparted. While the coronal plane flare of the medial distal tibia is evident on an AP radiograph (an approximate 20-cm radius of curvature, Figure 13.6A), there is also torsional contour of the medial face of the distal tibia (Fig. 13.6B) that must be addressed. Mast has recommended bending 25 degrees of torsion into the plate, then using a bending press to apply a mild concavity to the plate. As a general rule, (1) the torsional bend is more important to the final reduction than the concavity and (2) the stiffer the implant, the more precise the bend must be or else deformity may be imparted. If the indirect reduction has already been obtained with other adjuvant measures, the plate is fixed proximally and distally with a combination of locking and nonlocking screws (i.e., hybrid plate constructs). In general, we prefer the use of locking screws in the distal metaphysis and nonlocking screws proximally.

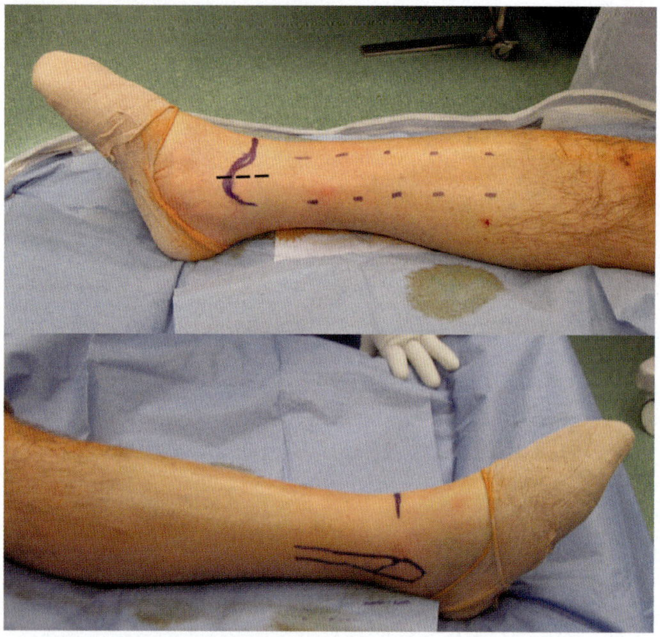

Figure 13.4 The anatomy is drawn out and a 2- to 3-cm incision at the tip of the medial malleolus is made for subcutaneous plate insertion.

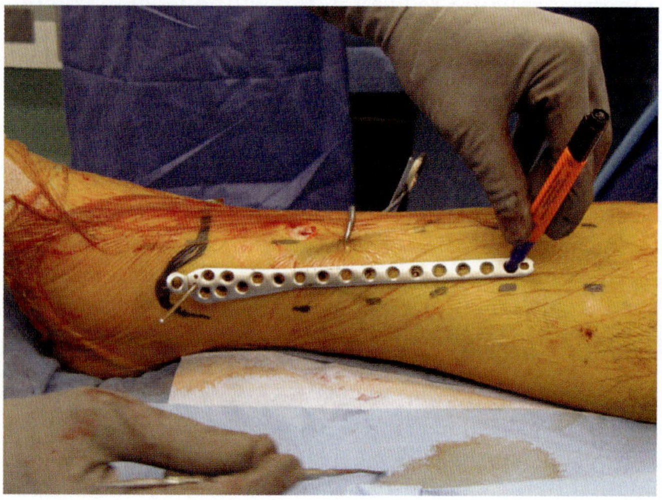

Figure 13.5 The plate itself can be used before its insertion to plan incisions. Alternatively, laying a similar plate over the inserted one, allows for marking the incisions.

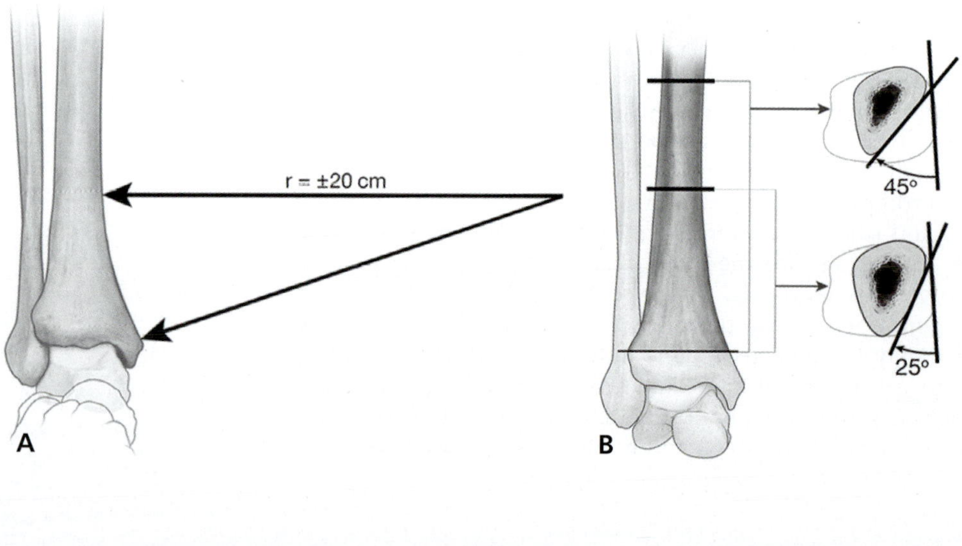

Figure 13.6 The distal tibia's bony anatomy includes **(A)** the flare of the medial supramalleolar at 20 cm, and **(B)** in internal torsion of 20 to 25 degrees.

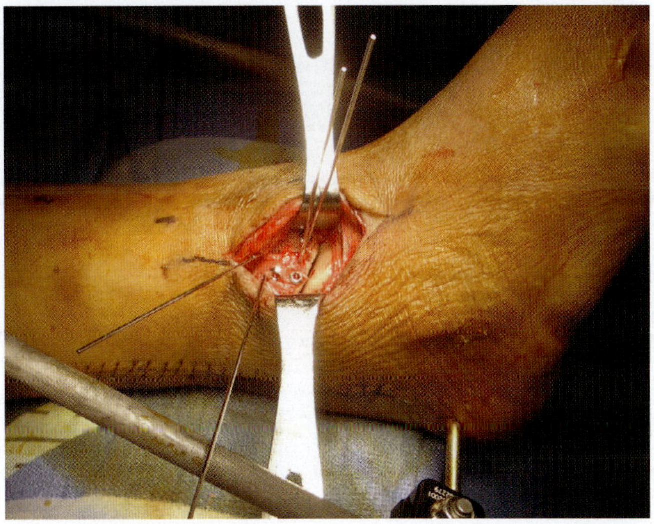

Figure 13.7 The anterolateral or Bohler approach to the ankle and distal tibia is demonstrated.

When the fracture pattern is simple and amenable to compression, we recommend obtaining distal fixation first then compressing the fracture with either a lag screw tangential to the fracture, with axial compression using an eccentrically drilled hole through the plate, or with the use of an articulated tensioning device. For comminuted fractures in which the plate will be used as a reduction aid, screw placement strategy is variable and depends on the fracture pattern and displacement vectors being reduced (see next section).

The anterolateral approach is particularly useful for pilon fractures with a simple anterolateral articular fracture lines. The incision is 3 to 4 cm in length and centered between the fibula and tibial crests generally in line with the fourth ray and directly over the tibiotalar joint (Bohler incision, Figure 13.7). Care must be exercised with the superficial dissection to avoid injury to the superficial peroneal nerve, which often crosses in the field. The extensor retinaculum is incised and isolated as a separate layer for closure to avoid tendon bowstringing. The underlying extensor digitorum brevis may be gently mobilized laterally in the distal aspect of the incision, if necessary. Capsulotomy exposes the anterolateral plafond, and exposure medially along the anterior surface is necessary to place screws through the anterior plate holes. Anterolateral plates from most manufacturers involve locking anterior to posterior options. After anatomic reduction of the articular surface, the plate can be slid proximally again in an extraperiosteal, submuscular tunnel along the lateral aspect of the tibia deep to the anterior compartment. Unlike the medial approach, the anterolateral MIPPO approach requires a separate proximal incision to identify and protect the deep neurovascular structures, which are intimately related to the anterolateral tibia at this level. These structures may be compressed under the plate, or injured by percutaneously applied screws if not carefully protected.[6] Because of the anterolateral leg muscles proximally, anterolateral plates are difficult to use as reduction aids, and are most often placed after other reduction techniques have been used.

Reduction Techniques

Fracture reduction and implant insertion, while leaving a small surgical "fingerprint," is the art that complements the science of fracture fixation. Indirect fracture reduction is used to avoid disruption of the fracture environment and to avoid soft tissue problems. Below we present our reduction methods for treating distal tibia fractures using MIPPO technique.

For fractures with intra-articular extension, direct or indirect reduction of major articular fragments is performed preceding metaphyseal fracture fixation. Open versus closed reduction of the joint is dictated by the injury pattern, soft tissue concerns, and patient factors. Indirect reduction of the articular surface may be attempted using percutaneously placed clamps, joysticks, lag screws, or manipulation with a freer elevator. MIPPO can then be performed. We feel strongly that anatomical reduction of the articular surface with rigid internal fixation using lag screws is the mainstay of treatment for articular injuries.

The authors use an algorithm for the reduction of metaphyseal distal tibia fractures to regain appropriate length, axial alignment, and rotation across the metaphyseal fracture.

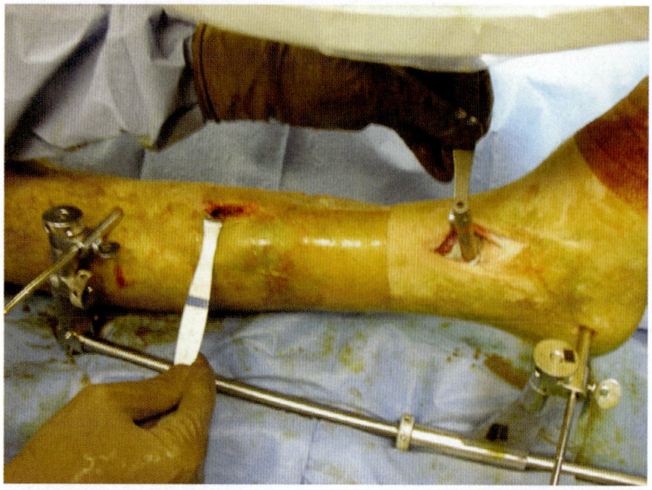

Figure 13.8 An external fixator in traction or femoral distractor is nearly universally helpful at gaining and holding length and gross reduction.

1. Traction using a pre-existing external fixator or a universal distractor is extremely helpful in gaining gross reduction in length, axial alignment, and rotation (Figs. 13.7 and 13.8). The femoral distractor is typically applied medially with 5-mm Schanz pins placed in the tibial shaft and posterior third of the calcaneus, and the threaded distraction rod positioned posterior to the axis of the leg. With the distractor applied in this manner and the limb elevated on a roll, plates can be inserted into a subcutaneous medial tunnel without obstruction. Often only minor corrections to this reduction will be necessary after "distraction," especially if surgery is done early when muscles are not contracted and hematoma is still unorganized.
2. Associated displaced fibula fractures are often reduced and repaired to aid in indirect reduction a for distal tibia fracture unless it is felt that fibular repair would place the soft tissues at unacceptable risk (Fig. 13.9).

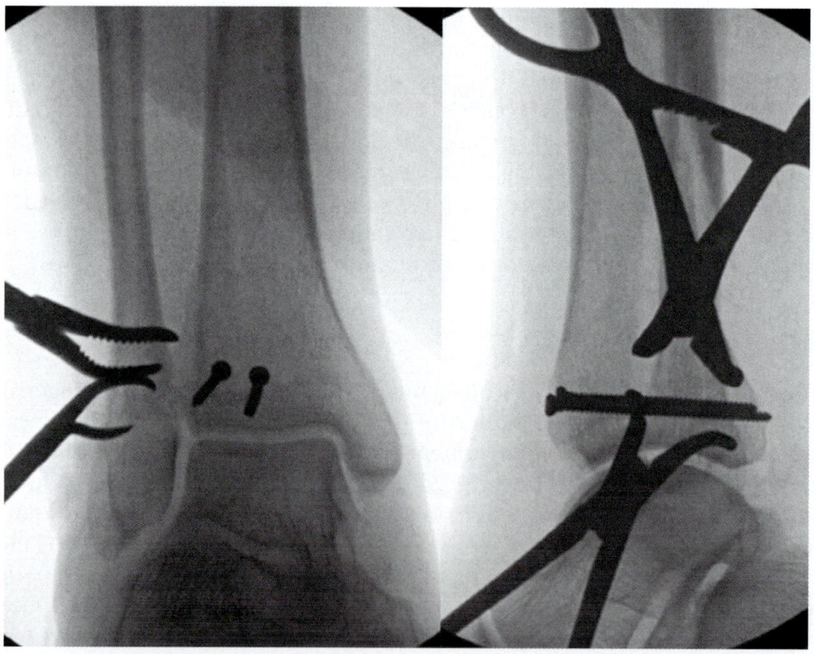

Figure 13.9 *Anatomic* reduction of an associated lateral malleolus fracture will aid reduction of the tibia and provide lateral column stability. In this case, the fibula was reduced and clamped aiding in the tibia's reduction. This was followed by fixation of the articular surface with percutaneous lag screws.

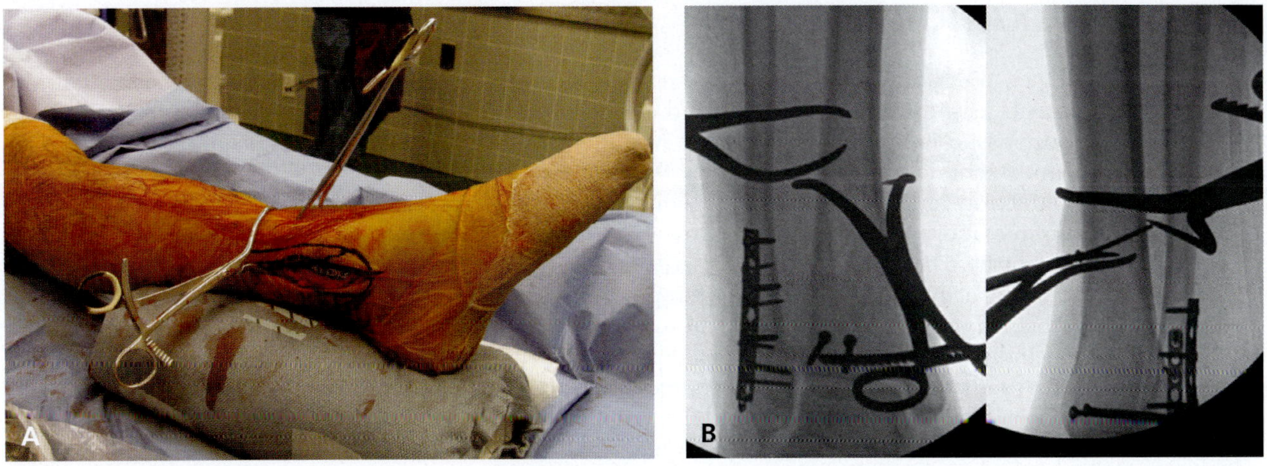

Figure 13.10 **(A)** Clinical photograph and **(B)** fluoroscopy show cautiously applied pointed clamps (e.g., Weber or modified Weber, as seen here); these are very helpful for gaining reduction. Positioning of the pointed tines must be carefully planned and we have found that gently "oscillating" the tips will help them effectively pass the soft tissues.

3. A towel roll or bump is simple and cost effective, and can easily be tailored intraoperatively to optimize sagittal plane correction by moving the roll proximally or distally (Figs. 13.3, 13.7, and 13.10).
4. Percutaneous clamps are frequently used for reduction of simple fracture patterns such as spiral or oblique fractures (Fig. 13.10A, B). The clamp can be used for fracture reduction, compressing the bone fragments together (minimizing fracture gap), and for reducing the bone to the plate. A percutaneous lag screw (i.e., 2.7-mm cortical) may be placed at the surgeon's discretion, and countersunk if the plate is to be placed in the area of lag screw insertion.
5. Well-contoured plates can be used as a reduction aid in the distal tibia. The plate is inserted and grossly realigned such that a cortical screw or percutaneously applied clamp (or other device) can be used to reduce the bone to the anatomically contoured plate (Fig. 13.11), thereby reducing the fracture.

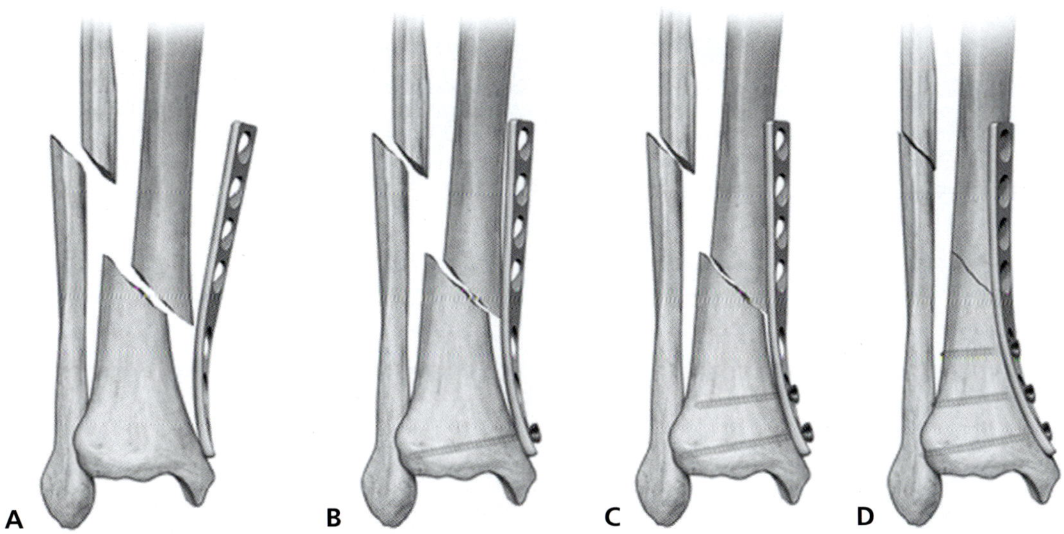

Figure 13.11 A well-contoured plate may be used as a reduction tool. After plate insertion **(A)**, the plate is affixed distally **(B)**. As screws are sequentially added more proximally **(C, D)**, the plate will act as a clamp pushing the proximal fragment laterally into improved position.

FIXATION

Open fractures should undergo early debridement and irrigation with subsequent debridements as indicated. Both open and closed fractures with significant deformity or associated soft tissue injury, where primary MIPPO would be "unsafe," should undergo temporary ankle-spanning external fixation.[7] We prefer to stabilize displaced fibula fractures with open reduction and internal fixation concurrent with external fixation *if* the fibula fracture is simple and appears likely to allow for anatomic reduction. Otherwise, ORIF of the fibula might best be performed in concert with the percutaneous plating of the tibia at the time of staged reconstruction. When a temporizing fixator is applied, internal fixation of the distal tibia is typically delayed until the soft tissues envelope is quiescent.[7,8]

Indirect fracture reduction, as described in the previous section, is performed in an effort not to disrupt the fracture environment and to minimize soft tissue problems. If the fibula has not been internally fixed, the fibula is typically addressed first to help indirectly with length and alignment of the distal tibia. A femoral distractor is then applied medially to the tibia and posterior third of the calcaneus using 5-mm Schanz pins. Care is taken to ensure that the pin sites will not interfere with planned percutaneous plate placement. The threaded distraction rod is placed so that it is positioned posteriorly and does not interfere with fixation.

Fractures with Intra-articular Extension

Indirect reduction of the articular fragments is performed as previously described using percutaneously applied clamps, joysticks, interfragmentary lag screws, or gentle manipulation with a freer elevator. The articular injury is rigidly stabilized with lag screws. Following this step, MIPPO is performed.

MIPPO of the Distal Tibia

Plate selection: Typically 3.5-mm anatomically contoured stainless steel locking medial tibial plafond plates are used (Fig. 13.12). We prefer to use hybrid fixation, using both nonlocking and locking screws to gain the advantages of both screw types. Other options include the use of 3.5-mm LCP or 3.5-mm reconstruction plates which must be prebent to fit the distal tibia anatomy. Plates of 4.5-mm have also been described, but are not typically used due to their prominence at the distal tibia where there is little soft tissue to cover the implant. Ideally, plates that are not anatomically specific are prebent and sterilized prior to the procedure with finer adjustments made intraoperatively.

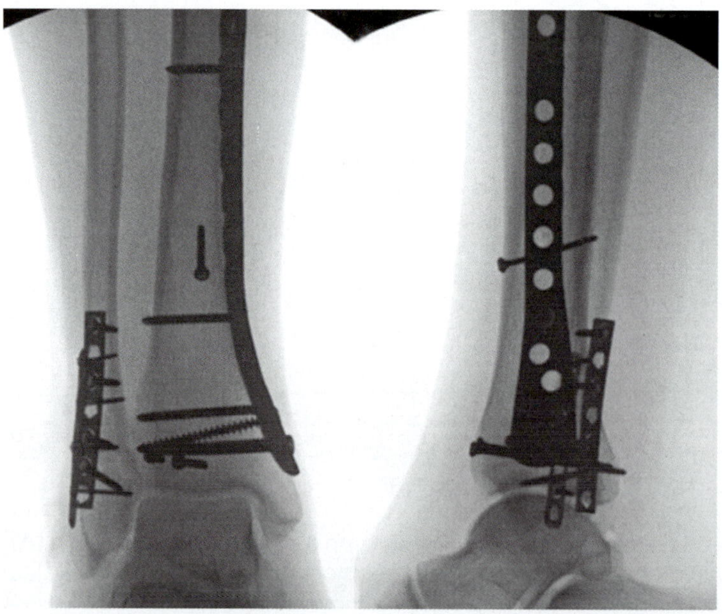

Figure 13.12 Fixation of the distal tibia and fibula is complete. The fractures are well aligned, a long plate is used with well-spaced screws.

The traditional approach involves making a 2.5- to 3-cm incision at the distal aspect of the medial malleolus. A subcutaneous tunnel is created and oriented proximally on the tibia. This tunnel is initially created with blunt instruments such as a Cobb elevator or Kelly clamp, or the plate itself may be used because most are spade tipped. It is important to note that the tunnel is subcutaneous, but not subperiosteal and the periosteum should be preserved. The fracture is reduced and in some cases the plate can be used to assist with fracture reduction, as described above. The optimal distance between the plate and the bone is less than 2 mm.[9] Screws are then placed through small stab incisions or through a more extended incision at the proximal end of the plate. Soft tissue handling is important and stretching or tearing of the skin must be avoided (Fig. 13.13). When possible, compression between major fragments is achieved through the use of interfragmentary screws through or outside the plate, or by compression plating technique using eccentric drill holes through the plate. If compression is

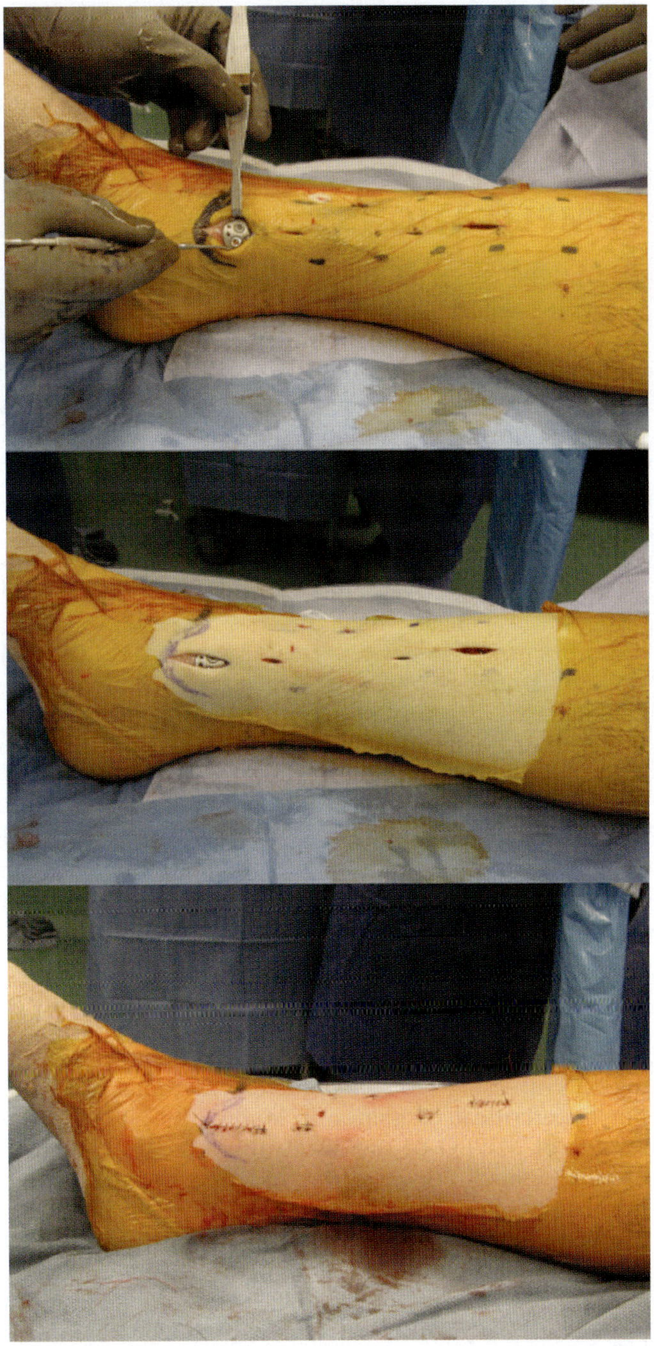

Figure 13.13 Careful incision placement, as well as retraction and use of instrumentation, is critical to minimize wound problems with MIPPO techniques.

not possible due to comminution, true bridge-plating technique can be done. We prefer long plates with screws that are well spaced. A minimum of two bicortical screws is necessary on both sides of the fracture, but the authors prefer a third screw due to its associated increase in axial stability.[10]

REHABILITATION/POSTOPERATIVE CARE

A bulky splint is placed on the lower extremity immediately following surgery. Postoperative drains are not typically used. The patient is made non–weight bearing with crutches and frequent elevation encouraged to minimize wound complications. The splint and sutures are removed at 2 weeks. For compliant patients, they are placed in a removable boot to prevent an equines contracture and instructed to begin ankle range-of-motion exercises. For patients where compliance may be a concern, they are placed into a short leg or patellar tendon-bearing cast until the 6-week follow-up, at which point they are converted to a removable boot. Clinical and radiographic examinations are performed at 2, 6, and 10 weeks after surgery and every 6 weeks thereafter until fracture healing. Weight bearing is typically initiated at 3 months with the presence of early clinical and radiographic signs of healing, although several studies have reported full unprotected weight bearing as early as 9 to 10 weeks.[11,12]

COMPLICATIONS

Both MIPPO and formal open extensile approaches to the distal tibia share the same set of complications—infection, wound breakdown, nonunion, and malalignment.[13] The relative occurrence of these complications; however, is variable between the two approaches. Because of the technical difficulty associated with MIPPO for the distal tibia, it is associated with a higher incidence of fracture malalignment. However, the biologic benefits of the technique—low rates of wound breakdown and infection—have been proven in recent series[4,14] when compared to open approaches, where disastrous soft tissue complications were previously reported.[15]

Nonunion and Delayed Union

Nonunions and delayed unions of the distal tibia are relatively common despite the method of treatment. An early meta-analysis by Zelle et al.[13] showed a 2% rate of nonunion in 105 distal tibia fracture patients treated with MIPPO. Nearly all of these were low-energy injuries, however, with only seven open fractures. In a subsequent series of high-energy injuries, Collinge et al.[14] reported a delayed union rate of 35%. Nine patients with high-grade open fractures or bone loss required eleven procedures to achieve union. Since then, larger series treating a more typical spectrum of injury show the nonunion rate for MIPPO of the distal tibia to be around 8%.[4] It is reasonable to educate the patient if host factors are present that indicate they may be at an increased risk for healing problems and may require an additional procedure to achieve union. We prefer to intervene early at 5 to 7 months if there is little evidence of progression of healing to perform bone grafting or conversion to intramedullary nail fixation if a portion of the fracture has healed making it amenable to nailing.[4,14]

Malalignment

Malalignment is commonly defined as >5 degrees angulation in any plane or shortening >1 cm. Using indirect reduction methods can result in malalignment if the surgeon is not hypercritical of anatomic landmarks and intraoperative radiographic images. Initial reports of MIPPO of the distal tibia noted malalignment to occur in up to 20% or more of all patients.[11] However, with advances in the technique and recognition of the problem, malalignment occurs less frequently. In recent series, a malunion rate of 5% to 8% of cases has been reported.[4,14,16] The authors cannot emphasize strongly enough the importance of critically assessing quality intra-operative fluoroscopy, and acting on malalignment at the time of index surgery to minimize this complication. Imaging of the contralateral extremity preoperatively provides a useful reference for comparison intraoperatively. Some surgeons

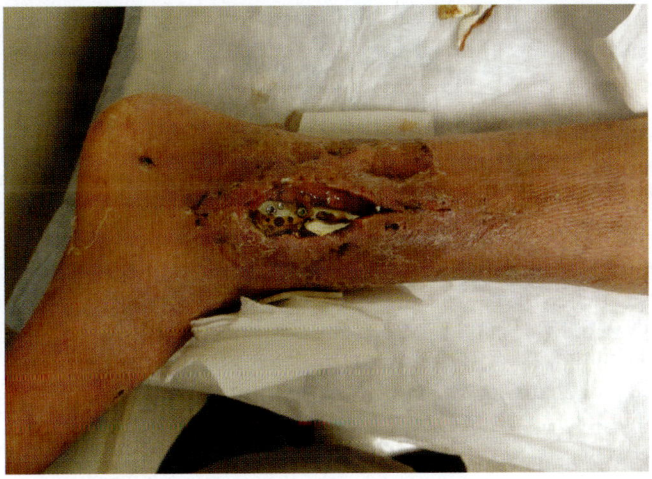

Figure 13.14 Wound problems and infection are less common with MIPPO techniques, but are no less severe. This patient required extensive debridement, subsequent free soft tissue transfer, and long-term intravenous antibiotic therapy.

have advocated prepping the uninjured extremity in the operative field to allow for direct intraoperative comparison, which helps ensure proper rotation is restored in comminuted fracture patterns.[17]

Infection/Wound Breakdown

Wound infections are relatively uncommon after MIPPO of distal tibia fractures—a key distinction compared to previous reports of extensile exposures to the distal tibia. This complication; however, should not be underestimated, as when it does occur, the bone and the plate are vulnerable. Thus, hardware and bone infections are associated with wound problems in this area and major soft tissue reconstructions are sometimes necessary (Fig. 13.14). Wound problems may be minimized by careful soft tissue handling and ensuring that the "percutaneous" incisions used allow easy, atraumatic plate, and screw passage. A small incision is not necessarily biologically friendly when improperly performed. Furthermore, one must be critical of half pin placement during external fixator placement if staging is done. Infections, including osteomyelitis, have been seen related to plate overlap with colonized pin sites from initial external fixation.

Implant Failure

The tibial plates and screws commonly used with the MIPPO technique can fatigue or loosen, especially in the setting of full weight bearing and delayed union. Implant failures or loss of fixation occurs in 0% to 8% of case series and typically occurs late (after 5 months).[4,14,18] It is important to recognize this complication early and treat with revision fixation and consideration for the use of bone grafting in cases of delayed or nonunion.

Implant Removal

Due to the subcutaneous nature of the medial border of the distal tibia, implant prominence can be bothersome. Also, patients may complain of pain at the proximal end of the plate, presumably where stress is concentrated. While few surgeons elect to routinely remove plates after fracture healing, they may need to be removed in up to 48% of cases.[19] We do not routinely remove the distal tibia plates unless patients have returned to full weight bearing and have both clinically and radiographically healed, and symptoms warrant removal.

OUTCOMES

Since MIPPO of the distal tibia is a relatively new technique, outcomes studies are limited with most describing only the occurrence of complications, secondary procedures, and ankle range of motion. The occurrence of complications and secondary procedures are described in the previous section. Ankle range of motion is usually minimally decreased with comparison to the uninjured sided (e.g., less than 5 degrees).[11,12]

Functional Outcome Measures

Collinge and Protzman[4] reported an average AOFAS of 85 in a consecutive case series of 38 patients with a spectrum of distal tibia fractures treated with MIPPO. When evaluating the outcomes of a cohort of high-energy metaphyseal distal tibia fractures, Collinge et al.[14] found an average AOFAS of 83 at 2 years. The only variable associated with poorer function on the AOFAS grading system in these studies was the occurrence of secondary procedures ($p < 0.05$). Similar averages using the Olerud and Molander ankle scores have been reported in the literature, ranging from 84 to 89 in three studies.[4,12,14]

When using the SF-36 at a minimum of 2 years, Collinge and Protzman[4] reported no significant differences in any category when compared to population norms except in the physical function category. Only one study has used the Musculoskeletal Functional Assessment (MFA) functional outcome measure.[14] In this study, patients with high-energy injuries had significantly diminished function in four of the ten MFA subsections—mobility, leisure/recreation, cognition/thinking, and employment.

REFERENCES

1. Vallier HA, Le TT, Bedi A. Radiographic and clinical comparisons of distal tibia shaft fractures (4 to 11 cm proximal to the plafond): Plating versus intramedullary nailing. *J Orthop Trauma.* 2008;22(5):307–311.
2. Vallier HA, Cureton BA, Patterson BM. Randomized, prospective comparison of plate versus intramedullary nail fixation for distal tibia shaft fractures. *J Orthop Trauma.* 2011;25:736–741.
3. Court-Brown CM, Gustilo T, Shaw AD. Knee pain after intramedullary tibial nailing: Its incidence, etiology and outcome. *J Orthop Trauma.* 1996;11:103–105.
4. Collinge C, Protzman R. Outcomes of minimally invasive plate osteosynthesis for metaphyseal distal tibia fractures. *J Orthop Trauma.* 2010;24:24–29.
5. Collinge C, Sanders R, DiPasquale T. Treatment of complex tibial periarticular fractures using percutaneous techniques. *Clin Orthop Relat Res.* 2000;375:69–77.
6. Wolinsky P, Lee M. The distal approach for anterolateral plate fixation of the tibia: An anatomic study. *J Orthop Trauma.* 2008;22(6):404–407.
7. Sirkin M, Sanders R, DiPasquale T, et al. A staged protocol for soft tissue management in the treatment of complex pilon fractures. *J Orthop Trauma.* 1999;13(2):78–84.
8. Patterson MJ, Cole JD. Two-staged delayed open reduction and internal fixation of severe pilon fractures. *J Orthop Trauma.* 1999;13(2):85–91.
9. Ahmad M, Nanda R, Bajwa AS, et al. Biomechanical testing of the locking compression plate: When does the distance between bone and implant significantly reduce construct stability? *Injury.* 2007;38(3):345–351.
10. Stoffel K, Dieter U, Stachowiak G, et al. Biomechanical testing of the LCP-how can stability in locked internal fixators be controlled? *Injury.* 2003;34(suppl 2):B11–B19.
11. Helfet DL, Shonnard PY, Levine D, et al. Minimally invasive plate osteosynthesis of distal fractures of the tibia. *Injury.* 1997;28:A42–A48.
12. Oh C, Kyung H, Park I, et al. Distal tibia metaphyseal fractures treated by percutaneous plate osteosynthesis. *Clin Orthop Relat Res.* 2003;408:286–291.
13. Zelle BA, Bhandari M, Espiritu M, et al. Treatment of distal tibia fractures without articular involvement: A systematic review of 1125 fractures. *J Orthop Trauma.* 2006;20:76–79.
14. Collinge C, Kuper M, Larsen K, et al. Minimally invasive plating of high-energy metaphyseal distal tibia fractures. *J Orthop Trauma.* 2007;21:355–361.
15. Teeny SM, Wiss DA. Open reduction and internal fixation of tibial plafond fractures. Variables contributing to poor results and complications. *Clin Orthop Relat Res.* 1993;292:108–117.
16. Khoury A, Liebergall M, London E, et al. Percutaneous plating of distal tibial fractures. *Foot Ankle Int.* 2002;23:818–824.
17. Ronga M, Shanmugam C, Longo UG, et al. Minimally invasive osteosynthesis of distal tibial fractures using locking plates. *Orthop Clin North Am.* 2009;40:499–504.
18. Hazarika S, Chakravarthy J, Cooper J. Minimally invasive locking plate osteosynthesis for fractures of the distal tibia-results in 20 patients. *Injury.* 2006;37:877–887.
19. Lau TW, Leung F, Chan CF, et al. Wound complication of minimally invasive plate osteosynthesis in distal tibia fractures. *Int Orthop.* 2008;32:697–703.

CHAPTER 14

Minimally Invasive Treatment of Ankle Fractures

Jodi Siegel

The goal in treating ankle fractures is to have a well-aligned mortise at union. Open reduction and internal fixation of unstable ankle fractures is the most frequent surgical intervention used to achieve an anatomic reduction and stable fixation. In certain circumstances, minimally invasive treatment options may be more appropriate. Compromised soft tissue envelopes or patients with significant medical comorbidities may benefit from these techniques.

EXTRAPERIOSTEAL PLATING OF PRONATION–ABDUCTION ANKLE FRACTURES

Indications

Pronation–abduction ankle fractures, as described by Lauge-Hansen,[1] are caused by translation rather than rotation. The medial side fails first under tension. The fibula fails last, typically resulting in a transverse fracture associated with lateral comminution several centimeters proximal to the joint. This fracture may be more effectively treated with extraperiosteal plating.

Patient Positioning

The patient is positioned supine on a standard operating room table with a small bump placed under the ipsilateral hip so that the knee is straight up and down.

Surgical Approaches

If a supracollicular medial malleolus fracture is present, it is repaired first as it will help restore congruence of the talus beneath the plafond, thereby assisting with reduction of the lateral malleolus.

Turning attention laterally, the ankle is positioned on bolsters placed at the level of the joint and not under the heel. Placing the bolters under the heel can cause anterior subluxation of the talus and cause a malreduction. The reduction maneuver is performed (see Reduction Techniques section). After assessing the reduction, a lateral incision is made over the posterior half of the fibula. Care is taken when dividing the subcutaneous tissue onto the periosteum, as the periosteum is located immediately subcutaneous. Sharp Weitlaner retractors can aid by applying tension to the skin causing the subcutaneous tissue to peel off the periosteum. Often there are rents in the periosteum due to the injury. Take care to leave the remaining periosteum intact; do not strip or further handle the fracture fragments. At this point, retractors should be removed as tension on the surrounding tissues can cause shortening of the fibula.

Reduction Techniques

Prior to the lateral incision, the ankle is placed on a bolster. The foot is adducted and medially translated to center the talus in the mortise. This aids in obtaining fibular length as the lateral ankle ligaments typically remain intact. Fluoroscopic images are used to determine

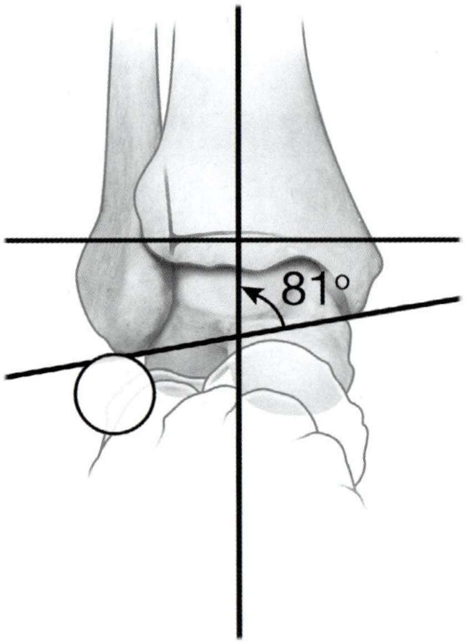

Figure 14.1 Assessing fibular length radiographically is aided by measuring the talocrural ankle, for which normal is reported at 83 ± 4 degrees.[2] The contralateral ankle can be used as a control. In addition, the "ball sign" is described as the smooth curve made by the distal tip of the fibula and the lateral process of the talus.[21]

fibular length (Fig. 14.1). Although the lateral cortex is comminuted, the medial cortex often involves a single fracture line and can be used to assess length. In addition, the talocrural angle is compared to the uninjured ankle to confirm fibular length.[2] Once the necessary reduction maneuver is confirmed, one can proceed with the approach.

After the extraperiosteal dissection is completed, a reduction is affected by manipulating the foot. A lateral fluoroscopic image is then obtained to ensure there is no angulation or translation of the fibula. Returning to the coronal plane imaging, a precontoured, underbent direct lateral fibular plate is placed directly lateral on the fibula. Take care to position the plate in the center of the bone by palpating the anterior and posterior borders of the fibular shaft as the intact soft tissues will preclude adequate visualization. A fluoroscopic lateral view will confirm appropriate position, which is essential as the plate must apply a direct medial force to accurately reduce the fracture. Any angulation at the fracture site must be corrected, often simply by adjusting the bolsters. Once appropriate position is confirmed, the plate is temporarily secured by Kirschner wires, provisional fixation pins, or a reduction clamp. Residual lateral translation will be corrected by the plate (Fig. 14.2). Bicortical nonlocking screws are then placed from proximal to distal, pushing the fibula (and the talus) medially to its position under the plafond. Fluoroscopic imaging confirms reduction.

The syndesmosis is then evaluated either by applying an abduction stress on the foot (if the medial malleolus is intact) or by using a clamp on a fibula to apply the stress (if the medial malleolus is a fracture that was repaired) and is reduced and stabilized if unstable.

Fixation

Precontoured direct lateral fibular plates or straight one-third tubular small fragment plates that are contoured to the shape of the distal fibula are ideal. Underbent, flexible plates allow the plate to correct and buttress the lateral translation of the fibula. Nonlocking, bicortical screws are placed from proximal to distal within the plate to allow the implant to effect a reduction.

Complications

Hardware irritation due to lateral plating is a common complaint from patients. Functional outcome scores are worse for patients with hardware-related pain, and implant removal does not guarantee resolution of pain.[3]

Accurately assessing and obtaining appropriate fibular length is mandatory to restore proper ankle mechanics.[4,5] Fibular shortening leads to lateral talar tilt and medial clear space widening. With only 1 mm of lateral talar shift, there is 42% decrease in contact area, thereby increasing the risk of post-traumatic arthritis.[5] Symptoms may present as late as 5 years after malunion with varying degrees of radiographic arthritis present.[6] Proper reduction of fibular length and rotation, leading to a reduced mortise, will prevent talar tilt and medial widening and decrease the risk of late arthritic pain.

Rehabilitation Protocol

Postoperatively, patients are placed into a short leg cast and kept non–weight-bearing for 6 weeks. If syndesmotic fixation is needed, weight-bearing may be deferred for 12 weeks. Active and passive range of motion is started at 4 to 6 weeks.

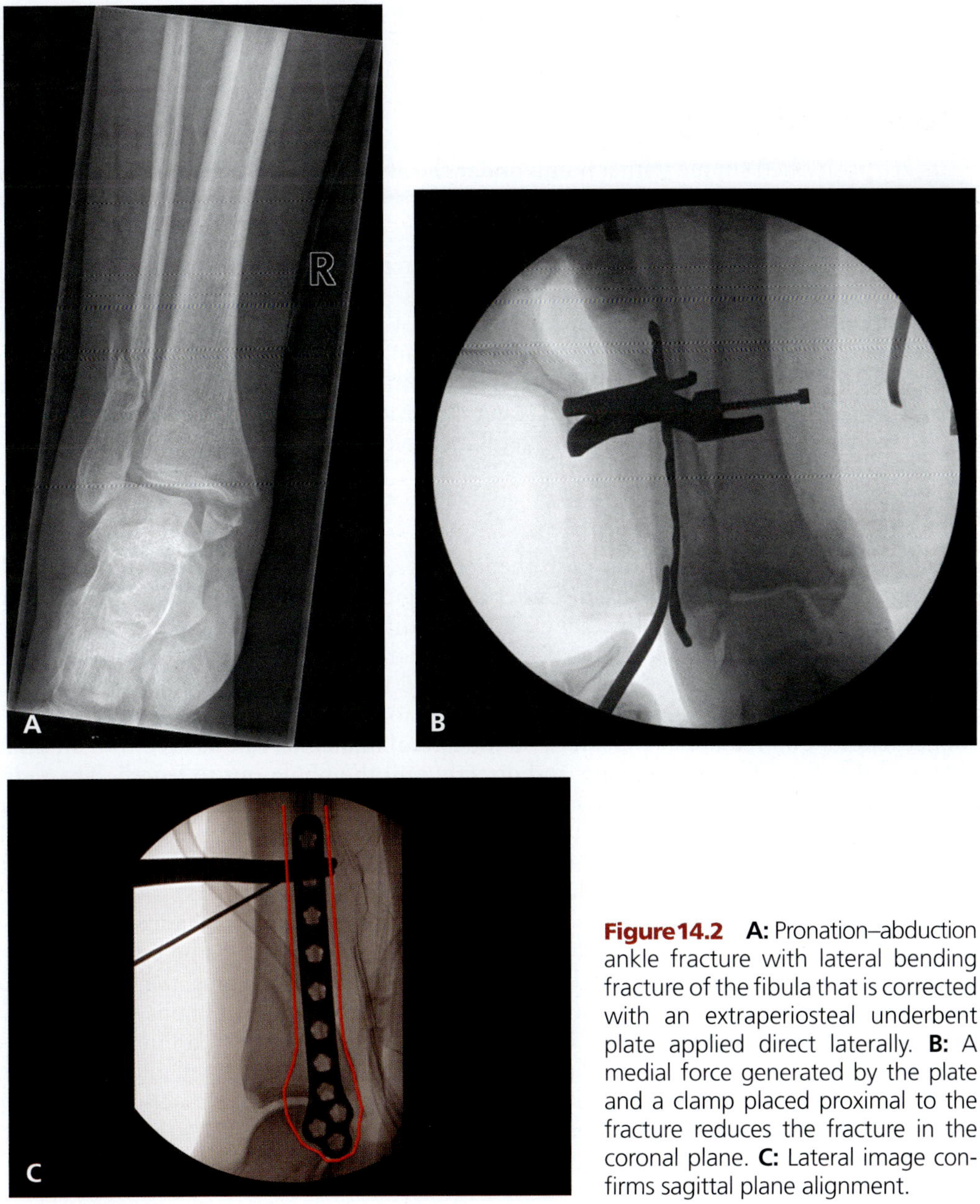

Figure 14.2 **A:** Pronation–abduction ankle fracture with lateral bending fracture of the fibula that is corrected with an extraperiosteal underbent plate applied direct laterally. **B:** A medial force generated by the plate and a clamp placed proximal to the fracture reduces the fracture in the coronal plane. **C:** Lateral image confirms sagittal plane alignment.

Outcomes

Historically, pronation–abduction ankle fractures have the highest nonunion rate and authors have recommended bone grafting after traditional fixation techniques.[7,8] A small series stabilized using this extraperiosteal technique reported union of all fractures within 10 weeks and no deep infections.[9]

SYNDESMOTIC-ONLY FIXATION FOR WEBER-C ANKLE FRACTURES

Indications

The Danis-Weber ankle fracture classification describes the level of the fibula fracture in relationship to the syndesmosis. Fibula fractures that occur above the syndesmosis, with an adequate segment of intact fibula for placement of at least two syndesmotic screws, can be repaired with syndesmotic-only fixation, provided adequate fibular length and mortise reduction is achieved.

Patient Positioning

Patients are positioned supine with a bump under the affected hip, which allows the leg to be easily internally rotated, granting access to the fibula.

Surgical Approaches

There is limited surgical exposure with this method of fixation. One small incision is made over the fibula at the level of the distal tibia physeal scar. An accompanying incision is made at the same level medially over the distal tibia for placement of a reduction clamp. A second small fibular incision is made proximal to the first lateral incision for insertion of the first screw. The second screw will be inserted through the lateral incision used for the reduction clamp.

Reduction Techniques

Place the affected ankle on a bolster with the heel free, which will prevent anterior translation of the talus relative to the plafond. Under c-arm guidance in the mortise plane, manipulate the foot while evaluating the medial clear space, distal tibia–fibula overlap, the incisura, the mortise, and the fibular length (Fig. 14.1). No method of foot manipulation works successfully in every case; however, internal rotation and inversion followed by application of the periarticular clamp across the distal tibiofibular joint is often successful. Percutaneous introduction of a pointed bone tenaculum on the lateral malleolus can be used to manipulate and control the distal fibular fragment and directly pull the fibula out to length. The reduction can be secured temporarily with a periarticular clamp or K-wires from the distal fibula into the tibia. If adequate fibular length cannot be achieved, then this technique should be abandoned and converted to a standard direct open reduction technique, as proper ankle mechanics cannot be restored with a shortened fibula.[4,5]

With the affected limb on a bump and a large bolster, there should be adequate access to the unaffected ankle so a perfect lateral image can be obtained and saved on one of the c-arm monitors. Alternatively, this may be done before prepping and draping the patient. After reduction of the syndesmosis, a perfect lateral of the injured ankle is obtained, defined as a "true talar dome" projection in which there is no double density seen. Careful evaluation of the fibula in relationship to the posterior malleolus on these two images will allow assessment of the reduction of the fibula on the tibia. It is a common pitfall to cause anterior or posterior translation of the fibula that is not recognized on the AP or mortise images (Fig. 14.3).

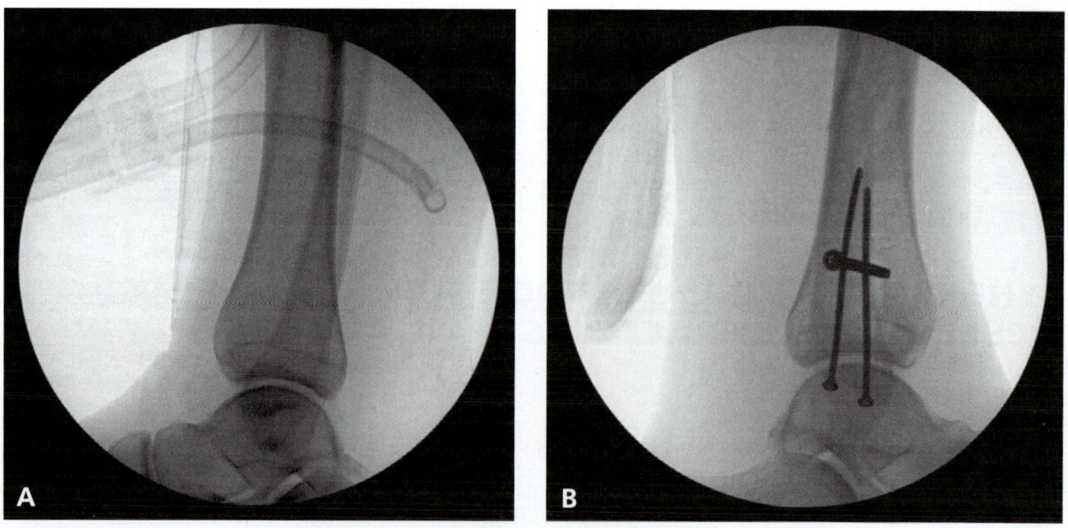

Figure 14.3 **A:** A perfect lateral fluoroscopic image of the uninjured ankle will indicate where the fibula should sit in relationship to the tibia. **B:** Obtaining this same perfect lateral image of the injured ankle will confirm if the fibula has been reduced to its proper position.

Fixation

With the fibula out to length and reduced to the distal tibia, screws are used to secure its position. The author prefers to use two tricortical 3.5-mm cortical screws placed as position screws. The second screw is placed in the wound originally made for the reduction clamp, which is removed after the first syndesmotic screw is placed.

Complications

Inaccurate reduction of the ankle with malreduction of the fibula relative to the tibia, inadequate restoration of fibular length, or rotational malreduction are the most often reported complications.[4,10–12]

Rehabilitation Protocol

The ankle is immobilized for 4 to 6 weeks. At that time, ankle range of motion is started. Patients are kept non–weight-bearing for 12 weeks. Syndesmotic screws are maintained in place for at least 12 weeks. The author offers screw removal at 12 weeks before initiating weight-bearing.

Outcomes

Tornetta et al.[13] reported 96% good or excellent outcomes at 3 years in 55 patients treated with percutaneous reduction and syndesmotic-only fixation of Weber-C ankle fractures. Alternatively, Pelton et al.[10] have abandoned closed reduction and percutaneous fixation due to high rates of malreduction. If there is any question regarding the accuracy of the reduction, the syndesmosis should be opened and the fibula should be directly reduced into the incisura, as accurate reduction is the most important predictor of functional outcome.[14]

INTRAMEDULLARY FIXATION OF LATERAL MALLEOLUS FRACTURES

Indications

Intramedullary fixation for most fibular fractures will not be adequate, so careful indications are vital when choosing this method. Axially unstable, comminuted fractures are generally not amenable to this technique since the implant will not be rigidly secured on bone sides of the fracture. Instead, transverse or length-stable fractures can successfully be treated with intramedullary fixation. Alternatively, in a salvage situation in a patient with a poor soft tissue envelope, this technique may provide the only option.

Patient Positioning

The patient is positioned supine with a bump under the ipsilateral hip. A bolster is placed under the affected leg, allowing the heel to be free and unsupported.

Surgical Approaches

Identify the longitudinal axis of the fibular canal either by palpation or with fluoroscopic guidance. Make a small incision in-line with the fibular shaft approximately 2 to 3 cm distal to the tip of the lateral malleolus. Dissect bluntly onto the tip of the malleolus. Confirm adequate position with AP and lateral fluoroscopic images. Open a starting portal with a 2.5-mm drill bit or a small sharp awl. The drill can be advanced to or across the fracture site if necessary, as guided by the preoperative template. An oscillating drill or a tap can be used to minimize risk of cortical perforation.[15]

Reduction Techniques

The fibula fracture should be reduced before obtaining the portal. Closed, indirect reduction techniques, including manipulation of the foot (typically into inversion and/or internal rotation) and indirect control of the subcutaneous bone, can be successful. Alternatively, a small incision followed by blunt dissection at the fracture site allows insertion of various elevators, K-wires, or a small bone tenaculum to assist with obtaining a reduction.

Fixation

Various implants have been used for intramedullary fibular fixation. Fully threaded 3.5-mm cortical screws and 2.5-mm humeral nail guidewires were used by one group.[15] Rush rods, flexible nails, smooth K-wires, and larger diameter, fully threaded screws have also been used.

Complications

The most commonly reported complications is loss of fibular height.[16] Due to percutaneous reduction and fixation, reported wound complications and hardware irritation are minimal.[16,17]

Rehabilitation Protocol

Patients are kept in a short-leg, non–weight-bearing cast for 4 to 6 weeks based on the soft tissue envelope and the compliance of the patient. Range of motion exercises are begun once the cast is removed. Weight-bearing is then advanced as tolerated at 6 weeks.

Outcomes

Ray et al.[16] reported good-to-excellent functional outcomes in 84% (16 of 19) of patients with union rates of 95.5% at an average of 8.2 weeks. Bankston et al.[17] reported 100% union rate, no deep infections, no hardware-related pain from the intramedullary screw, and only one malunion attributed to early ambulation with an associated syndesmotic injury.

POSTERIOR MALLEOLUS FRACTURES

Indications

Most authors agree that posterior malleolus fractures that comprise greater than 25% to 30% of the joint should be surgically repaired.[18,19] Percutaneous reduction followed by percutaneous anterior-to-posterior lag screws is a treatment option when the fracture fragment is minimally displaced. Typically, these fragments are more successfully reduced with minimally invasive techniques if treated within the first few days after injury.

Patient Positioning

Patients are positioned supine, with a bump placed under the ipsilateral hip so that the knee is pointing straight up and down. After routine skin preparation and draping, the leg is placed on sterile bolsters that allow the ankle and distal tibia to hang free. This allows access posterolaterally for the clamp, fixation of any other fractures, and easy fluoroscopic imaging.

Surgical Approaches

Fixation of the posterior malleolus can be done either alone, as with isolated posterior malleolus fractures, when associated with tibial shaft fractures, or in combination with fixation of the other malleoli. If a fibula fracture is being repaired, the clamp may be applied through the same incision. Whether through a previous incision or through a poke-hole incision big enough to accommodate a clamp, the clamp tine is passed between the peroneal tendons

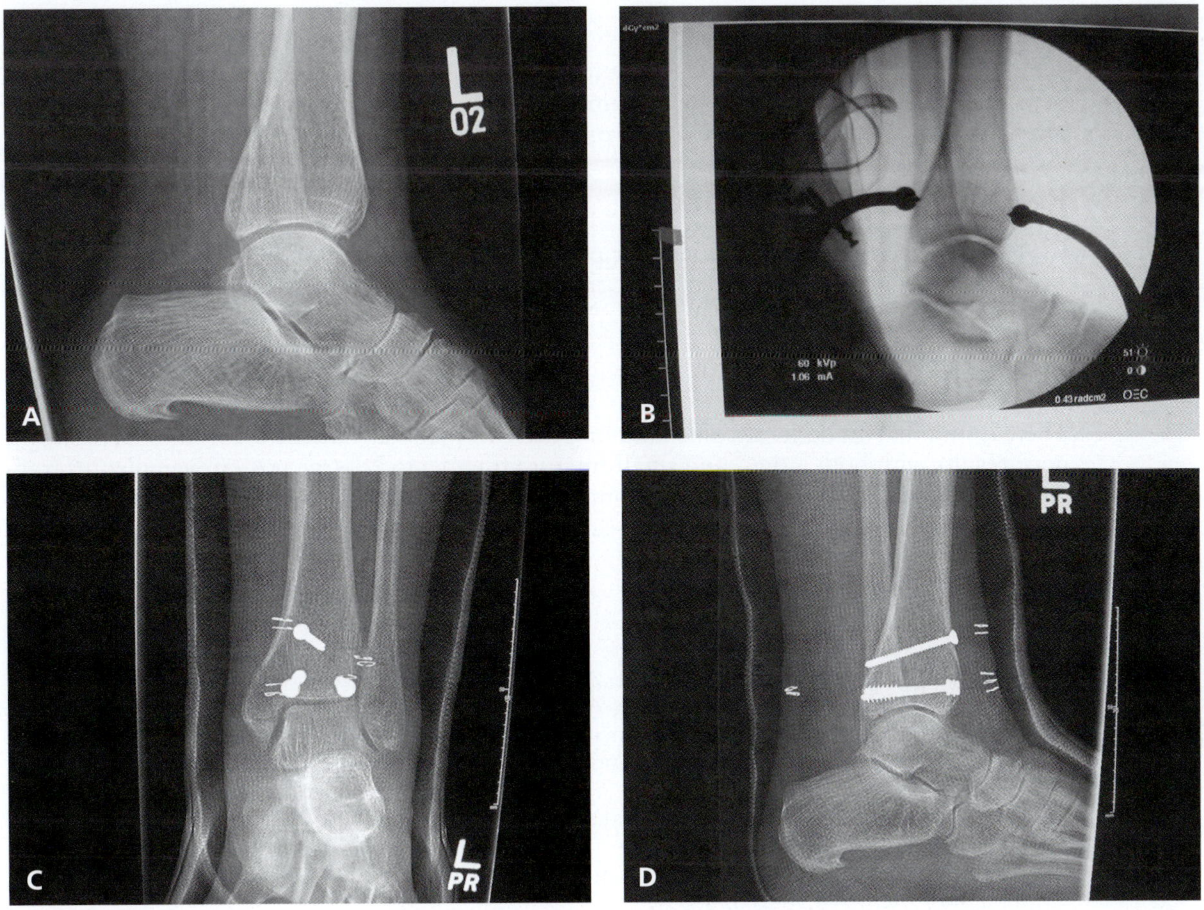

Figure 14.4 **A,B:** Injury lateral **(A)** and intraoperative fluoroscopic lateral **(B)** showing placement of reduction clamp and restoration of smooth surface of the tibial plafond. **C,D:** Postoperative AP and lateral radiographs showing restoration of the ankle mortise and reduction of the posterior malleolus fracture. (Courtesy of P. Tornetta, MD.)

and the Achilles tendon, and through the flexor hallicus longus muscle belly after blunt dissection. The anterior line of the clamp is placed onto the distal tibia through a percutaneous incision and after blunt dissection, taking care not to injure the nearby neurovascular and tendinous structures. Typically, the fracture line dictates the most appropriate location for the clamp anteriorly, which most commonly involves an anteromedial-to-posterolateral vector. After placement of some of the fixation and removal of the clamp, an additional screw can be placed through the incision used for the clamp.

Reduction Techniques

With a large reduction forceps placed on the fragment posteriorly, the fragment can be manipulated into its fracture bed and then held in place. A perfect lateral fluoroscopic image will allow evaluation of reduction of the articular surface (Fig. 14.4).

If the posterior malleolus fracture is associated with a lateral malleolus fracture, reduction of the fibula and restoring its length will aid in reduction of the posterior malleolus, but fibular reduction alone does not ensure anatomic reduction of the posterior malleolus.

Fixation

Routine anterior-to-posterior lag screws are placed percutaneously. Partially threaded 4-mm, 4.5-mm, 5-mm screws or fully threaded 3.5-mm screws placed through gliding holes can be used. Most authors would recommend at least three screws, if possible.In addition, consider using washers for the screws placed at the level of the joint to avoid penetration of the screw heads into the metaphyseal bone.

Complications

Care must be taken not to injure the nearby neurovascular and tendinous structures anteriorly. Blunt dissection followed by placement of a drill guide directly on the bone will minimize risk of damage to the structures crossing the distal tibia and ankle anteriorly.

Rehabilitation Protocol

Patients are placed into a short leg cast post-operatively and immobilized for 4 to 6 weeks. At that time, ankle and subtalar joint range of motion is started. Patients are kept non–weight-bearing for 8 to 12 weeks.

Outcomes

There is minimal modern outcome data on posterior malleolus fractures. Studies have shown poor results with both large[19] and small fracture fragments.[20] Large posterior malleolus fragments treated open yielded better outcomes than those undergoing closed treatment.[19]

REFERENCES

1. Lauge-Hansen N. Fractures of the ankle. II. Combined experimental-surgical and experimental-roentgenologic investigations. *Arch Surg.* 1950;60(5):957–985.
2. Phillips W, Schwartz H, Keller C, et al. A prospective, randomized study of the management of severe ankle fractures. *J Bone Joint Surg Am.* 1985;76(1):67–78.
3. Brown O, Dirschl D, Obremskey W. Incidence of hardware-related pain and its effects on functional outcomes after open reduction and internal fixation of ankle fractures. *J Orthop Trauma.* 2001;15(4):271–274.
4. Sproule J, Khalid M, O'Sullivan M, et al. Outcome after surgery for Maisonneuve fracture of the fibula. *Injury.* 2004;35(8):791–798.
5. Ramsey P, Hamilton W. Changes in tibiotalar area of contact caused by lateral talar shift. *J Bone Joint Surg Am.* 1976;58(3):356–357.
6. Yablon I, Leach R. Reconstruction of malunited fractures of the lateral malleolus. *J Bone Joint Surg Am.* 1989;71(4):521–527.
7. Limbird R, Aaron R. Laterally comminuted fracture-dislocation of the ankle. *J Bone Joint Surg Am.* 1987;69(6):881–885.
8. Ebraheim N, Mekhail A, Gargasz S. Ankle fractures involving the fibula proximal to the distal tibiofibular syndesmosis. *Foot Ankle Int.* 1997;18(8):513–521.
9. Siegel J, Tornetta P. Extraperiosteal plating of pronation–abduction ankle fractures. *J Bone Joint Surg Am.* 2007;89(2):276–281.
10. Pelton K, Thordarson D, Barnwell J. Open versus closed treatment of the fibula in Maissoneuve injuries. *Foot Ankle Int.* 2010;31(7):604–608.
11. Gardner M, Demetrakopoulos D, Briggs S, et al. Malreduction of the tibiofibular syndesmosis in ankle fractures. *Foot Ankle Int.* 2006;27(10):788–792.
12. Miller A, Carroll E, Parker R, et al. Direct visualization for syndesmotic stabilization of ankle fractures. *Foot Ankle Int.* 2009;30(5):419–426.
13. Tornetta P, Creevy W, Surdam J. Syndesmotic-only fixation for Weber C ankle fractures. Paper presented at: *Orthopaedic Trauma Association* San Diego, CA; 2001.
14. Weening B, Bhandari M. Predictors of functional outcome following transsyndesmotic screw fixation of ankle fractures. *J Orthop Trauma.* 2005;19(2):102–108.
15. Evans J, Gardner M, Brennan M, et al. Intramedullary fixation of fibular fractures associated with pilon fractures. *J Orthop Trauma.* 2010;24(8):491–494.
16. Ray T, Nimityongskul P, Anderson L. Percutaneous intramedullary fixation of lateral malleolus fractures: Technique and report of early results. *J Trauma.* 1994;36(5):669–675.
17. Bankston B, Anderson L, Nimityongskul P. Intramedullary screw fixation of lateral malleolus fractures. *Foot Ankle Int.* 1994;15(11):599–607.
18. Hartford J, Gorczyca J, McNamara J, et al. Tibiotalar contact area. Contribution of posterior malleolus and deltoid ligament. *Clin Orthop Rel Res.* 1995;(320):182–187.
19. McDaniel W, Wilson F. Trimalleolar fractures of the ankle. An end result study. *Clin Orthop Rel Res.* 1977;(122):37–45.
20. Jaskulka R, Ittner G, Schedl R. Fractures of the posterior tibial margin: Their role in the prognosis of malleolar fractures. *J Trauma.* 1989;29(11):1565–1570.
21. Weber B, Simpson L. Corrective lengthening osteotomy of the fibula. *Clin Orthop Rel Res.* 1985;(199):61–67.

CHAPTER 15

Calcaneus

Patrick Yoon

INDICATIONS

Fracture Characteristics

Traditionally, percutaneous treatment of calcaneus fractures has been reserved for tongue-type fractures. In this type of fracture, there is direct bony continuity between the posterior aspect of the calcaneal tuberosity and the posterior facet of the subtalar joint, and the entire posterior facet is depressed as one contiguous fragment. This makes it possible to reduce the posterior facet by manipulating the tuberosity with a pin and using the Essex-Lopresti technique.[1–3] A successful maneuver results in correction of both Bohler's and Gissane's angles, reduction of heel axial alignment into neutral or slight valgus, restoration of the normal relationship between the posterior facet of the calcaneus with the corresponding articular surface of the talus, and reduction in the calcaneal width.

There are certain other clinical situations in which this and other percutaneous techniques can be used successfully in the treatment of joint-depression calcaneus fractures. Individual surgeon experience as well as careful patient selection are both important factors in using this technique successfully. Although some authors use these techniques routinely for all Sanders II and III fractures, whether they be joint-depression or tongue-type[4] or even *all* displaced calcaneus fractures,[5–7] it should be noted that other authors use them only for Sanders II fractures.[8,9] Others reserve these techniques for patients who would not normally be candidates for extensile open procedures due to smoking or other comorbidities. When these techniques are used for non–tongue-type fractures, an anatomic reduction is more difficult to achieve. There is a steep learning curve, and the surgeon must be adept at obtaining and interpreting intraoperative fluoroscopic lateral, Harris, and Broden's views. Subtalar arthroscopy to confirm a percutaneous reduction[8,9] is also a useful adjunct. No matter which method one chooses to obtain and confirm the percutaneous reduction, this technique is more challenging than performing an extensile incision and directly manipulating the fracture and visually confirming the reduction.

There is no universal agreement as to which fractures are best treated percutaneously. A spectrum of opinions exists as to how far the indications can be safely and effectively stretched. In the author's opinion the further the indications are widened, the less anatomic the results one will have to consider acceptable. Given these limitations, there are some individual fracture patterns in which percutaneous treatment can result in successful correction of deformity. These patterns include the following.

1. *Tongue-type fractures* in which there are direct anterior-to-posterior continuity between the entire posterior aspect of the tuberosity and the entire posterior facet. These fractures are the classic indication for percutaneous treatment (Fig. 15.1).
2. *Partial tongue-type fractures* in which there is a sagittal plane split in the posterior facet continuing into the tuberosity, but continuity remains between a portion of the tuberosity and the posterior facet. This continuity should be confirmed with sagittal CT reconstructions (Fig. 15.2) or with the coronal reconstructions. As with tongue-type fractures, the partial tongue fragment is always lateral with respect to the sustentacular, or constant, fragment. Percutaneous treatment for these fractures is more amenable if the partial tongue fragment is large compared to the constant fragment. For example, a Sanders IIB would be easier to reduce than a Sanders IIA as there is a larger fracture fragment with which to work. It is important to note that only the portion of the posterior fragment that is in direct continuity with the tuberosity is reducible with the Essex-Lopresti technique.

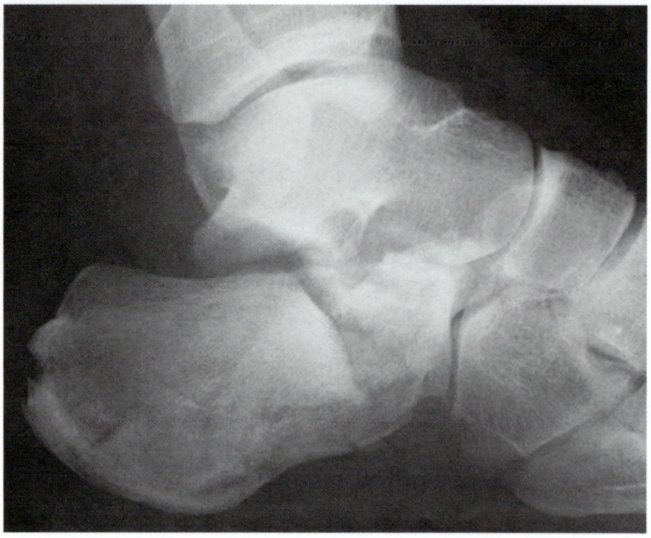

Figure 15.1 Tongue-type fracture.

3. *Joint-depression fractures with minimal displacement between the tuberosity and the depressed posterior facet fragment.* In these situations, whatever displacement there is between the posterior facet and the tuberosity is simply accepted, and the two fragments are reduced together using an Essex-Lopresti maneuver as if they are one fragment (Fig. 15.3).
4. *Sanders IIB and IIC joint-depression–type fractures.* Joint-depression fractures in which the fragment is large enough to be maneuverable with a percutaneous joystick or tamp. The larger the fragment, the easier and more successful percutaneous reduction attempts will be (Fig. 15.4).
5. *Displaced extra-articular tuberosity fractures* not involving the posterior facet (Fig. 15.5).

Patient Characteristics

Patients with fractures that may optimally be treated with a standard extensile open incision may be candidates for percutaneous treatment if an open approach would pose an undue risk for wound necrosis or deep infection. This may include patients with diabetes mellitus, tobacco use, peripheral vascular disease, or severely traumatized lateral skin.

Contraindications

Because the incisions are small stab wounds the surgeon does not have to wait for swelling to diminish; in fact, if percutaneous reduction is to be performed it should be done as soon

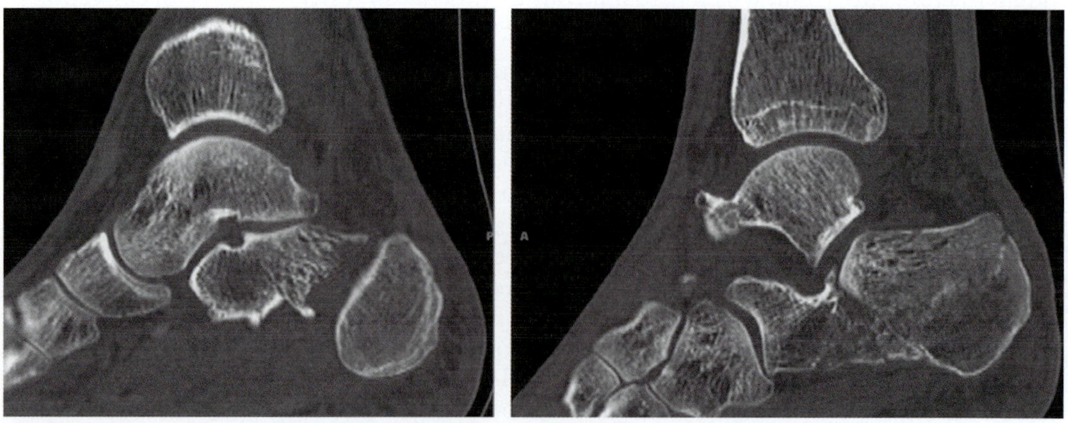

Figure 15.2 Partial tongue-type fracture.

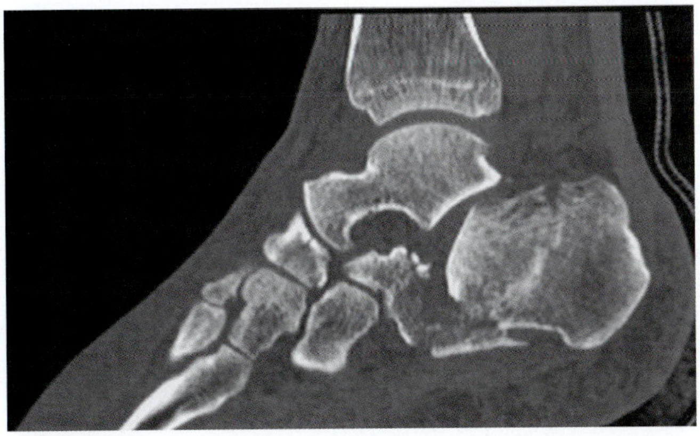

Figure 15.3 Joint-depression fracture with minimal displacement between the tuberosity and the depressed posterior facet fragment.

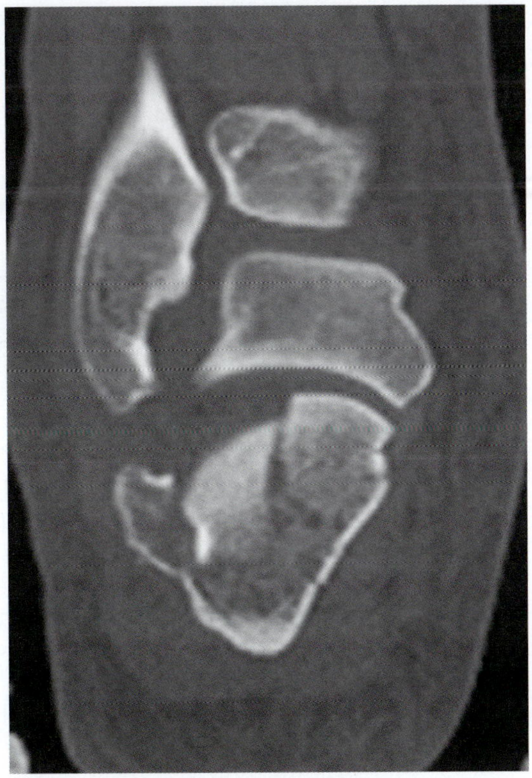

Figure 15.4 Sanders IIB fracture with adequate size of depressed posterior facet.

as possible once the patient is medically stable. Furthermore, fractures with delayed presentation will be more difficult to reduce percutaneously due to organized hematoma interposed at the fracture site. Because the fracture site is not directly exposed, hematoma, bone fragments, or other debris may prevent an adequate reduction and are more difficult to move after 5 to 7 days.[3] Some authors have reported success with protocols extending percutaneous treatment up to 14 or 19 days[8,9] though presentation after 10 days was a factor in 3 of the 5 failures of percutaneous treatment in one series.[9] The author has no strict cutoff for percutaneous treatment but recommends it be performed as soon as possible; operative fractures more than 1 week old are preferably treated with an open technique.

Figure 15.5 Displaced extra-articular tuberosity fragment. These fractures can be reduced percutaneously or through the often associated open wound.

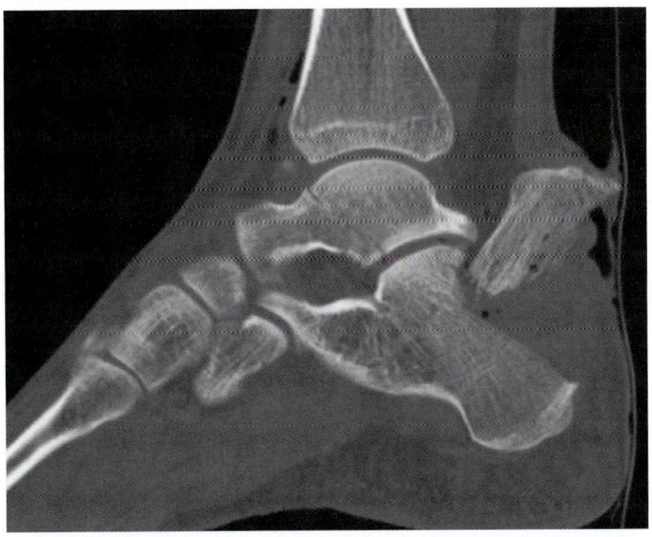

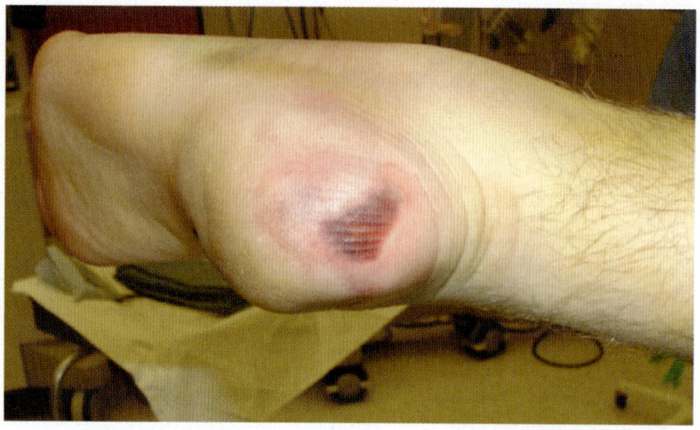

Figure 15.6 Skin necrosis on the posterior heel 1 week after an unreduced, displaced tongue-type fracture.

Particular attention should be given to tongue-type fractures when the tongue fragment tents the posterior heel skin; if not promptly reduced this can cause varying amounts of soft tissue compromise including full-thickness skin necrosis in one study.[10] For this reason, the author recommends emergent reduction for tongue-type fractures that tent the posterior skin (Fig. 15.6). If the fracture cannot be surgically treated immediately, the fracture should be splinted with the ankle in equinus to minimize the posterior skin embarrassment.[10]

Sanders IV fractures have a poorer prognosis with osteosynthesis regardless of the type of approach and are particularly difficult with a percutaneous approach. Several reports on the percutaneous treatment of calcaneus fractures have shown inferior results with Sanders IV fractures[5,6] and some authors restrict this technique to Sanders II fractures only.[9] The author recommends that caution be used when contemplating percutaneous treatment for Sanders III and IV fractures. Although extenuating clinical circumstances may make this a reasonable alternative, anatomic reduction is less likely, creating a higher risk of subtalar arthritis and the need for subtalar fusion.[11]

PATIENT POSITIONING

For unilateral fractures, the patient lies in the lateral position with the operative side up. (For bilateral fractures, patients are placed in the prone position with the leg currently being operated on externally rotated.) Hip positioners (Stulberg hip positioners, Innomed, Savanna, GA) are used to support the anterior superior iliac spine anteriorly and the sacrum posteriorly. This is preferable to a beanbag because it facilitates mobilization of the leg. The author uses a lateral foam positioning device (Bone Foam, Bone Foam, Inc, Plymouth, MN) to create a flat operative surface for the up (operative) limb and to protect the down (nonoperative) limb. A thigh tourniquet is placed although it is not routinely inflated. The entire lower extremity up to the thigh tourniquet is prepped and draped to facilitate knee flexion and hip rotation. C-arm is brought in from the posterior aspect of the calcaneus. The three required images are as follows.

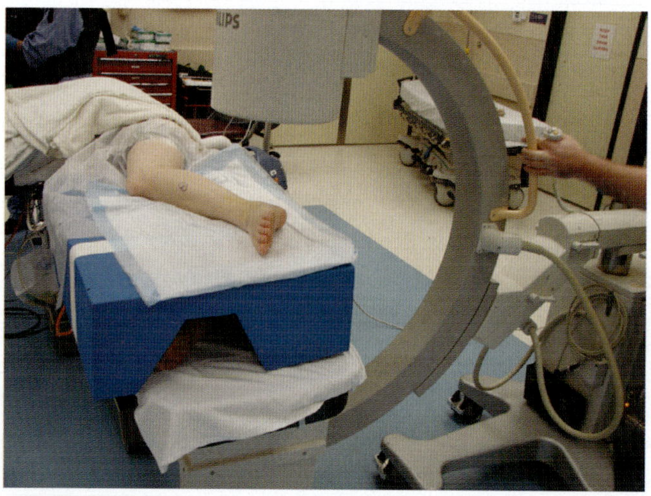

Figure 15.7 Intraoperative positioning for a lateral view.

1. *Lateral view.* The lateral views are obtained with the image source below the table and the image intensifier above the patient (Fig. 15.7).

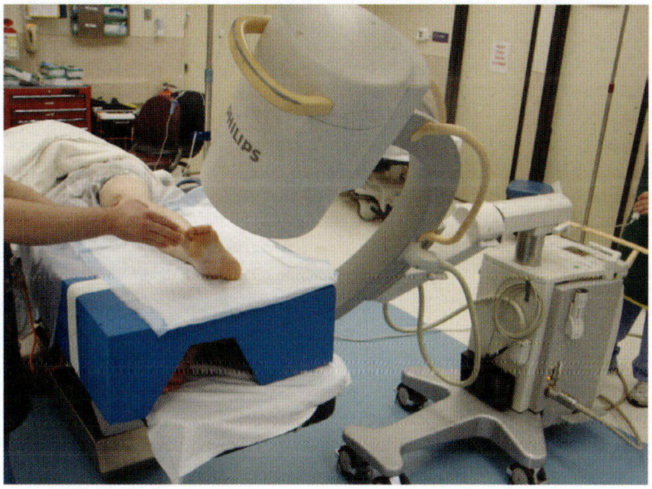

Figure 15.8 Intraoperative positioning for a Broden's view.

2. *Broden's views*. The Broden's views are taken by externally rotating the extremity. With the foot in internal rotation, images are taken with varying amounts (10 to 40 degrees) of caudad angulation of the beam. These are used to visualize various portions of the posterior facet (Fig. 15.8).
3. *Axial (Harris) view.* This view is taken by returning the foot to its resting position, lateral side pointing upward, and then tilting the entire c-arm sideways so that the image source is at the foot of the table and the image intensifier is just behind the buttock or upper thigh. A sterile sheet is used to cover the image source at the foot of the table. The image is then taken at a 45-degree angle to the calcaneal tuberosity by shooting from the foot of the table, through the calcaneus, and then posteriorly and proximally toward the image intensifier (Fig. 15.9).

During the reduction maneuver, flexion of the knee facilitates distal translation of the calcaneal tuberosity (and thereby elevation of the posterior facet) for tongue-type fractures. As this tends to place the operative limb posteriorly, it will help to have the nonoperative limb positioned slightly anteriorly to avoid superimposing c-arm images (Fig. 15.10).

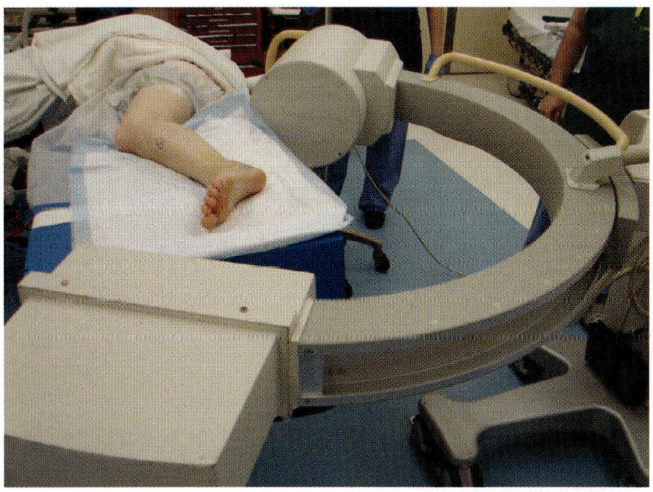

Figure 15.9 Intraoperative positioning for a Harris, or axial, view.

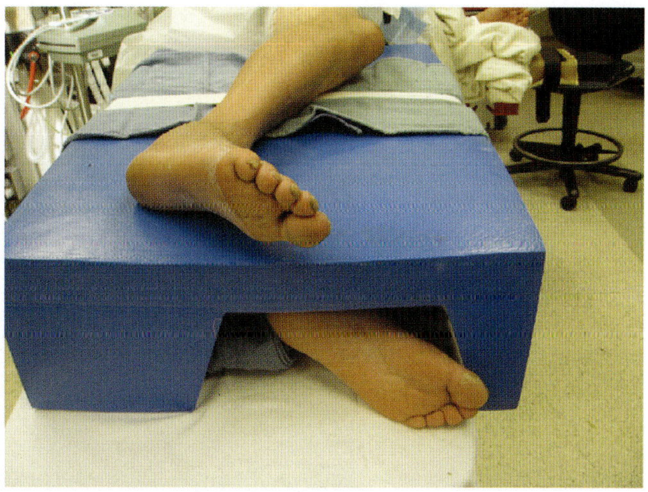

Figure 15.10 The operative foot **(right)** lies posteriorly since the knee is flexed, to relax the gastrocnemius. To keep the well leg **(left)** from getting in the way of the lateral c-arm images, a towel is used to push it forward gently.

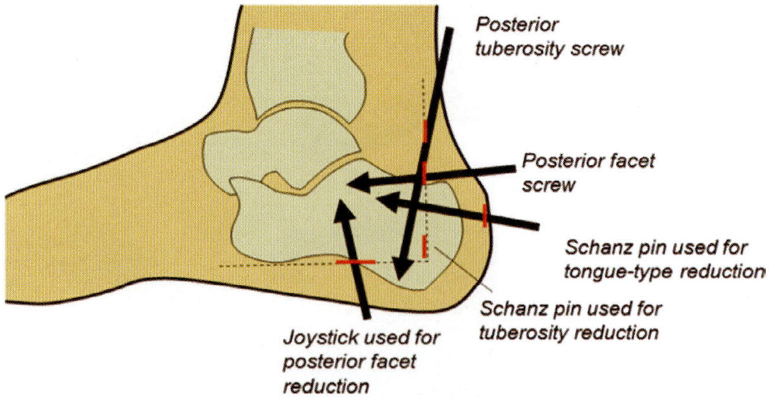

Figure 15.11 Five of the commonly used stab incisions for percutaneous reduction. Note that all except the posterior-to-anterior Schanz pin wound can be made in line with the L-shaped extensile lateral incision in the event of failure of percutaneous reduction.

SURGICAL APPROACHES

Before making any incisions the standard L-shaped extensile lateral incision[12,13] is drawn on the lateral heel with a sterile pen in the event the percutaneous technique needs to be converted to an open procedure. The author typically makes multiple, small percutaneous stab incisions for this type of procedure. When practical, it is helpful to make these incisions in line with the L-shaped drawing (Fig. 15.11). If percutaneous attempts to reduce the posterior facet are unsuccessful, the stab wounds can be incorporated into the extensile incision. The typical stab incisions used are as follows: (1) Just lateral/anterior to the tendo Achilles, proximal to the tuberosity, through which superior-to-inferior screw is placed to secure a tongue fragment to the plantar portion of the tuberosity. (2) Slightly inferior to this, just superior to the top of the tuberosity, through which the posterolateral-to-anteromedial posterior facet screw(s) are placed. (3) At the posterior–inferior corner of the tuberosity, through which a Schanz pin is typically placed. These three stab wounds are typically along the vertical limb of an extensile L-shaped incision. (4) Along the inferior border of the calcaneus, through which joysticks or tamps can be inserted to elevate the posterior facet. (5) Not all the incisions can always be incorporated into the L-shaped template. For example, the posterior-to-anterior screws for a tongue-type fragment are typically made on the posterior aspect of the heel.

Occasionally, if the surgeon is having difficulty reducing, accessing, or visualizing a smaller depressed posterior facet fragment, a small sinus tarsi window can be used to directly approach the posterior facet. This is typically a 3- to 5-cm incision made in line with an imaginary line drawn from the tip of the fibula to the base of the fourth metatarsal (Fig. 15.12).

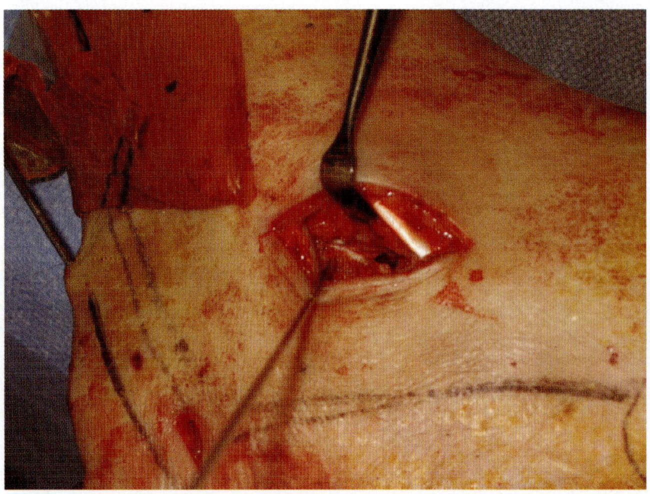

Figure 15.12 A small sinus tarsi window can be made to visualize the posterior facet reduction. The peroneal tendons are retracted superiorly and inferiorly. A K-wire is holding the posterior facet reduction.

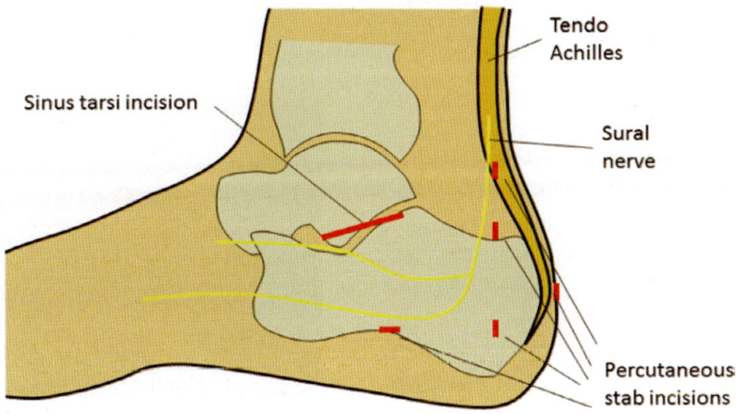

Figure 15.13 Structures at risk during percutaneous reduction.

After incising the skin, care should be taken to protect a branch of the sural nerve, which typically crosses close to this region obliquely in a posterior/inferior to anterior/superior direction (Fig. 15.13). This incision can be extended to varying degrees anteriorly or posteriorly to access more of the subtalar joint. Various fixation devices such as screws alone or small plates can be placed directly along the lateral aspect of the posterior facet through this incision.

REDUCTION TECHNIQUES

A partially threaded 5-mm Schanz pin is useful for many of these fractures. The author typically uses a Schanz pin in three locations: From posterior to anterior in the tongue fragment as a joystick for the Essex-Lopresti maneuver, from superior to inferior in the tuberosity to lever the tuberosity away from the impacted posterior facet, and from lateral to medial to translate the tuberosity medially and pull the tuberosity out of varus (Fig. 15.14). Other useful instruments include a bone tamp, a small periosteal elevator, and Kirschner wires. Specialized equipment in selected circumstances includes a small joint arthroscope to perform subtalar arthroscopy or an inflatable balloon tamp (InflateFX, Medtronic Spine, Minneapolis, MN).

1. *Tongue-type fractures*
   a. First, a small longitudinal incision is made in the midline of the posterior aspect of the heel directly posterior to the tongue fragment. For a partial tongue-type fracture, which lies lateral, the incision is made just lateral to the Achilles tendon. A 5-mm Schanz pin is inserted from posterior-to-anterior into the tuberosity, toward the posterior facet stopping just deep to the articular surface. C-arm is used to confirm

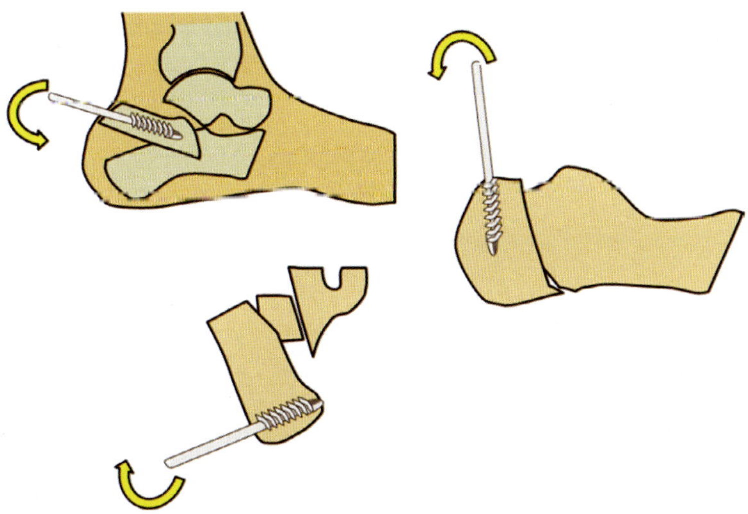

Figure 15.14 Techniques to use a Schanz pin to reduce the tuberosity: As a joystick for tongue-type fractures, as a joystick to lever a tuberosity fragment posteriorly, and as a lateral-to-medial joystick to pull the heel out of varus.

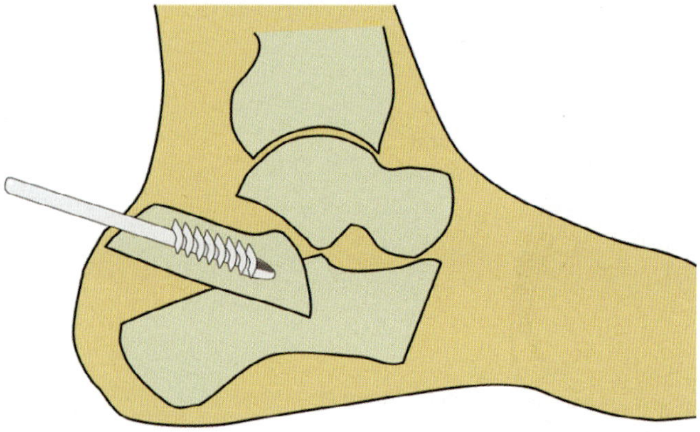

Figure 15.15 Insertion of a Schanz pin into a tongue fragment, staying just short of the subchondral bone of the posterior facet.

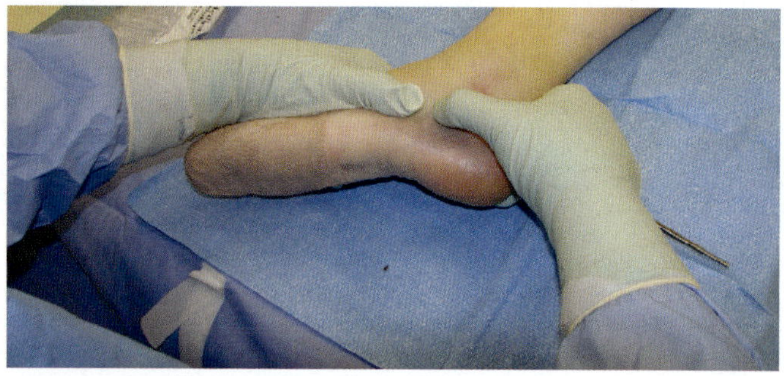

Figure 15.16 Hand positioning for the modern adaptation of the Essex-Lopresti maneuver. For a left foot, the surgeon's right hand grasps the heel and the Schanz pin; both thumbs are over the fracture site and serve as a fulcrum.

accurate placement. Note that for partial tongue-type fractures, this can be rather difficult, and the author recommends obtaining a Broden's view as well to confirm that the Schanz pin remains in the tongue fragment and has not exited medially or laterally (Fig. 15.15).

b. The reduction maneuver is now performed. It is similar to that described by Essex-Lopresti (though his was in the prone position)[1] and Tornetta.[2,3] The index through small fingers of one hand are placed around the Schanz pin, and the other hand grasps the forefoot (Fig. 15.16). Both thumbs are placed over the lateral side of the calcaneus at the fracture site. The fracture is then unlocked by bending the foot into varus at the fracture site by pushing both hands downward toward the table. This exaggerates the deformity to unlock the posterior facet. Next, with the thumbs still over the fracture site as a fulcrum, both hands are then pulled plantarward—the hand on the Schanz pin pulls the tuberosity inferiorly using the pin. As the tuberosity is pushed inferiorly, the posterior facet is elevated superiorly in a reciprocal direction (Fig. 15.17). Both hands are then used to pull the foot into abduction with the thumbs again over the fracture site, which pushes the posterior facet medially toward the sustentaculum. Manual compression from the medial and lateral sides of the calcaneus is used to narrow the heel width.

c. A c-arm lateral image is then obtained to confirm that the posterior facet and the tuberosity are reduced. The lateral view is scrutinized to ensure that the articular surfaces of the posterior facet of the calcaneus and the talus are parallel. In the case of a partial tongue-type fracture, Broden's views are also checked to confirm reduction of the posterior facet, ensuring that the displaced lateral fragment has been elevated to the level of the reduced medial fragment.

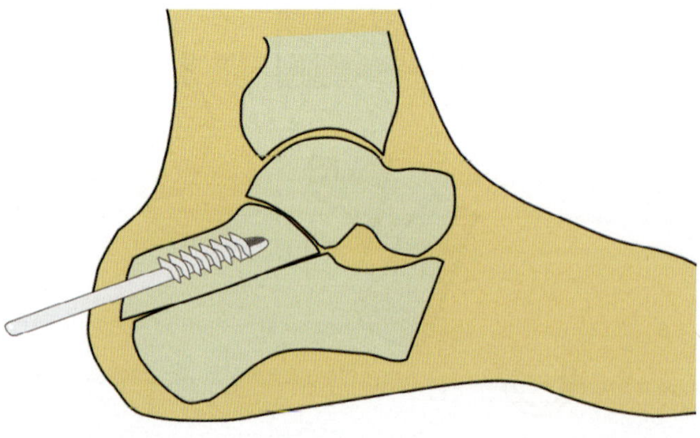

Figure 15.17 Depressing the Schanz pin elevates the posterior facet after it has been unlocked.

2. *Partial tongue-type fractures*
   a. The Schanz pin is advanced into the lateral part of the tuberosity from posterior to anterior, taking care to stay within the lateral part of the facet that is connected to the tuberosity. Accurate pin placement should be confirmed with c-arm lateral and Broden's views.
   b. The pin is pushed plantarward, thus elevating the posterior facet. For a Sanders IIA or IIB fracture, the reduction can be confirmed through a small sinus tarsi window, by examining the lateral and Broden's views, or with subtalar arthroscopy. For a Sanders III fracture, the third fragment is still depressed as it lies between the partial tongue fragment and the sustentaculum and must be addressed as per the techniques described under Item 4 below, Sanders IIB and IIC joint-depression fractures. Once reduced, the fragment is stabilized with a lateral to medial posterior facet screw; this may be followed by posterior-to-anterior screws from the tuberosity to the anterior process, and/or a superior-to-inferior screw to stabilize the tuberosity.
3. *Joint-depression fractures with minimal displacement between the tuberosity and the depressed posterior facet fragment*
   a. If the displacement between the tuberosity and the posterior facet is minimal, the two fragments can be reduced together using the same technique. A Schanz pin is advanced into the tuberosity, across the fracture site, and into the depressed posterior facet fragment.
   b. The two fragments, now effectively united as one, are then reduced together using the Schanz pin as described in the previous section for tongue-type and partial tongue-type fractures.
4. *Sanders IIB and IIC joint-depression fractures*
   a. The tuberosity is usually addressed first. In joint-depression fractures the posterior facet is embedded to varying extents in the calcaneal body and can be covered by overhanging tuberosity. By pulling the tuberosity posteriorly, the calcaneus is lengthened and the posterior facet can then be elevated. There are different ways to achieve this depending on the fracture pattern. For most fractures a terminally threaded bicortical Schanz pin on a T-handle chuck is placed into the posteroinferior corner of the calcaneal tuberosity from lateral to medial. This pin is used to distract the tuberosity from the sustentacular fragment in a posterior–inferior direction and to tilt the tuberosity out of varus (Fig. 15.18A, B). It can also be used to correct the lateral translation by pushing it medially. Significant force is applied to this pin; to lessen the chance of pulling out, "rebar" K-wires can be placed directly superior and inferior to this pin from the posterior aspect of the heel to minimize pullout. They are removed at the end of the procedure along with the Schanz pin. Occasionally, a femoral distractor or external fixator placed medially with one pin in the tibia and one pin in the medial calcaneal tuberosity is needed to correct the varus malalignment. This is removed at the conclusion of the procedure. Once the tuberosity has been reduced, it is held in place with K-wires provisionally fixing it to the sustentacular fragment and anterior process. Occasionally fractures are

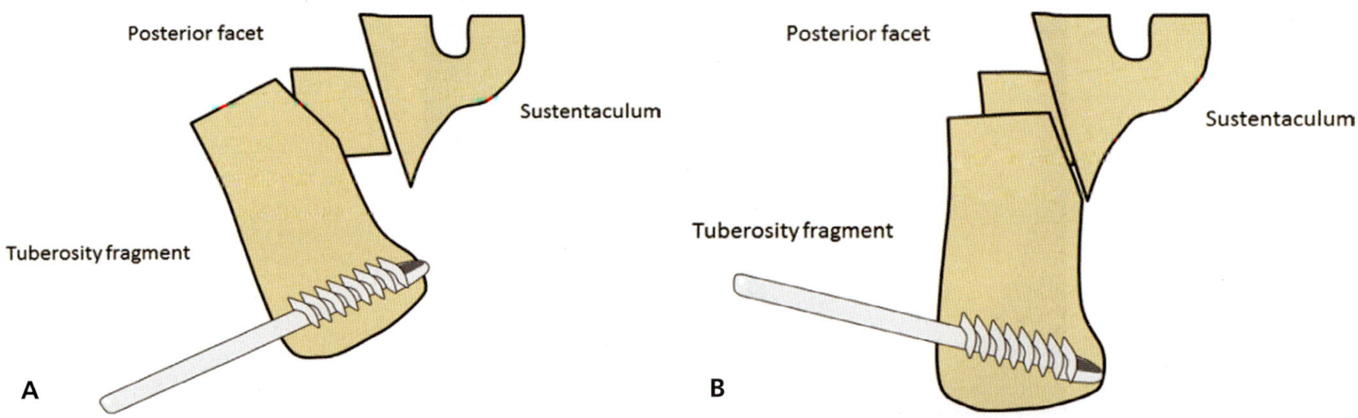

Figure 15.18 Reduction of the tuberosity. **A:** Inserting a Schanz pin lateral to medial in the posteroinferior aspect of the tuberosity. **B:** The pin is pulled posteriorly and inferiorly, pushed medially, and tilted into valgus.

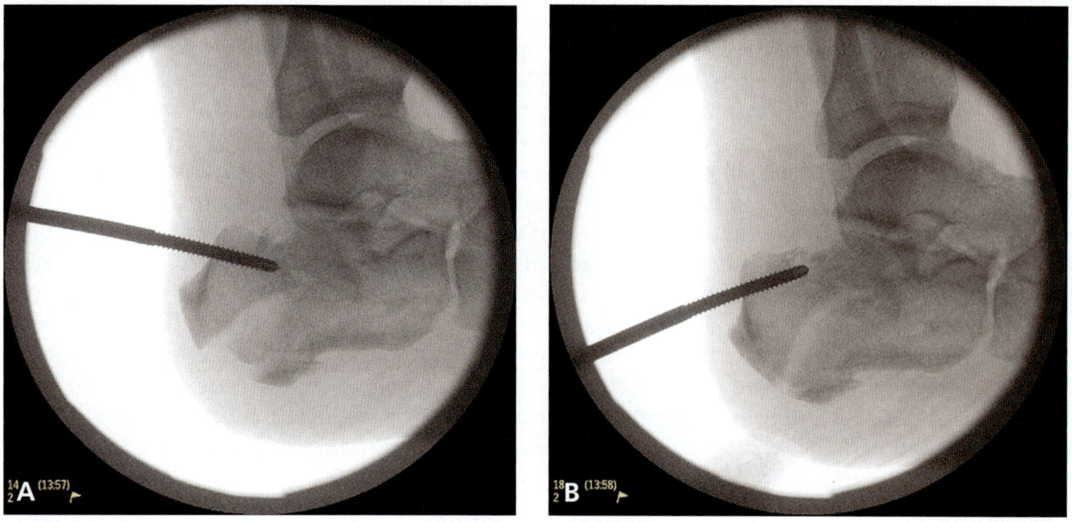

Figure 15.19 Reduction of a split tuberosity fragment in a Sanders IIB joint-depression fracture. **A:** Insertion of a Schanz pin as a joystick, stopping short of the posterior facet. **B:** Reduction of the superior half of the tuberosity and the posterior facet.

seen where the tuberosity is not a single piece but there is also a split between the dorsal and plantar fragments. A Schanz pin is inserted into the superior half of tuberosity and used to reduce this to the plantar half; the two pieces are then fixed together with a dorsal-to-plantar partially threaded screw (Fig. 15.19A, B).

b. Next, the joint-depression fragment is addressed. A small transverse incision is made plantar to the posterior facet. The author typically makes this in line with the plantar limb of the extensile lateral incision (Fig. 15.11), which allows a small bone tamp or periosteal elevator to be inserted below the facet (Fig. 15.20). This is often the most difficult part of the procedure as the fragment be small, challenging to find, and impacted into the surrounding body. This difficulty is compounded for fractures more than a week old. The author recommends using the Broden's views to localize the fragment and to guide the elevator as the most effective way to perform the reduction (Fig. 15.21A–C). In some cases it may be useful to use an inflatable balloon tamp to elevate the joint-depression fragment (Fig. 15.22A, B).

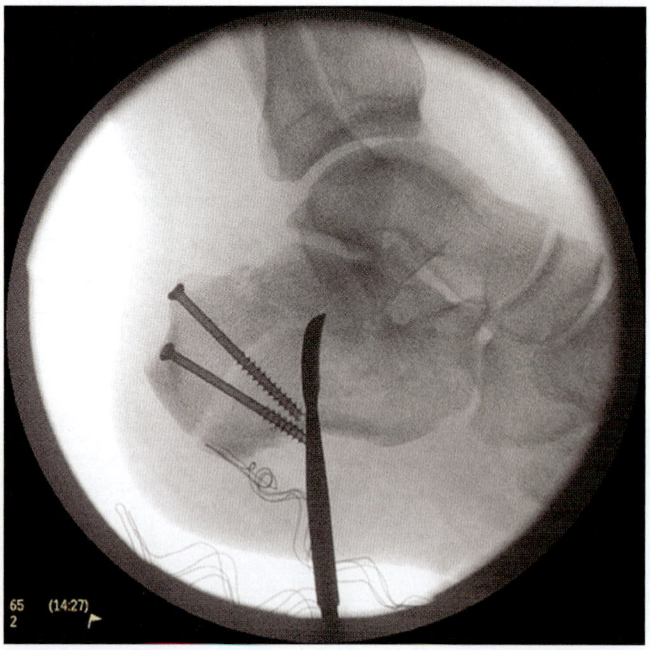

Figure 15.20 The same fracture as in Figure 15.19A, B. After fixing the split tuberosity with partially threaded cannulated screws, a periosteal elevator inserted through percutaneous wound along the plantar limb of an extensile incision is used as a tamp to complete the posterior facet reduction.

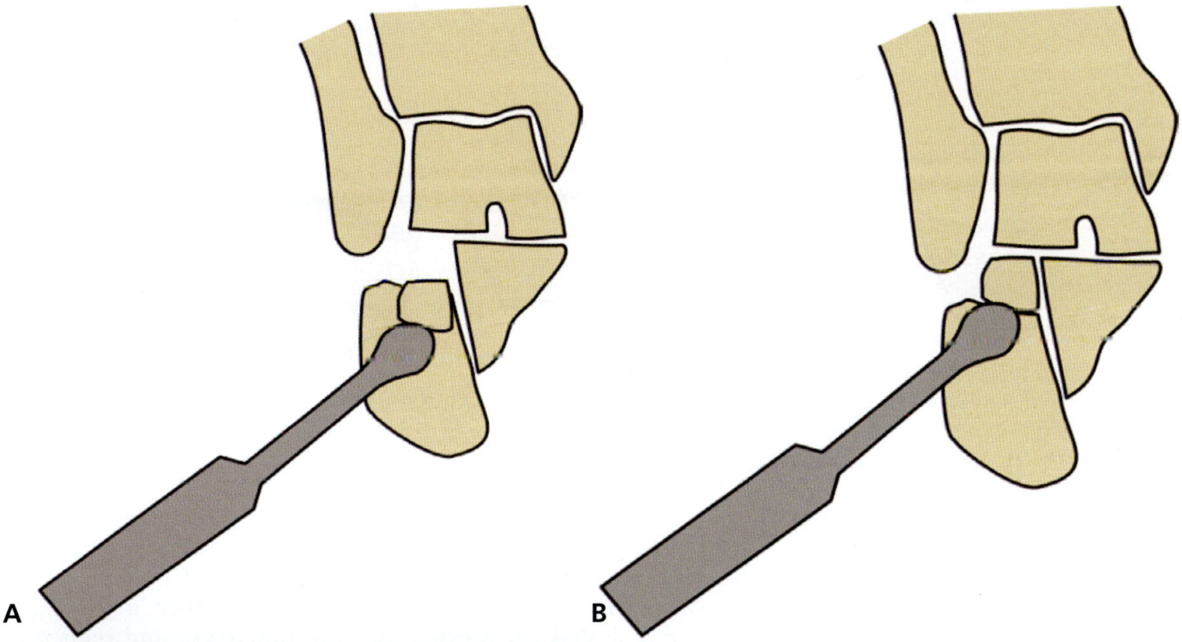

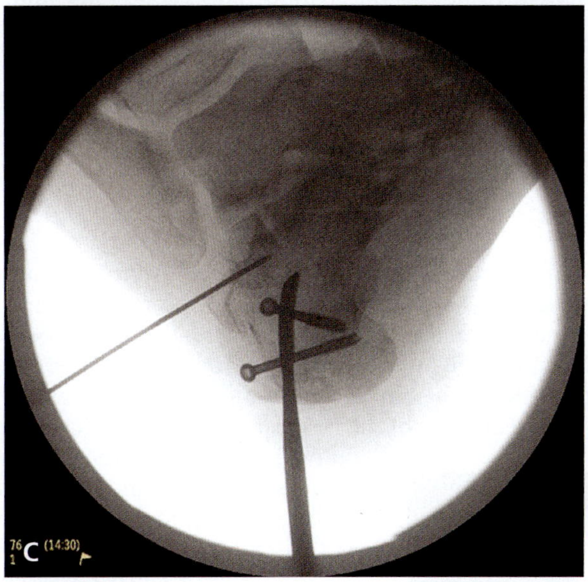

Figure 15.21 Tamp position checked with a Broden's view to confirm location under the depressed part of the posterior facet. **A:** Pre-reduction. **B:** Post-reduction. **C:** Fluoroscopically.

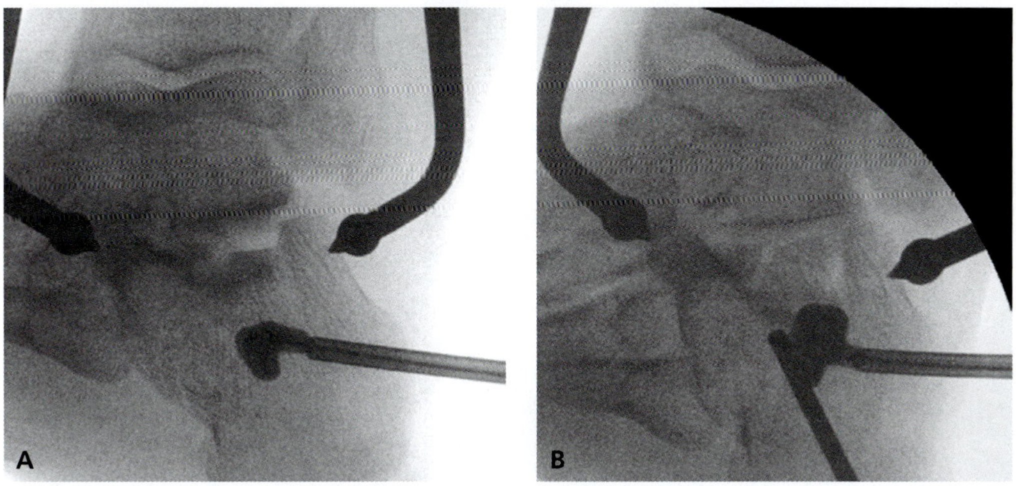

Figure 15.22 Use of an inflatable balloon tamp to elevate the depressed middle fragment of a posterior facet in a Sanders III joint-depression fracture. **A:** Pre-reduction Broden's view. **B:** Post-reduction Broden's view. A large reduction forceps is placed on the lateral wall and on the sustentaculum tali through percutaneous incisions to prevent the balloon from displacing the fragments laterally.

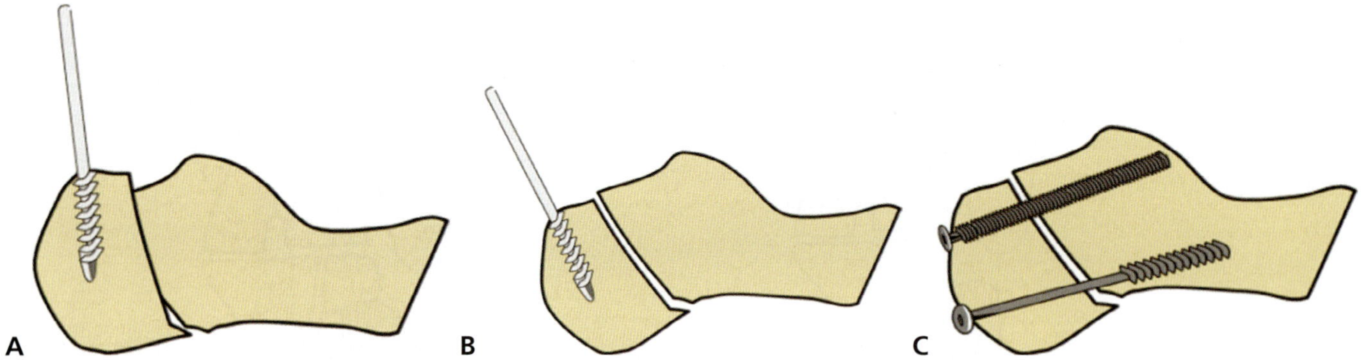

Figure 15.23 Reduction of an extra-articular displaced tuberosity fragment with the use of a Schanz pin. This maneuver will work if the tuberosity is not in a significant amount of varus. **A:** Pre-reduction. **B:** Post-reduction. **C:** Fully threaded screws placed superiorly to keep the top the calcaneus distracted, and partially threaded screws inferiorly to lag the inferior surface together.

5. *Displaced extra-articular tuberosity fractures*
   a. If there is significant varus malalignment of a displaced tuberosity fragment, a lateral-to-medial Schanz pin should be inserted into the tuberosity and reduction of the axial heel alignment should proceed as for a joint-depression–type injury described previously.
   b. If there is no axial heel malalignment and the tuberosity is only displaced superiorly then a superior-to-inferior Schanz pin may be inserted to push the tuberosity plantarward followed by insertion of screws (Fig. 15.23A–C).

FIXATION

Fixation is performed with multiple cannulated screws. The author prefers 4-mm or 5-mm cannulated screws with reduced heads to decrease hardware prominence, and to use a larger number of smaller screws rather than a smaller number of larger screws. The posterior-to-anterior screws are generally in the 70–80 mm range and are fully threaded; unless there are secondary fracture lines in the anterior process, these screws are usually placed first as they hold the tuberosity reduced which assists with reduction of the posterior facet. However, sagittal plane fractures in the anterior process should be stabilized first with a lateral-to-medial screw as this will improve purchase of the long anterior process screw. Next, partially threaded screws are used to compress the posterior facet fragment to the constant fragment from medial to lateral (Fig. 15.24). If directed correctly into the sustentaculum tali, these screws are in the 45 mm range. For tongue and partial tongue fractures, partially threaded screws are also used to stabilize the posterior aspect of the tuberosity in a superior-to-inferior direction (Fig. 15.25). Additional fully threaded position screws may be added for stability to maintain calcaneal length and axial alignment; the

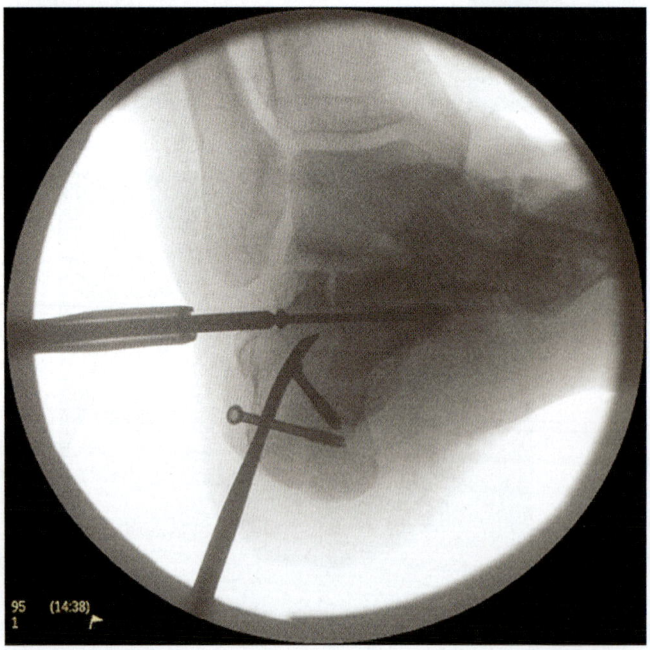

Figure 15.24 Intraoperative Broden's view of a Sanders IIB joint-depression fracture with a threaded screw placed from lateral to medial in the posterior facet to compress the fragments together.

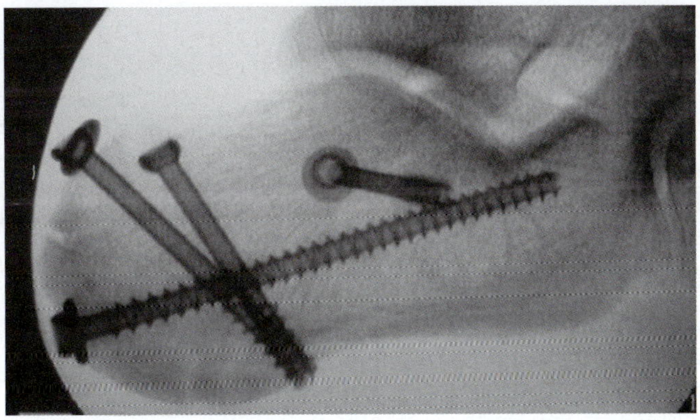

Figure 15.25 Tongue-type fracture with partially threaded superior-to-inferior screws in the posterior of the tuberosity to reduce and stabilize the superior half to the inferior half after the Essex-Lopresti maneuver was performed. Note the lateral-to-medial posterior facet screw as well as the fully threaded long posterior-to-anterior screw.

long posterior-to-anterior screws into the anterior process ideally should skim the inner cortex of the medial wall of the calcaneus to act as a strut to maintain medial column length and axial alignment (Fig. 15.26A, B). It may be useful to use a fully threaded "kickstand" screw to support the posterior facet from below. Figures 15.27 to 15.29 summarize typical screw configurations for tongue-type, partial tongue-type, and joint-depression fractures.

Of all of the screws, the placement of the medial-to-lateral posterior facet screw is the most crucial. There is a narrow corridor for this screw; it should be adjacent to subchondral bone while remaining out of the subtalar joint but still within the good bone stock of the sustentaculum tali (Fig. 15.30). If a screw hits this target successfully, it will commonly be in the 35 to 45 mm range, depending on the degree of obliquity. This screw typically is placed in a posterolateral-to-anteromedial direction since the posterior facet sits posterior to the middle facet and sustentaculum.

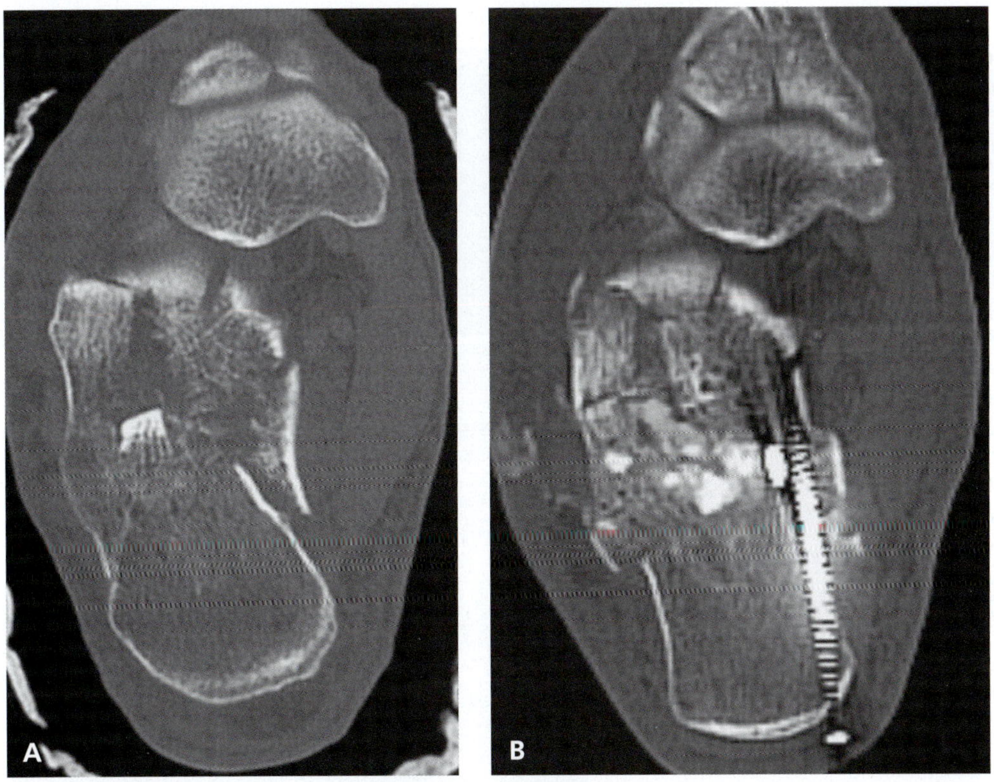

Figure 15.26 Axial CT scan showing correction of heel varus. **A:** Pre-op. **B:** Post-op. Note the medial fully threaded posterior-to-anterior screw aiming toward the sustentacular fragment, skimming the medial wall to support and prevent medial column failure into varus.

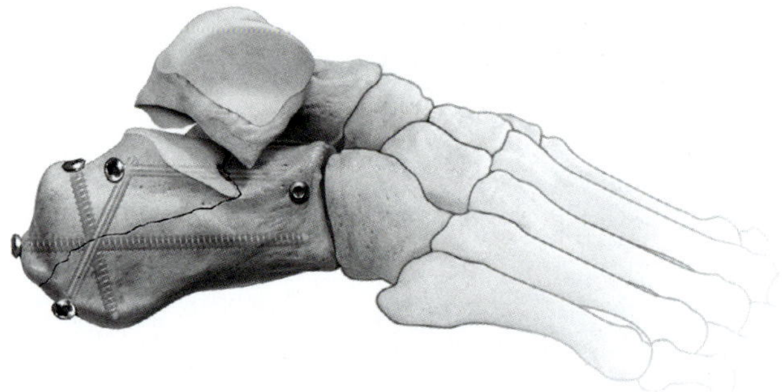

Figure 15.27 Composite sketch of various trajectories of percutaneous screws. The lateral-to-medial posterior facet screw is angled posterior to anterior to engage the sustentaculum tali, which lies anterior to the posterior facet. The screw is partially threaded or placed by lag technique to compress the posterior facet fragments. The fully threaded inferior-to-superior kickstand screw helps to support the posterior facet from below. The long fully threaded posterior-to-anterior screw into the anterior process maintains axial alignment and can support a tongue-type fracture. The lateral-to-medial screw in the anterior process stabilizes any fracture that may be present prior to placement of a long posterior-to-anterior screw to improve that screw's purchase. The partially threaded superior-to-inferior screw stabilizes the superior tuberosity when it is a separate fragment from the plantar tuberosity.

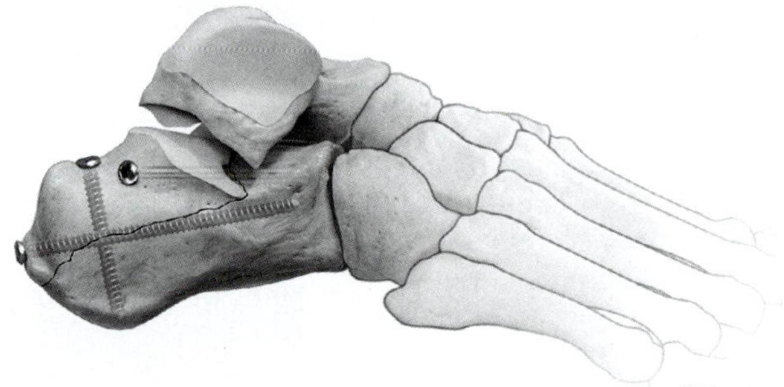

Figure 15.28 Typical screw configuration for a tongue-type fracture.

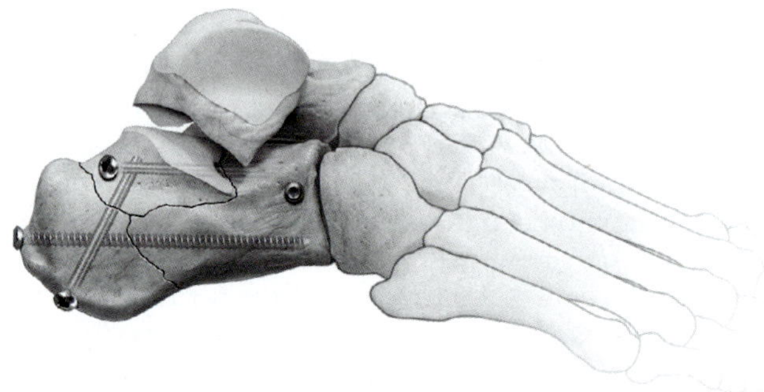

Figure 15.29 Typical screw configuration for a joint-depression–type fracture. More screws are often needed; for example, two screws may be placed to support the posterior facet. In addition, multiple screws from posterior to anterior in the body or the tuberosity may be necessary.

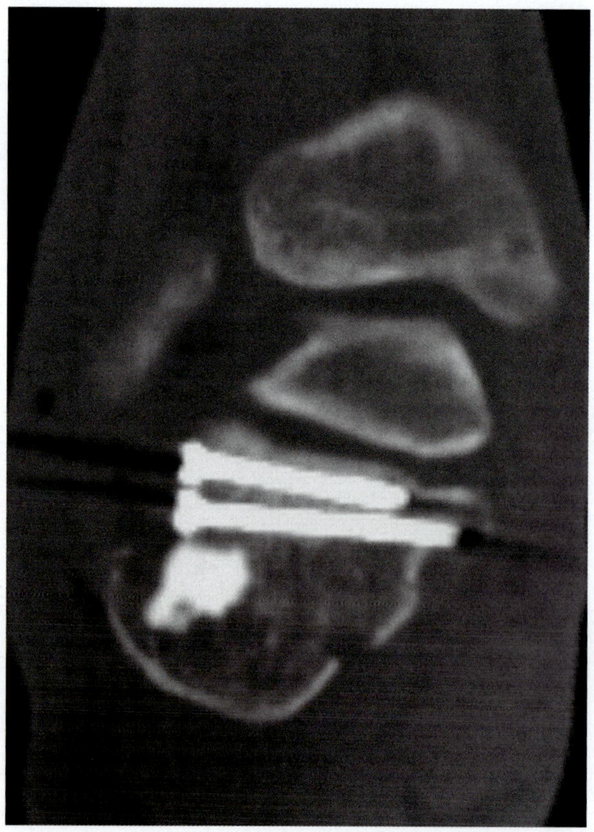

Figure 15.30 There is a narrow working zone for the posterior facet screw. It must stay out of the subtalar joint while still hitting the sustentaculum tali.

Injectable calcium phosphate ceramic may be injected to fill the void left by elevation of the posterior facet. In a randomized controlled trial of 52 fractures in 47 patients, Johal et al.[14] found that the use of resorbable calcium phosphate (α-BSM, Etex Corporation, Cambridge, MA) during ORIF of displaced intra-articular fractures reduced the loss of Bohler's angle at 6 months.

In rare circumstances the entire posterior facet and calcaneal body will fracture off the sustentaculum tali, leaving that latter structure reduced to the subtalar joint and the rest of the calcaneus displaced. This is a variant of a subtalar dislocation in which a small portion of the calcaneus (the sustentaculum only) remains reduced to the talus. The surgeon should resist the temptation to "reduce" the sustentaculum to the body; rather, it is the body that should be reduced to the sustentaculum. In these cases one or two screws from lateral to medial should adequately stabilize the posterior facet to the sustentaculum after reduction, assuming no other fractures are present.

COMPLICATIONS

Intraoperative Complications

Although generally associated with less surgical risks than an extensile open procedure, some intraoperative complications with percutaneous treatment of calcaneus fractures can occur.

1. *Failure to achieve percutaneous reduction* can occur in fractures with delayed presentation or with significantly impacted posterior facet fragments. When percutaneous methods fail to elevate the depressed fragment and the skin condition is amenable, the approach is converted to extensile lateral open and standard ORIF techniques are used. If the skin condition does not permit a safe open reduction, the incisions are closed, a dressing and splint are applied, and an open procedure is staged.
2. *Injury to neurovascular structures or tendons.* The peroneal tendons are susceptible to injury given their path within the sinus tarsi approach. Careful dissection and gentle retraction of the tendons can help to avoid injury. The sural nerve is at risk with placement of the lateral-to-medial screws that fix the posterior facet. Although irritation is common, injury can be minimized by careful blunt dissection and by using a drill sleeve. Should dysesthesias occur, medications and topical agents may be useful postoperatively. Medially, the flexor hallucis longus tendon is susceptible to injury with an errant inferiorly placed lateral-to-medial posterior facet screw (Fig. 15.31).
3. *Intra-articular screw penetration.* Intraoperative c-arm images should be carefully examined for intra-articular screws. A Broden's view and lateral foot view must be scrutinized for violation of the subtalar joint and should redirected more inferiorly. For the calcaneocuboid joint, oblique and lateral foot views should be evaluated. Since it is a saddle-shaped joint, it can be difficult to tell if a screw is intra-articular and the author recommends erring

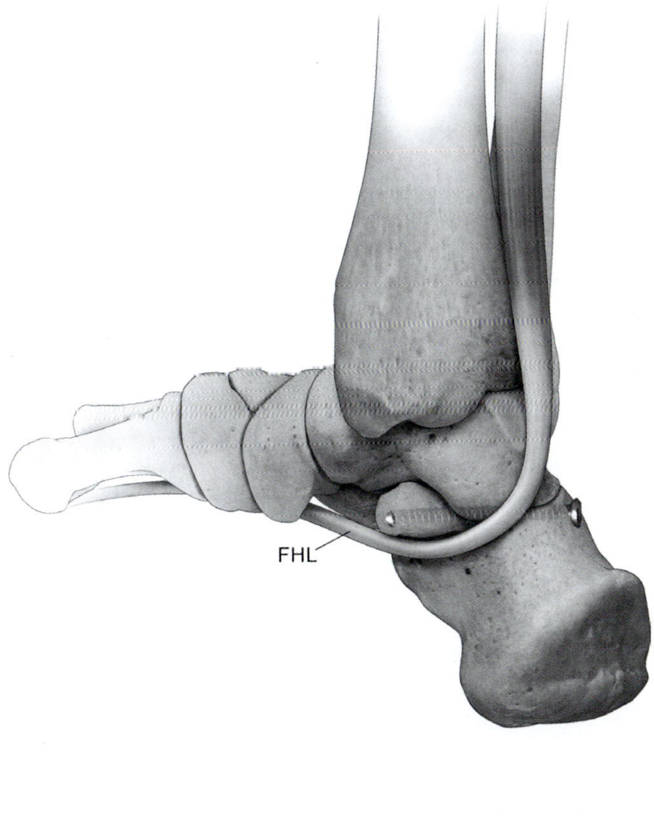

Figure 15.31 Care must be taken to avoid injury to the FHL tendon which lies just inferior to the sustentaculum tali. Contracture of the hallux IP joint can result from errant screw placement.

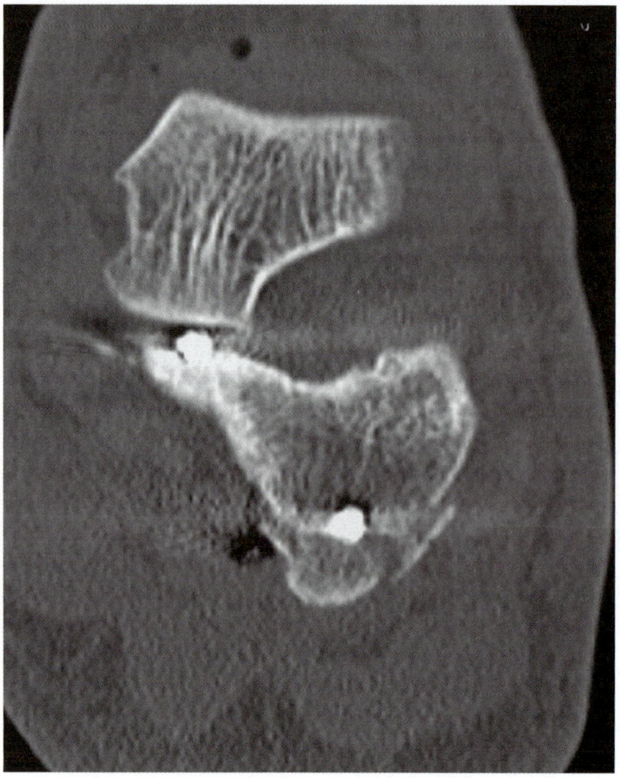

Figure 15.32 The tip of a posterior facet screw can be seen aiming superiorly and lying within the middle facet of the subtalar joint.

on the side of safety. If there is any question postoperatively, the author recommends getting a postoperative CT scan (Fig. 15.32).

4. *Poor screw purchase.* When poor intrinsic bone stock or fracture comminution results in poor fixation, screws will need to be redirected or fracture fragments will first need to be stabilized with an additional fixation, resulting in interdigitation of screws or functioning like rebar. Careful examination of the preoperative CT scan to localize these regions is crucial in hopes to avoid this issue. In general, these problems are seen more frequently with the posterior-to-anterior screws when there is comminution of the anterior process. This can be mitigated by prior stabilization of the anterior process fracture with lateral-to-medial screws. There are unfortunately some cases where there is simply no good bone stock; in these cases it may be necessary to pass temporary K-wires across the fracture fragments, through the subtalar joint, and into the talus to achieve adequate stabilization.

Postoperative Complications

These can include superficial infection, deep infection, secondary loss of reduction, nonunion, post-traumatic arthritis, and symptomatic hardware requiring removal.

1. *Infection,* when it occurs, is generally superficial and usually does not require a return trip to the operating room. Several series have reported zero infections and wound dehiscence.[4,8,9] It is notable that three series that used K-wires outside of the skin[5,6] reported superficial infection rates of 7% and 9.8%. In the early part of his series in which Steinman pins were left outside of the skin, Tornetta[3] reported a 12.2% incidence of pin site drainage (5 of 41 patients), all of which resolved with oral antibiotics and early pin removal at 6 weeks. There were no cases of osteomyelitis. Superficial infection can usually be managed with dressing changes, oral antibiotics, and close observation. Although deep infection rates in expert hands can be as low as 1.8% for extensile open approaches,[15] they have also been reported to be as high as 27% by other authors, and wound necrosis is reported to be in the 8% to 9% range.[12] Both deep infection and

wound necrosis are rare with percutaneous techniques. Stulik et al.[5] had a deep infection rate of 1.7% which required operative debridement. Westberg et al.[11] reported a deep infection rate of 2.8%. Deep infection is treated with operative debridement of the wound and an antibiotic regimen tailored to the culture results. The author often places antibiotic-impregnated cement beads followed by staged repeat debridement(s) in cases of severe infection and bone loss.

2. *Loss of reduction.* This is a reported complication with both open and percutaneous approaches and does not significantly differ between the two. There is usually a small loss of Bohler's angle that occurs during the healing period between the initial post-op x-ray and the x-ray taken at final healing.[7,11] In the author's experience a mild 4- to 7-degree loss of Bohler's angle occurs over this time frame.[11] If there is a significant, early loss of reduction in conjunction with increased displacement at the articular surface or intra-articular penetration of a screw, the patient should be considered for return to the operating room for revision reduction and fixation.
3. *Nonunion* is an infrequently reported complication with calcaneus fractures. The surgeon should be suspicious for deep infection and obtain acute phase reactants laboratory markers and send cultures at the time of any revision surgery. Successful treatment has been reported using staged protocols, debriding any infection if present, followed by bone grafting and subtalar arthrodesis either in situ or with a bone block distraction.[16]
4. *Post-traumatic arthritis* usually involves the subtalar joint and can lead to the need for a subtalar fusion. It is generally expected that there will be some amount of post-traumatic arthritis of the subtalar joint.[5,6] However, even when post-traumatic subtalar arthritis is present, it is not always symptomatic. Stulik et al.[5] reported 85.7% of their patients had radiographic evidence of subtalar arthritis but only 12.9% of patients had pain referable to the subtalar joint.
5. *Symptomatic hardware* appears to be more common with percutaneous techniques than with the extensile lateral incision. This is attributed to most screws being inserted from posterior to anterior which can leave screw heads palpable on the back of the heel and interfere with shoewear. They may be removed once the fracture has healed. In the author's experience screws are removed about 30% of the time[11]; Tomesen et al.[17] reported a 47% rate of hardware removal.
6. Malunion, to varying degrees of severity, occurs commonly and may be more common than ORIF for Sanders III and IV fractures.[5,6,11] This can result in a variety of clinical problems that include heel widening, loss of height with resulting anterior ankle joint impingement with dorsiflexion, subfibular impingement, peroneal tendinopathy or dislocation, and varus malalignment of the hindfoot. Clare et al. described three types of calcaneal malunions. Type I malunions had a large lateral wall exostosis. Type II malunions had a lateral wall exostosis and post-traumatic subtalar joint arthritis. Finally, Type III malunions had both the above features as well as significant hindfoot varus malalignment.[18] The authors reported favorable results using a protocol that treated the Type I malunions with an exostectomy of the widened lateral calcaneal wall and peroneal tenolysis, the Type II malunions with the same treatment plus a subtalar arthrodesis, and the Type III malunions with the above treatments as well as a Dwyer-type calcaneal osteotomy.

REHABILITATION PROTOCOL

Rehabilitation is facilitated with adequate postoperative pain management. The author typically administers a popliteal fossa block for postoperative pain relief. This often results in excellent anesthesia for 18 to 24 hours postoperatively; during this time, although sensation may be altered, active motion is often preserved. The patient is initially non–weight-bearing on the operative extremity. The foot is placed in a well-padded Robert-Jones splint in the operating room to reduce swelling. This is removed at approximately 2 weeks postoperatively to check the wounds and remove the sutures. The patient is given a removable boot, is allowed to shower, and is started on range of motion exercises three times a day for 20 minutes at a time. Range of motion includes both dorsiflexion/plantarflexion and inversion/

eversion exercises. The patient may loop a towel under the forefoot and manually assist with ankle dorsiflexion, and may also use the hallux to trace the letters of the alphabet to assist with inversion/eversion. These exercises should be performed with a pillow or towel roll under the distal calf to prevent pressure on the heel. To prevent claw toes from becoming a problem after calcaneus fractures,[19] the author recommends performing plantarflexion stretching exercises at the lesser toe MTP joints or using Budin splints.

The author permits weight-bearing at 12 weeks postoperatively in a boot. After 1 month of weight-bearing in a boot the patient may return to a regular shoe. Other authors permit weight-bearing earlier. In a series of 15 patients, Thordarson et al.[20] reported no loss of reduction when weight-bearing was permitted at 3 to 6 weeks when Norian SRS cement was used to support the fixation. In a series of 36 fractures, Schildhauer et al.[21] likewise reported no loss of reduction when weight-bearing was begun at 3 to 6 weeks, again when SRS cement was used.

Patients may require the use of foot orthoses with normal shoewear. This may include silicone heel cups or over-the-counter or custom arch supports.

OUTCOME

A successful percutaneous reduction should result in restoration of calcaneal height (Bohler's angle), neutral hindfoot alignment, reduction in heel width, and alignment of the articular surface of the posterior facet with step-off <2 mm. If the fracture is not a Sanders IV and if an anatomic reduction is achieved, the patient should be able to ambulate with mild or no limp, return to employment, and wear normal footwear. Although the majority of patients can achieve these goals, many patients still have some ongoing pain, whether mild or severe. Furthermore, there are many patients with an anatomic reduction and poor functional results, and some patients with suboptimal reduction who have excellent function.

Review of published results of percutaneous fracture fixation indicates that when an anatomic reduction is achieved with large fracture fragments that are relatively easy to reduce and to hold, results are generally good. Tornetta[2] reported results on 26 consecutive patients with tongue-type calcaneus fractures treated with an Essex-Lopresti reduction. Three were unsuccessful leaving 23 patients followed for an average of 2.9 years. There were 50% excellent, 36% good, 13% fair, and no poor results by the Maryland foot score. There were four patients with pin drainage that resolved with pin removal and no deep infections. This prompted a change in the protocol toward cannulated screws. In a separate publication reporting the results when this series was expanded to 46 patients, Tornetta[3] reported 41 successful percutaneous reductions. Seven of the fractures were type 2B tongue-type fractures, in which the posterior facet is not one contiguous piece. Using the Maryland Foot score, there were 50% excellent, 35% good, 15% fair, and no poor results. In 2002 Gavlik et al.[8] reported results of 15 patients followed for a mean of 15 months after arthroscopically assisted percutaneous treatment of Sanders II calcaneus fractures. They report mean AOFAS and Maryland foot scores of 93.7 and 95.8, respectively, and all patients were "satisfied" and wearing normal shoewear.

When these techniques are applied to patients with more severe injuries, the outcomes are worse.[5,6] Tomesen et al.[17] reported their results of 39 displaced intra-articular fractures with a mean 5.5-year follow-up. Their study included Sanders II, III, and IV fractures. Mean AOFAS and SF-36 scores were 84 and 76, respectively. Although they were unable to correlate Sanders classification with outcome, the study may have been underpowered to detect a difference. Because of the technical difficulties in obtaining adequate reduction and the potential for poorer results with more severe fractures, the author recommends caution when performing percutaneous reduction for Sanders III and IV calcaneus fractures.

REFERENCES

1. Essex-Lopresti P. The mechanism, reduction technique, and results in fractures of the os calcis. *Clin Orthop*. 1993;290:3–16.
2. Tornetta P III. The Essex-Lopresti reduction for calcaneal fractures revisited. *J Orthop Trauma*. 1998;12(7):469–473.

3. Tornetta P III. Percutaneous treatment of calcaneal fractures. *Clin Orthop Relat Res.* 2000;375: 91–96.
4. Abdelgaid SM. Closed reduction and percutaneous cannulated screws fixation of displaced intra-articular calcaneus fractures. *J Foot Ankle Surg.* 2012;18:164–179.
5. Stulik J, Stehlik J, Rysavy M. Minimally-invasive treatment of intra-articular fractures of the calcaneum. *J Bone Joint Surg Br.* 2006;88-B(12):1634–1641.
6. Walde TA, Sauer B, Degreif J, et al. Closed reduction and percutaneous Kirschner wire fixation for the treatment of dislocated calcaneal fractures: Surgical technique, complications, clinical and radiological results after 2-10 years. *Arch Orthop Trauma Surg.* 2008;128:585–591.
7. DeWall M, Henderson CE, McKinley TO, et al. Percutaneous reduction and fixation of displaced intra-articular calcaneus fractures. *J Orthop Trauma.* 2010;24(8):466–472.
8. Gavlik JM, Rammelt S, Zwipp H. Percutaneous, arthroscopically-assisted osteosynthesis of calcaneus fractures. *Arch Orthop Trauma Surg.* 2002;122:424–428.
9. Rammelt S, Amlang M. Percutaneous treatment of less severe intraarticular calcaneal fractures. *Clin Orthop Relat Res.* 2010;468:983–990.
10. Gardner MJ, Nork SE, Barei DP, et al. Secondary soft tissue compromise in tongue-type calcaneus fractures. *J Orthop Trauma.* 2008;22(7):439–445.
11. Westberg JR, Yoon P, Moeller AT, et al. Open vs. percutaneous fixation of joint depression, tongue-type, and partial tongue-type calcaneus fractures, Mid-America Orthopaedic Association 30th Annual Meeting, Bonita Springs, FL, April 20, 2012.
12. Barei DP, Bellabarba C, Sangeorzan, et al. Fractures of the calcaneus. *Orthop Clin North Am.* 2002;3(1):263–285.
13. Benirschke SK, Sangeorzan BJ. Extensive intra-articular fractures of the foot: Surgical management of calcaneal fractures. *Clin Orthop Relat Res.* 1993;292:128–134.
14. Johal HS, Buckley RE, Le ILD, et al. A prospective randomized controlled trial of a bioresorbable calcium phosphate paste (α-BSM) in treatment of displaced intra-articular calcaneal fractures. *J Trauma.* 2009;67(4):875–882.
15. Harvey EJ, Grujic L, Early JS, et al. Morbidity associated with ORIF of intra-articular calcaneus fractures using a lateral approach. *Foot Ankle Int.* 2001;22(11):868–873.
16. Molloy AP, Myerson MS, Yoon P. Symptomatic nonunion after fracture of the calcaneum: Demographics and treatment. *J Bone Joint Surg Br.* 2007;89-B:1218–1224.
17. Tomesen T, Biert J, Frolke JP. Treatment of displaced intra-articular calcaneus fractures with closed reduction and percutaneous screw fixation. *J Bone Joint Surg Am.* 2011;93-A(10):920–928.
18. Clare MP, Lee WE III, Sanders RW. Results of a treatment protocol for calcaneal fracture malunions. *J Bone Joint Surg Am.* 2005;87-A(5):963–973.
19. Yoon P. Compartment syndrome of the foot. *Tech Orthop.* 2012;27(1):58–61.
20. Thordarson DB, Bollinger M. SRS cancellous bone cement augmentation of calcaneal fracture fixation. *Foot Ankle Int.* 2005;26(5):347–352.
21. Schildhauer TA, Bauer TW, Josten C, et al. Open reduction and augmentation of internal fixation with an injectable skeletal cement for the treatment of complex calcaneal fractures. *J Orthop Trauma.* 2000;14(5):309–317.

BIBLIOGRAPHY

1. Bajammal S, Tornetta P, III, Sanders D. Displaced intra-articular calcaneal fractures. *J Orthop Trauma.* 2005;19(5):360–364.
2. Buckley R, Tough S, McCormack R, et al. Operative compared with nonoperative treatment of displaced intra-articular calcaneal fractures. *J Bone Joint Surg Am.* 2002;84-A(10):1733–1744.

Index

NOTE: Page numbers followed by "*f*" indicate figures; those followed by "*t*" indicate tables.

A

B

C

D

R

S

T

U

V

W